Michael Eriksen
Judith Mackay
Hana Ross

THE TOBACCO ATLAS

FOURTH EDITION

Completely Revised and Updated

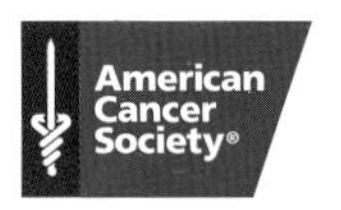

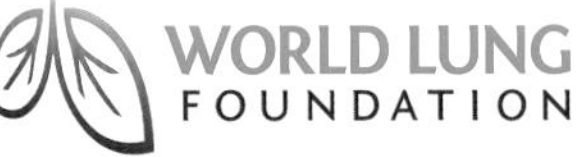

Published by the American Cancer Society, Inc.
250 Williams Street
Atlanta, Georgia 30303 USA
www.cancer.org

ISBN-10: 1-60443-093-1
ISBN-13: 978-1-60443-093-6

Library of Congress Cataloging-in-Publication Data

Mackay, Judith.
The tobacco atlas / Judith Longstaff Mackay, Michael Eriksen, Hana Ross. — 4th ed.
p. cm.
Includes bibliographical references and index.
ISBN 978-1-60443-093-6 (pbk. : alk. paper) — ISBN 1-60443-093-1 (pbk. : alk. paper)
1. Tobacco use—Maps. 2. Tobacco industry—Maps. 3. Medical geography—Maps.
I. Eriksen, Michael P. II. Ross, Hana. III. Title.
G1046.J94M3 2012
362.29'60223—dc23
2012001286

Developed for the American Cancer Society by
Bookhouse Group, Inc.
Atlanta, Georgia
www.bookhouse.net

Managing Editors: Debra Daugherty, Sarah Fedota, and Steve Hamill
Design: Language Dept. (www.languagedept.com)
Contributing Editor: John M. Daniel
Copy Editor: Bob Land

Printed in Korea

SECOND PRINTING, *The Tobacco Atlas*, Fourth Edition
The second printing of *The Tobacco Atlas* includes several updates and edits.
To learn more about the differences between the first and second printing,
please visit www.TobaccoAtlas.org/blog.

Suggested Citation:
Eriksen M, Mackay J, Ross H. *The Tobacco Atlas*. Fourth Ed. Atlanta, GA: American Cancer Society; New York, NY: World Lung Foundation; 2012. Also available at www.TobaccoAtlas.org

The fourth edition of *The Tobacco Atlas* marks its tenth anniversary.
***The Tobacco Atlas* can be found online at www.TobaccoAtlas.org.**
The online version of the *Atlas* provides additional resources and information unique to the online interactive version.

CONTENTS

CONTENTS

CONTENTS

"The battle is far from being over. Unless the prevalence of smoking is reduced substantially, the number of smokers will increase in the world in the next several decades, mostly due to population expansion in low- and middle-income countries. Measures to tackle the epidemic remain seriously under-funded."

Margaret Chan, Director-General, WHO, 2012

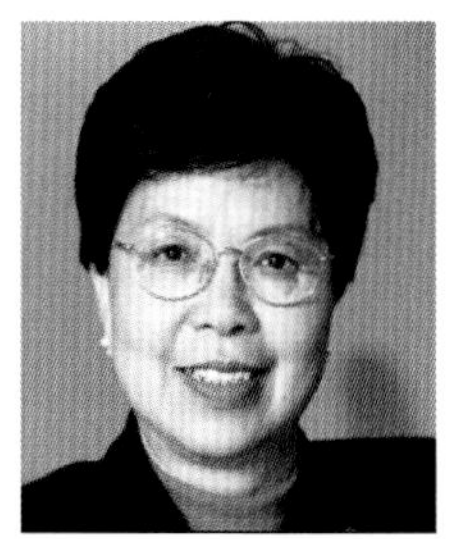

The first and pioneering edition of *The Tobacco Atlas* was published by the World Health Organization in 2002. The words of previous WHO Director-General Dr. Gro Harlem Brundtland still resonate today: "Let us all speak out: Tobacco is a killer. It should not be advertised, subsidized or glamorized." Her foreword in the first edition was a clarion call to develop the WHO Framework Convention on Tobacco Control (WHO FCTC), which at the time was several years in the future, and to build a "vibrant alliance with other UN agencies, NGOs, the private sector, academic/research institutions, and donors."

Many of these ambitions have been achieved, for example:

- 2005: The WHO FCTC entered into force.
- Today the WHO FCTC has 174 Parties.
- 2011: The United Nations High-Level Meeting on noncommunicable diseases (NCDs) prevention and control recognized tobacco control as a key factor in reducing the rise of NCDs. WHO provides the secretariat for taking the meeting's Political Declaration forward, liaising with other UN agencies to develop voluntary targets for 2025.

To help countries fulfill some of their WHO FCTC obligations, WHO has highlighted the good and best buys for reducing tobacco use—the *MPOWER* package of six cost-effective measures that reduce the demand for tobacco. As a result of decisive action taken by many countries around the world, 1.1 billion people have become covered over the past two years by at least one of these measures newly applied at the highest level.

All four editions of *The Tobacco Atlas* have utilized published data from WHO sources, especially from the WHO *Report on the Global Tobacco Epidemic*, and the newly available tobacco attributable mortality data. In addition, the atlases contain data from the Global Tobacco Surveillance System (GTSS): the Global Youth Tobacco Survey (GYTS), Global School Personnel Survey (GSPS), Global Health Professions Student Survey (GHPSS), and Global Adult Tobacco Survey (GATS), a joint venture between WHO and the United States Centers for Disease Control and Prevention (CDC)—an example of a successful partnership in monitoring the tobacco epidemic.

The battle is far from being over. Unless the prevalence of smoking is reduced substantially, the number of smokers will increase in the world in the next several decades, mostly due to population expansion in low- and middle-income countries. Measures to tackle the epidemic remain seriously under-funded. As the subtle promotion of their lethal products under the appearance of "socially responsible causes or business practices" is becoming exposed, the tobacco industry has adopted newer and bolder tactics to undermine and counteract tobacco control measures by means of legal challenges to tobacco control legislation, as well as using bilateral trade agreements to challenge strong laws. Big tobacco can afford to hire the best lawyers and PR firms that money can buy. Big money tries to speak louder than any moral, ethical, or public health argument and wants to trample even the most damning scientific evidence. I urge all countries to stand firm together and not to bow to pressure. We must never allow the tobacco industry to get the upper hand.

I would like to see a united world that no longer accepts the detrimental health and economic effects of tobacco, recognizing that tobacco control and the full implementation of the WHO FCTC are good for the health and wealth of nations.

Margaret Chan
Director-General, World Health Organization

"I encourage advocates, policymakers, health-care professionals, journalists, and commentators to carefully review the contents of *The Tobacco Atlas* and use the information to push for action."

Michael Bloomberg, Philanthropist and Mayor of New York City, US, 2012

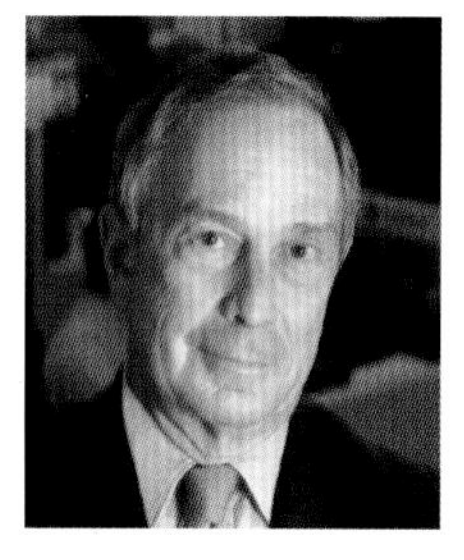

Every six seconds, someone somewhere in the world dies because of tobacco use. Unless concerted global action is taken, that rate of death will accelerate. At the recent United Nations High-Level Meeting on noncommunicable diseases (NCDs) in New York City, government leaders acknowledged tobacco use to be the single most preventable cause of death in the modern world, yet no firm targets were set to help tackle this global pandemic.

We must take action now. If we don't, tobacco will claim 1 billion lives during this century. But the good news is that solutions exist to combat this deadly pandemic. The *MPOWER* package of proven measures outlines six effective steps countries can take now to reduce tobacco use. The *MPOWER* policies have been increasingly implemented by governments over the past several years. The *MPOWER* strategy involves: Monitoring tobacco use and prevention policies; Protecting its people from tobacco smoke; Offering help to those who want to quit; Warning about the dangers of tobacco; Enforcing bans on tobacco advertising, promotion, and sponsorship; and Raising taxes on tobacco.

While significant progress has been made in recent years, there is still much more work to be done. Most countries could do much more to inform their citizens adequately about the illness and death caused by tobacco, particularly through the use of mass media and graphic health warnings. Taxes on tobacco products must be increased and plain packaging introduced. These are all proven, cost-effective strategies to help reduce tobacco consumption.

In just five years of the Bloomberg Initiative to Reduce Tobacco Use, we have witnessed extraordinary global progress: 21 countries have passed 100 percent smoke-free laws, there has been a 400 percent increase in the proportion of people protected from secondhand smoke, more than 300 tobacco laws have been drafted or consultations provided, and 7,000 public health professionals have been trained in tobacco control. Bloomberg Philanthropies supports these efforts through partner organizations such as the World Health Organization, the Campaign for Tobacco-Free Kids, the World Lung Foundation, the CDC Foundation, and the Johns Hopkins Bloomberg School of Public Health.

In the global fight against tobacco, information is one of our most powerful weapons. *The Tobacco Atlas* is an invaluable resource for collating our current knowledge about tobacco and demonstrating the true nature of this global pandemic. For example, *The Tobacco Atlas* notes that more than 89 percent of the world's population remain unprotected by comprehensive smoke-free laws. We can use the *Atlas* to educate consumers and health-care professionals about the risks of tobacco use, to rebut misinformation, to share successful tobacco control strategies, and to push for legislation that optimally protects the world's citizens from the harms of tobacco use.

I encourage advocates, policymakers, health-care professionals, journalists, and commentators to carefully review the contents of *The Tobacco Atlas* and use the information to push for action. We can change the course of this pandemic. Effective tobacco control more than any other single measure could help reduce the toll of NCDs and prevent tobacco-related deaths. We can protect our citizens, our economy, our planet, and future generations, but we need to act now.

Michael Bloomberg

Philanthropist and Mayor of New York City, US

"With the tenth anniversary of *The Tobacco Atlas*, it's a good time to reflect on the accomplishments we've made in this fight and to hone in on ways we can continue to make progress."

John R. Seffrin and Peter Baldini, US, 2012

Tobacco is the only legal product that when used as directed, is lethal. Its influence extends into all corners of the globe, threatening lives and livelihoods and endangering the health and prosperity of developed and developing nations alike. Left unchecked, tobacco is predicted to kill more than 8 million people globally each year by 2030—and to take a staggering 1 billion lives in this century.

The good news is we know how to stop this deadly epidemic —and we have proven successes doing so. We simply must educate, raise awareness, and implement these strategies worldwide. With the tenth anniversary of *The Tobacco Atlas*, it's a good time to reflect on the accomplishments we've made in this fight and to hone in on ways we can continue to make progress. We have seen many tobacco control milestones in the past decade, but there is still much to do, particularly in low- and middle-income countries, home to 85 percent of the world's population.

A substantial victory came in 2003 with the World Health Organization's unanimous adoption of the Framework Convention on Tobacco Control (WHO FCTC). Since then, the majority of eligible countries have taken a stand against tobacco, ratifying this first global public health treaty. Building on this work, WHO in 2008 introduced its *MPOWER* model, offering strategies to implement and manage tobacco control, and providing a proven road map for policymakers, advocates, and public health practitioners.

In September 2011, the tobacco fight took on new prominence as global leaders came together in New York for the first-ever United Nations High-Level Meeting on noncommunicable diseases (NCDs). At this historic gathering, world leaders unanimously approved an action plan for fighting NCDs that has the potential to meaningfully impact the tobacco battle. This plan calls for greater international collaboration and for programs that help combat tobacco, such as tobacco-free workplaces.

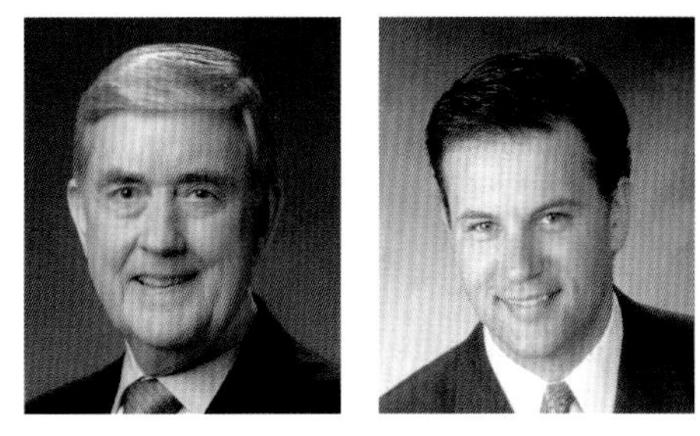

These milestones are impressive, yet so are the challenges and opportunities ahead. While smoking rates have been slowly declining in the United States and many other high-income nations during the past 25 years, they have been increasing in low- and middle-income nations, which are also the least prepared to deal with the effects of tobacco-related disease. In 2011, tobacco use killed approximately 6 million people worldwide, with 80 percent of those deaths occurring in low- and middle-income nations. Now is the time for concerted action to save lives and stop this growing plague—we simply cannot wait.

With cross-sector commitment and collaboration, emerging economies can flourish rather than falter, and millions upon millions of lives can be saved, not lost to tobacco-related deaths. This all-new fourth edition of *The Tobacco Atlas* will, we believe, be an essential tool as people worldwide seek to understand—and to help turn back—the rising tide of suffering and death caused by tobacco. In another 10 years, it is our hope we will be telling the story of our greatest victory—a world well on its way to conquering tobacco for good.

John R. Seffrin
CEO, American Cancer Society, US

Peter Baldini
Executive Director, World Lung Foundation, US

SINCE THE RELEASE OF THE FIRST *TOBACCO ATLAS* IN 2002, MUCH PROGRESS HAS BEEN MADE IN GLOBAL EFFORTS TO ADVANCE TOBACCO CONTROL, BUT FAR TOO MUCH REMAINS TO BE DONE. IN FACT, THE 10 YEARS SINCE 2002 HAVE LIKELY BEEN THE MOST PRODUCTIVE PERIOD IN TOBACCO CONTROL HISTORY.

During the past 10 years, there have been significant multilateral, philanthropic, governmental, and civil society successes. For example, in 2002, the World Health Organization Framework Convention on Tobacco Control (WHO FCTC) was still being discussed by the Intergovernmental Negotiating Body and not yet approved by the World Health Assembly. With the support of civil society and especially low- and middle-income countries, a strong WHO FCTC was approved. Today, the WHO FCTC is one of the most widely adopted treaties in United Nations history, with 174 Parties to the Convention covering over 85 percent of the world's population.

In September 2011, the UN held an unprecedented high-level meeting on the prevention and control of noncommunicable diseases, with a clear recognition that combating tobacco use is central to success. Countries agreed that the battle against noncommunicable diseases can never be won unless we succeed in reducing tobacco use—the only risk factor that is common to all four of the major chronic diseases—cancer, heart disease, chronic lung disease, and diabetes. The resultant political declaration from the high-level meeting calls on government leaders to recognize that the economic harm caused by tobacco use is unsustainable, and to implement effective tobacco control interventions consistent with the WHO FCTC.

In 2002, while a few high-income countries were investing domestically in tobacco control, there was very little investment in tobacco control particularly in low-income countries. This situation was dramatically reversed by the investment of $500 million by philanthropists Michael Bloomberg and Bill Gates. Their unprecedented investment was inspired by their belief that implementing effective tobacco control programs could save lives at a level equivalent to or surpassing a similar investment in HIV or malaria programs. Consistent with this investment, effective tobacco control interventions were packaged and promoted globally in the low- and middle-income countries under the rubric of WHO *MPOWER*. Now, there were resources and evidence-based programs in which to invest.

For investments to be sustained and programs refined, there must be systems in place to document the problem and to measure outcomes. Since the time of the first *Tobacco Atlas*, and as part of the Global Tobacco Surveillance System (GTSS), the Global Adult Tobacco Survey (GATS) was established and implemented in the countries with the greatest tobacco burden, and the Global Youth Tobacco Survey (GYTS) was expanded to assess the tobacco-use behaviors of over 2 million children in over 150 countries. The GYTS has now been conducted multiple times in the same countries, so we are now able to monitor important trends in youth tobacco use — something that had previously been lacking.

In addition to these global success stories, there are scores of examples throughout the world in which individual countries have stepped up to implement the provisions of the WHO FCTC, and have, in many instances, surpassed their obligations. Marketing bans, clean indoor-air laws, graphic warning labels, tax increases, and litigation holding the tobacco industry accountable for the harm it has caused are becoming the norm rather than the exception. Perhaps the most notable recent effort has been the Australian government requiring the plain packaging of cigarettes. While this law is being challenged by the tobacco industry, Australia's bold step has invigorated global tobacco control efforts and will likely result in similar plain-packaging efforts throughout the world.

While much has been accomplished, much remains to be done. Tobacco use continues to kill millions of people a year, and the tobacco industry continues to operate in a relatively unfettered manner. Moreover, the success that has been achieved in tobacco control is somewhat uneven among countries, and sustained progress is never guaranteed. The tobacco industry is shrewd and effective in its ability to influence public policy —including legal, economic, and trade tactics—in a way that harms the public health.

It is the authors' hope that the fourth edition of *The Tobacco Atlas* will serve as a tool to remind decision-makers and civil society alike that, while progress has been great, the industry is unrelenting in its efforts to sell more products, irrespective of the harm it inflicts on its customers. We must be equally unrelenting in our efforts to advance tobacco control and, to the extent possible, confine tobacco use to a mistake associated with the 20th century.

Michael Eriksen

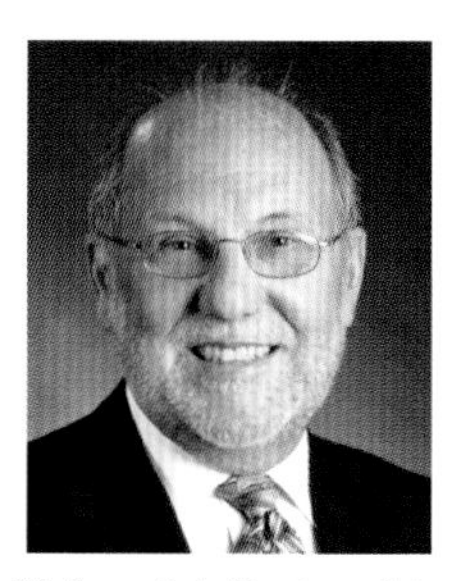

Michael Eriksen is a professor in and the founding director of the Institute of Public Health at Georgia State University. He is also director of Georgia State University's Partnership for Urban Health Research and Center of Excellence in Health Disparities Research. Prior to his current positions, Eriksen served as a senior advisor to the World Health Organization in Geneva and was the longest-serving director of the Centers for Disease Control and Prevention's Office on Smoking and Health (1992–2000). Previously, Eriksen was director of behavioral research at the M.D. Anderson Cancer Center. He has recently served as an advisor to the Bill & Melinda Gates Foundation, the Robert Wood Johnson Foundation, the American Legacy Foundation, and the CDC Foundation.

Eriksen has published extensively on tobacco prevention and control and has served as an expert witness of behalf of the US Department of Justice and the Federal Trade Commission in litigation against the tobacco industry. He is editor-in-chief of *Health Education Research* and has been designated as a Distinguished Cancer Scholar by the Georgia Cancer Coalition. He is a recipient of the WHO Commemorative Medal on Tobacco or Health and a Presidential Citation for Meritorious Service, awarded by President Bill Clinton. Eriksen is a past president and Distinguished Fellow of the Society for Public Health Education, and has been a member of the American Public Health Association for over 35 years.

Judith Longstaff Mackay

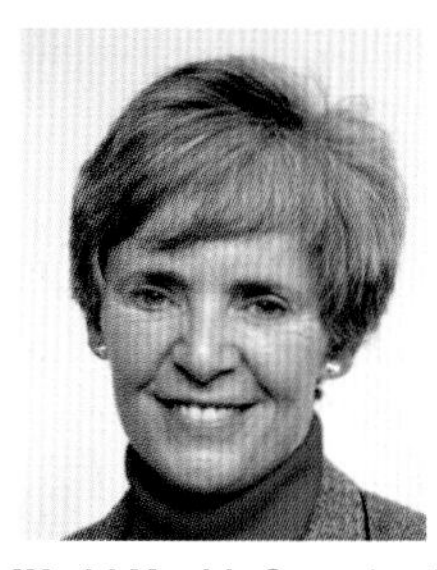

Judith Longstaff Mackay is a medical doctor based in Hong Kong. She is senior advisor to the World Lung Foundation, senior policy advisor to the World Health Organization, and director of the Asian Consultancy on Tobacco Control. She holds professorships at the Chinese Academy of Preventive Medicine and the Department of Community Medicine at the University of Hong Kong. After an early career as a hospital physician, she moved to public health. She is a Fellow of the Royal Colleges of Physicians of Edinburgh and of London. She has authored or coauthored 10 health atlases, published 200 papers, and addressed more than 450 conferences on tobacco control.

Mackay has received many international awards, including the WHO Commemorative Medal, Royal Awards from the United Kingdom's Queen Elizabeth II and Thailand's King Bhumibol Adulyadej, the Fries Prize for Improving Health, the Luther Terry Award for Outstanding Individual Leadership, the US Surgeon General's Medallion, the Founding International Achievement Award from the Asia Pacific Association for the Control of Tobacco, and the Lifetime Achievement Award from the International Network of Women Against Tobacco. She was selected as one of *Time*'s 60 Asian Heroes (2006) and one of *Time*'s 100 World's Most Influential People (2007), and is the recipient of the British Medical Journal Group's first Lifetime Achievement Award (2009). She has been identified by the tobacco industry as one of the three most dangerous people in the world.

Hana Ross

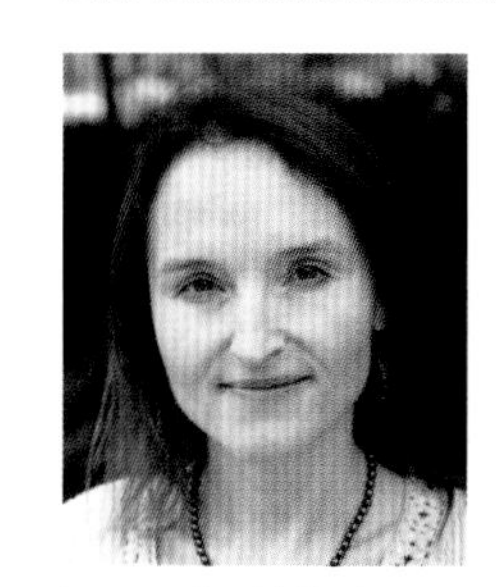

Hana Ross has more than 12 years' experience in conducting research on the economics of tobacco control and in management of research projects in low- and middle-income countries, including projects funded by the World Bank, the World Health Organization, the Rockefeller Foundation, the Open Society Institute, the Robert Wood Johnson Foundation, the European Commission, the Bloomberg Global Initiative, and the Bill & Melinda Gates Foundation. Ross joined the American Cancer Society's Intramural Research Department in 2006 and currently serves as a managing director of the International Tobacco Control Research Program. She has published more than 50 articles and independent reports on issues related to tobacco taxation, cigarette prices, costs of smoking, illicit trade, youth access laws, and other economic aspects of tobacco control. She also coauthored the third edition of *The Tobacco Atlas*. Her current research projects focus on the economic impact of tobacco control interventions in South-East Asia, the former Soviet republics, Eastern and Central Europe, and Africa. She is also interested in the economic impact of smokeless tobacco use, behavioral economics, and the overall economic impact of noncommunicable diseases. Ross currently supports several capacity-building research projects, primarily focusing on South-East Asia and Africa. She earned her BA and MA at the Prague School of Economics, and in 2000 she received her PhD in economics from the University of Illinois at Chicago.

MANY PEOPLE HAVE HELPED IN THE PREPARATION OF THIS *ATLAS*.

We would especially like to thank our principal researchers: Carrie Whitney, Georgia State University; Kimberly Sebek, World Lung Foundation (WLF); and Michal Stoklosa, American Cancer Society (ACS). Other researchers include Evan Blecher and Alex Liber, International Tobacco Control Research, American Cancer Society; and Hailey Dong, Tiffany Joseph, and Ichhya Pant, Georgia State University.

Sincere thanks to the American Cancer Society and the World Lung Foundation for their generous financial and overall support of the fourth edition of *The Tobacco Atlas*. We would like to especially thank Debra Daugherty, ACS, and Stephen Hamill, WLF, for their extensive involvement in and organization of this project, as well as Nathan Grey, ACS, and Sandra Mullin, WLF, for their leadership. Additionally, we would like to thank Len Boswell, Otis W. Brawley, Bob Chapman, John M. Daniel, Jacqui Drope, Jay Evans, Thomas Glynn, Soumya Hombaiah, Vanika Jordan, J. Leonard Lichtenfeld, Ann McMikel, Gail Richman, and Brenda Wilson, ACS. We would also like to acknowledge Georgia State University and the Georgia Cancer Coalition for their professional and financial support. We are also grateful to Bloomberg Philanthropies for their tremendous support of the *Atlas*.

The World Health Organization (WHO) and the Centers for Disease Control and Prevention (CDC) worked extensively to provide global data in an effort to make the *Atlas* as up-to-date and complete as possible. Many thanks to WHO for the early release of the *WHO Report on the Global Tobacco Epidemic, 2011 Report* and data, and to the CDC for the release of Global Youth Tobacco Survey and Global Health Professions Student Survey data.

Additional thanks to WHO and CDC for reviewing the full manuscript of the *Atlas* in order to provide feedback and comments during the editing process. We are especially grateful to Douglas Bettcher, Alison Commar, Anne-Marie Perucic, Armando Peruga, Sameer Pujari, Kerstin Schotte, Edouard Tursan d'Espaignet, and Ayda Yurekli with the Tobacco Free Initiative, World Health Organization; as well as to Samira Asma, Linda Anton, Eugene Lam, Kyung Ah Lee, Nichol Lowman, Krishna Palipudi, Italia Rolle, Raydel Valdez Salgado, and Mikyong Shin of the Global Tobacco Control, Office on Smoking and Health, Centers for Disease Control and Prevention.

We acknowledge the contribution that the first, second, and third editions of the *Atlas* have made to the tenth anniversary edition. Over the past decade, the *Atlas* has been shaped by the World Health Organization, the original publisher; Myriad Editions, the packager for the first and second editions; Omar Shafey, lead author of the third edition; and other contributors.

We would like to thank Jenn Cash, Tanya Quick, Lizania Cruz, and Urcella Di Pietro at Language Dept. who designed the fourth edition of *The Tobacco Atlas*. Their creativity and attention to detail resulted in a spectacular and unique tenth anniversary edition.

Our appreciation goes to Sarah Fedota for her luminous work as managing editor.

FOR THEIR ADVICE ON SPECIFIC CHAPTERS AND DATA, WE WOULD LIKE TO THANK THE FOLLOWING INDIVIDUALS:

01 DEATHS

Edouard Tursan d'Espaignet, Tobacco Free Initiative, World Health Organization, Switzerland
Majid Ezzati, School of Public Health, Imperial College, London, United Kingdom
Alan Lopez, School of Population Health, University of Queensland, Australia
Colin Mathers, Evidence and Information for Policy Cluster, World Health Organization, Switzerland
Richard Peto, Clinical Trial Service Unit, University of Oxford, United Kingdom

02 HARM FROM SMOKING

Jonathan Samet, Institute for Global Health, University of Southern California, US

03 SECONDHAND SMOKING

Italia Rolle, Office on Smoking and Health, Centers for Disease Control and Prevention, US
Jonathan Samet, Institute for Global Health, University of Southern California, US

04 TYPES OF TOBACCO USE

Margaretha Haglund, Tankesmedjan Tobaksfakta, Tobaksfakta, Sweden

05 NICOTINE DELIVERY SYSTEMS

Gregory Connolly, Center for Global Tobacco Control, Harvard University School of Public Health, US

06 CIGARETTE CONSUMPTION

Emmanuel Guindon, Propel Centre for Population Health Impact, University of Waterloo, Canada

07 MALE TOBACCO USE

Edouard Tursan d'Espaignet, Tobacco Free Initiative, World Health Organization, Switzerland

08 FEMALE TOBACCO USE

Edouard Tursan d'Espaignet, Tobacco Free Initiative, World Health Organization, Switzerland

09 BOYS' TOBACCO USE

Laura Kann, National Center for Chronic Disease Prevention and Health Promotion, Centers for Disease Control and Prevention, US
Terry Pechacek, Office on Smoking and Health, Centers for Disease Control and Prevention, US
Leanne Riley, Chronic Diseases and Health Promotion, World Health Organization, Switzerland
Italia Rolle, Office on Smoking and Health, Centers for Disease Control and Prevention, US

10 GIRLS' TOBACCO USE

Laura Kann, National Center for Chronic Disease Prevention and Health Promotion, Centers for Disease Control and Prevention, US
Terry Pechacek, Office on Smoking and Health, Centers for Disease Control and Prevention, US
Leanne Riley, Chronic Diseases and Health Promotion, World Health Organization, Switzerland
Italia Rolle, Office on Smoking and Health, Centers for Disease Control and Prevention, US

11 SMOKELESS TOBACCO

Krishna Palipudi, Office on Smoking and Health, Centers for Disease Control and Prevention, US

12 HEALTH PROFESSIONALS

Italia Rolle, Office on Smoking and Health, Centers for Disease Control and Prevention, US
Wick Warren, Division of Violence Prevention, Centers for Disease Control and Prevention, US

13 COSTS TO SOCIETY

Sarah McGhee, Department of Community Medicine, School of Public Health, University of Hong Kong, Hong Kong, SAR

14 CIGARETTE PRICES

Frank Chaloupka, Institute for Health Research and Policy, University of Illinois at Chicago, US

15 AFFORDABILITY OF CIGARETTES

Frank Chaloupka, Institute for Health Research and Policy, University of Illinois at Chicago, US

16 GROWING TOBACCO

Tom Capehart, Economic Research Service, US Department of Agriculture, US

17 MANUFACTURING CIGARETTES

Sarah Barber, Health Sector Development, World Health Organization, WPRO, Philippines
Matthew Kohrman, Department of Anthropology, Stanford University, US

18 TOBACCO COMPANIES

Teh-Wei Hu, University of California, Berkeley, US
Wang Ke-an, Think Tank Research Center for Health Development, China
Monique Muggli, International Legal Consortium, Campaign for Tobacco-Free Kids, US

19 ILLICIT CIGARETTES

Luk Joossens, Association of European Cancer Leagues and Belgian Foundation Against Cancer, Belgium

20 TOBACCO MARKETING

Becky Freeman, School of Public Health, Sydney Medical School, University of Sydney, Australia
Italia Rolle, Office on Smoking and Health, Centers for Disease Control and Prevention, US

21 UNDUE INFLUENCE

Monique Muggli, International Legal Consortium, Campaign for Tobacco-Free Kids, US

22 RIGHTS AND TREATIES

Marty Otanez, Department of Anthropology, University of Colorado, Denver, US

23 PUBLIC HEALTH STRATEGIES

Kenneth Warner, University of Michigan School of Public Health, US

24 SMOKE-FREE AREAS

Jim Middleton, Clear the Air, Hong Kong, SAR

25 QUITTING SMOKING

Sophia Chan, Department of Nursing Studies, University of Hong Kong, Hong Kong, SAR
Geoffrey Fong, University of Waterloo, Canada

26 MASS MEDIA CAMPAIGNS

Melanie Wakefield, Centre for Behavioural Research in Cancer, Victoria Cancer Council, Australia

27 PRODUCT LABELING

Rob Cunningham, Canadian Cancer Society, Canada

28 MARKETING BANS

Simon Chapman, School of Public Health, University of Sydney, Australia
Stanton Glantz, Center for Tobacco Control Research and Education, University of California, San Francisco, US
James Sargent, Dartmouth Medical School and Norris Cotton Cancer Center, Dartmouth University, US

29 TOBACCO TAXES

Frank Chaloupka, Institute for Health Research and Policy, University of Illinois at Chicago, US

30 LEGAL CHALLENGES AND LITIGATION

Richard Daynard, School of Law, Northeastern University, US
Patricia Lambert, International Legal Consortium, Campaign for Tobacco-Free Kids, US

31 THE FUTURE

Robert Beaglehole, University of Auckland, New Zealand
Ruth Bonita, University of Auckland, New Zealand

HISTORY OF TOBACCO

Robert Proctor, Department of History, Stanford University, US

GLOSSARY

Natasha Herrera, Smoking Cessation and Research Clinic, Centro Médico Docente la Trinidad, Venezuela

RESEARCH SAYS:

“…when you strip it down to what matters, there is really only one thing anyone needs to know about tobacco: It kills people.”

Arlene King, Chief Medical Officer of Health, Canada, 2010

SINCE THE FIRST EDITION OF *THE TOBACCO ATLAS* A DECADE AGO,

50 Million

ADDITIONAL PEOPLE HAVE BEEN KILLED AS A RESULT OF USING TOBACCO.

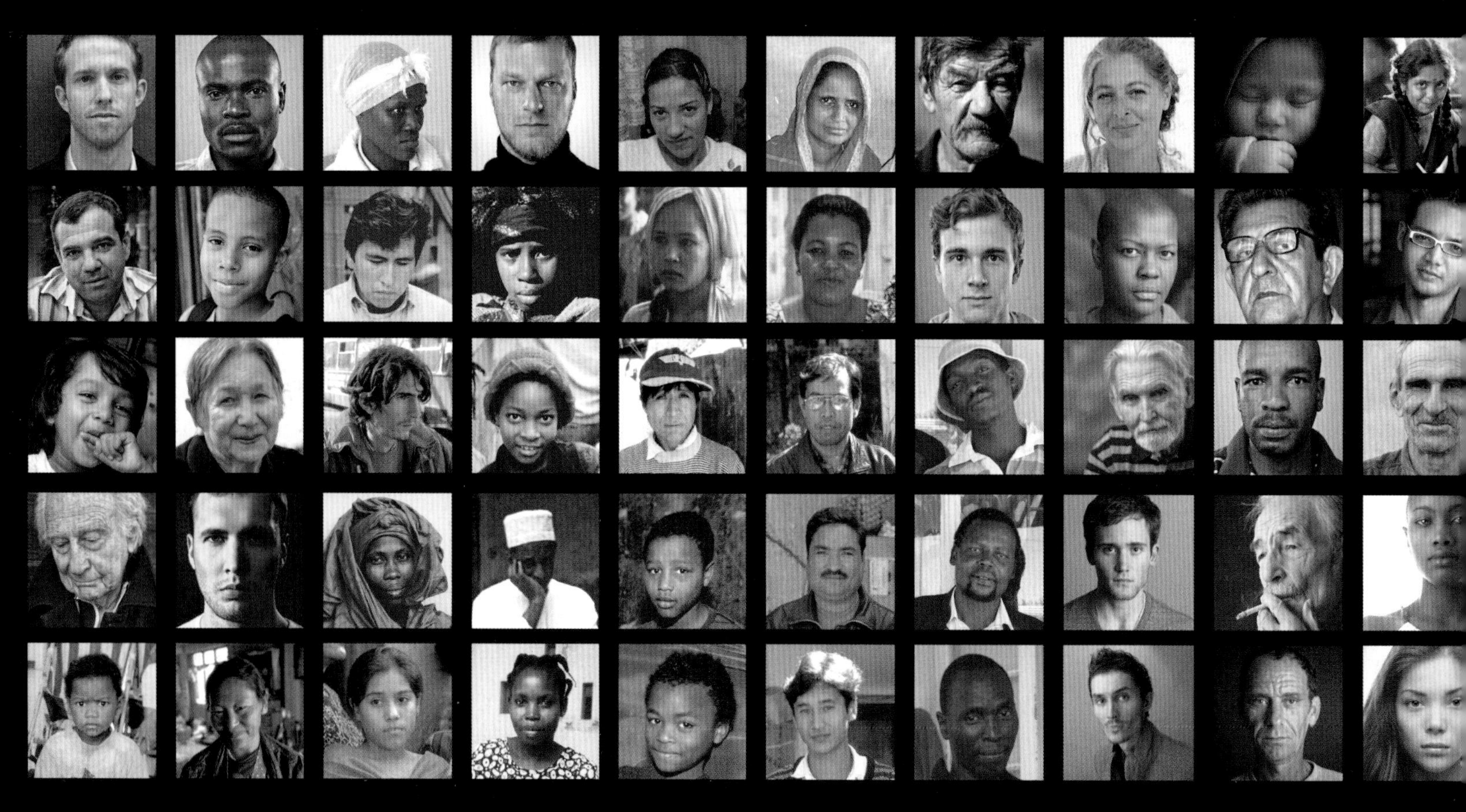

From December 2002 to November 2011

HARM

1 FACE = 500,000 LIVES

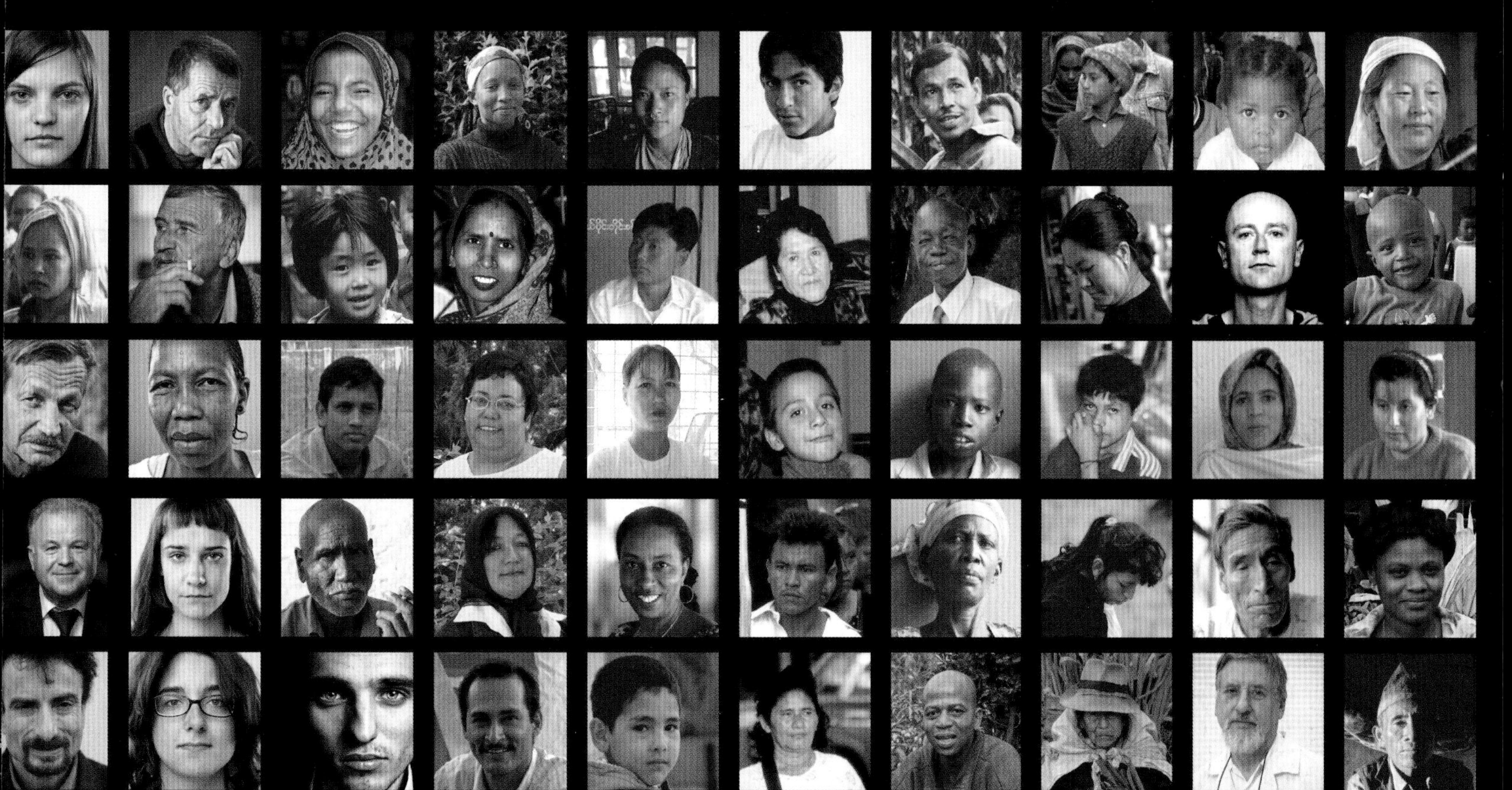

Male Deaths

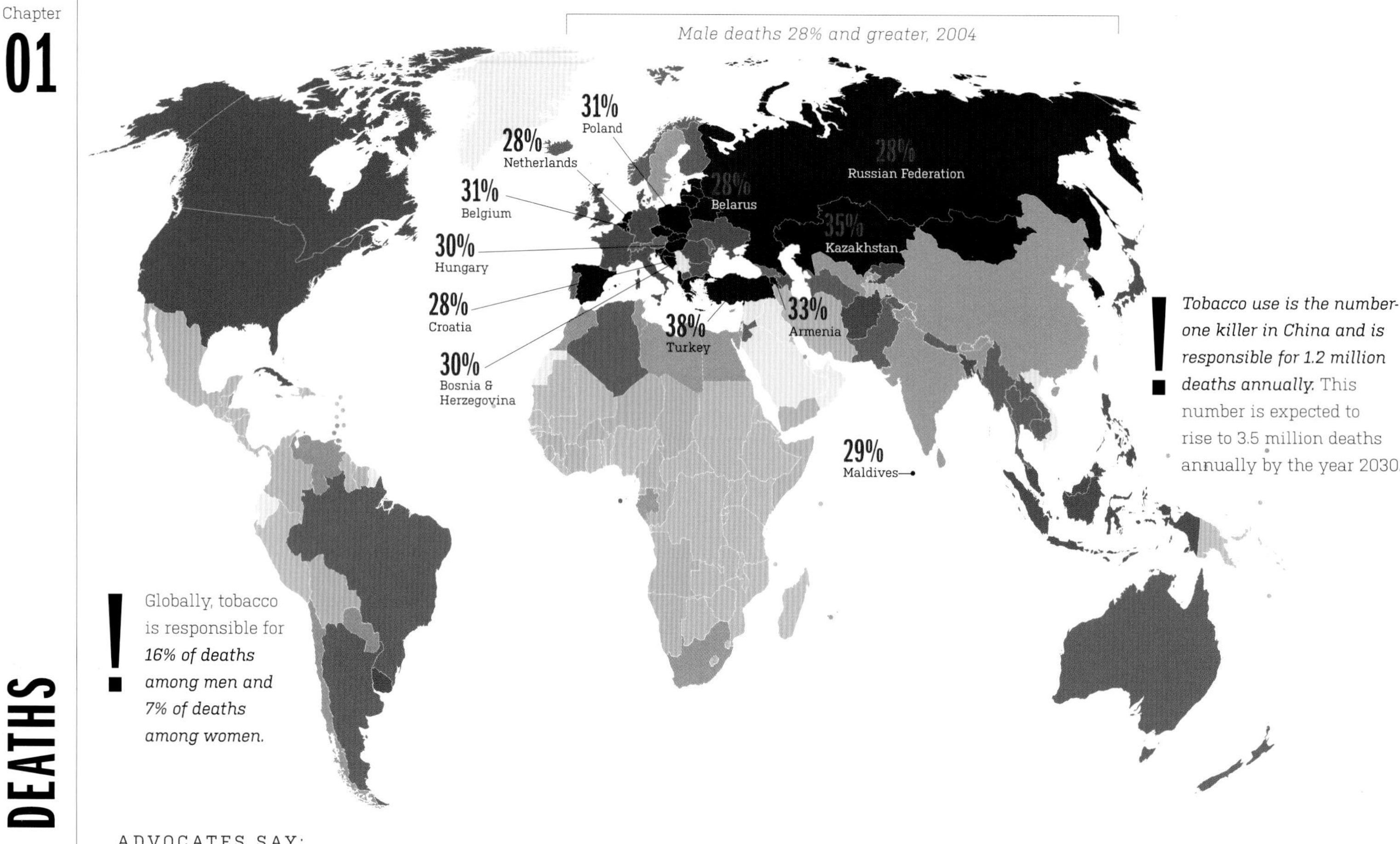

! *Tobacco use is the number-one killer in China and is responsible for 1.2 million deaths annually.* This number is expected to rise to 3.5 million deaths annually by the year 2030.

! Globally, tobacco is responsible for *16% of deaths among men and 7% of deaths among women.*

ADVOCATES SAY:

"Dying from smoking is rarely quick… and never painless."

Anti-smoking campaign, New York City, US, 2011

In 2011, tobacco use killed almost 6 million people, with nearly 80% of these deaths occurring in low- and middle-income countries. Tobacco use in any form is dangerous and is the single most preventable cause of death. Up to half of all lifetime smokers will ultimately die of a disease caused by smoking, and men and women with comparable smoking patterns exhibit similar patterns of death.

Tobacco use is a major risk factor for death from heart attacks and strokes. Worldwide, smoking causes almost 80% of male and nearly 50% of female lung cancer deaths. Smoking increases the risk of tuberculosis (TB) infection, and 40 million smokers with TB are expected to die between 2010 and 2050. By the year 2030, 8 million people will die annually from tobacco use.

SINCE THE FIRST PUBLICATION OF *THE TOBACCO ATLAS* A DECADE AGO, THE GLOBAL NUMBER OF DEATHS CAUSED BY TOBACCO HAS NEARLY TRIPLED, FROM 2.1 MILLION TO ALMOST 6 MILLION ANNUALLY.

Deaths from smoking are directly related to smoking prevalence and exposure to secondhand smoke. Smoking prevalence is higher among men than women. Smoking rates have the potential to increase among women, particularly young women, and this is a great public health concern. Additionally, women are often the victims of secondhand smoke exposure, illness, and death, particularly in countries with a high male and low female smoking prevalence. Worldwide, approximately

Projected Deaths
Caused by Tobacco Use During the 21st Century
Total 1 Billion

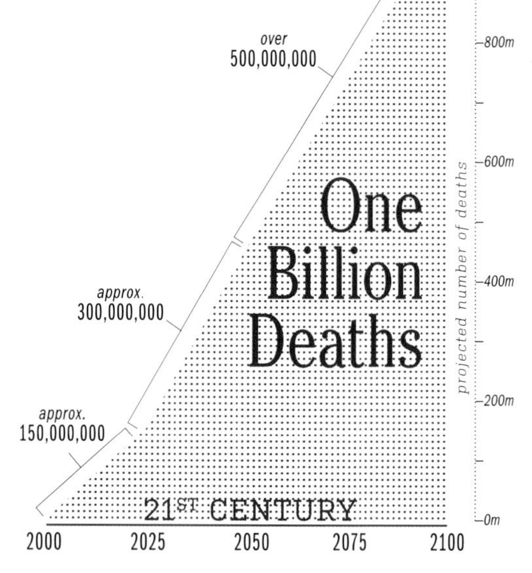

Female Deaths

Female deaths 20% and greater, 2004

20% Canada

23% United States of America

20% Iceland

21% Denmark

20% United Kingdom

22% Ireland

25% Maldives

In the developed countries of the European Union, an average of *22 years of life are lost with the death of each middle-aged smoker.*

"Every one in 8.6 Thais died [in 2009] of a smoking-related cause. We have to deal with the tobacco industry, as this can't go on."

Prakit Vathesatogkit, Action on Smoking and Health Foundation in Thailand, 2011

Percent of Deaths Due to Tobacco

2004

Below 5%

5%-9.9%

10%-14.9%

15%-19.9%

20%-24.9%

25% and Above

No Data

Countries labeled with percentages have the ***HIGHEST PROPORTION*** *of tobacco-attributable mortality*

%

600,000 nonsmokers died in 2011 from involuntary exposure to secondhand smoke. Exposure to secondhand smoke most commonly occurs in the home, workplace, and public areas and is especially risky for infants, children, pregnant women, and fetuses.

TOBACCO CAUSED 100 MILLION DEATHS DURING THE TWENTIETH CENTURY, AND IF CURRENT TRENDS CONTINUE, APPROXIMATELY 1 BILLION PEOPLE WILL DIE DURING THE TWENTY-FIRST CENTURY BECAUSE OF TOBACCO USE. Deaths caused by tobacco use are entirely preventable, and measures must be taken world-wide to prevent one person from dying every six seconds because of tobacco use and exposure.

Projected Global Tobacco-Caused Deaths

By cause, 2015 baseline scenario

Totals might not sum due to rounding.

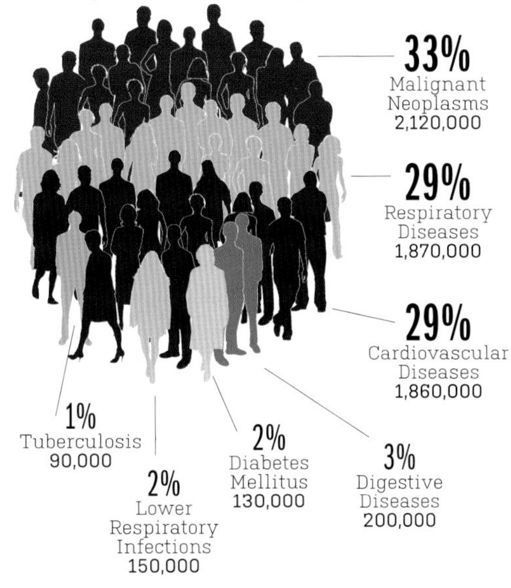

Male Cancer Mortality

Poland, ages 35–69, 1965–2010

In Poland, cancers caused by smoking were responsible for more deaths in middle-aged men than all other cancers combined.

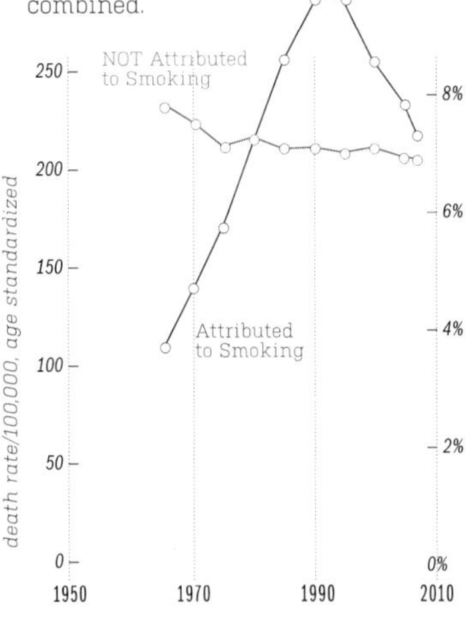

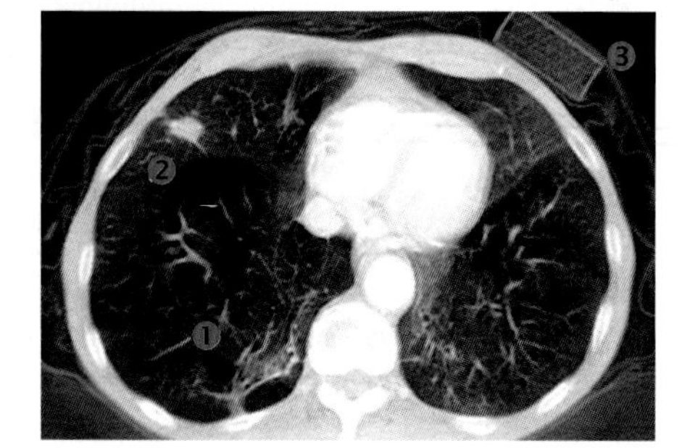

Smoking Causes Lung Cancer
A CAT scan of a patient showing
(1) emphysema, (2) a lung cancer tumor, and
(3) a pack of cigarettes in his shirt pocket.

Tobacco use diminishes health throughout an individual's lifetime, and these effects accumulate throughout adulthood, resulting in preventable illness and, all too often, premature death. Nicotine is most efficiently delivered through smoking, resulting in death to nearly half of lifetime users. Over the years, other nicotine products have entered the market in a cloud of controversy and debate. Tobacco companies have introduced products marketed in a manner that implies they are "safer," but **RESEARCH INDICATES THAT THERE IS NO COMPLETELY SAFE FORM OF TOBACCO.** Smoking cigarettes, including cigarettes with low tar as measured by a machine, has been scientifically proven to harm nearly every organ in the body and to increase morbidity and mortality. Smokeless tobacco products increase the risk of oral cancers, and smokers of cigars, pipes, water pipes, kreteks, and bidis also experience serious adverse health consequences.

Smoking is particularly harmful to pregnant women and their fetuses. Smoking during pregnancy is dangerous to the mother and can cause growth retardation, low birth weight, and possibly death of the fetus.

The harm caused by today's tobacco use will extend for decades into the future, which is made more tragic by the fact that the negative effects of tobacco are entirely preventable. Quitting tobacco use greatly reduces illness by immediately providing short-term benefits and lowering the risk of all diseases caused by smoking.

THE INDUSTRY SAYS:

"We recognize that cigarettes are an addictive product. That doesn't mean you can't stop smoking. **But nicotine is not the issue. It's the other compounds** that are created —they're called volatile compounds— that are created in smoke. They're the ones who create the harm, and they're the ones we're working on in terms of our reduced risk products."

Louis Camilleri, CEO, Philip Morris International, 2011

Deadly Chemicals
in Tobacco Smoke

Tobacco smoke contains more than ***7,000 chemicals*** and compounds. Hundreds of these are toxic, and at least ***69 are cancer-causing.***

Tobacco Smoke Includes	As Found in
Acetone	Paint Stripper
Acetylene	Welding Torches
Arsenic	Ant Poison
Benzene	Napalm
Butane	Lighter Fluid
Cadmium	Car Batteries
Carbon Monoxide	Car Exhaust Fumes
DDT	Insecticide
Formaldehyde	Embalming Fluid
Hydrogen Cyanide	Lethal Execution by Gas
Lead	Old Paint, Leaded Gasoline
Methanol	Rocket Fuel
Nicotine	Cockroach Poison
Phenol	Toilet-Bowl Disinfectant
Polonium 210	Nuclear Weapons
Toluene	Industrial Solvent
Vinyl Chloride	Plastics

RESEARCH SAYS:

"To date, no tobacco products have been scientifically proven to reduce the risk of tobacco-related disease, improve safety, or cause less harm than other tobacco products."

Food and Drug Administration, US, 2011

How Tobacco Harms You

Eyes
Blindness (macular degeneration)
Cataracts
Stinging, excessive tearing and blinking

Ears
Hearing loss
Ear infection

Nose
Cancer of nasal cavities and paranasal sinuses
Impaired sense of smell

Heart
Coronary thrombosis (heart attack)
Atherosclerosis; damage and occlusion of coronary vasculature

Chest & Abdomen
Possible increased risk of breast cancer
Esophageal cancer
Gastric, colon, and pancreatic cancer
Abdominal aortic aneurysm, peptic ulcer (stomach, duodenum, and esophagus)

Hands
Peripheral vascular disease; poor circulation (cold fingers)

Male Reproduction
Infertility; sperm deformity; loss of motility; reduced number
Impotence

Skeletal System
Osteoporosis
Hip fracture
Susceptibility to back problems
Bone-marrow cancer

Circulatory System
Buerger's disease (inflammation of arteries, veins, and nerves in the legs)
Acute myeloid leukemia

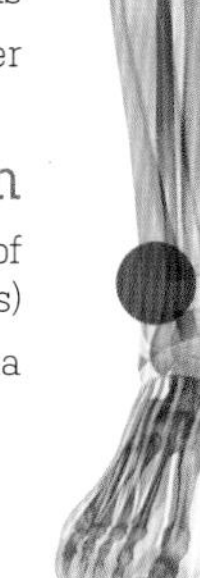

Brain & Psyche

Stroke (cerebrovascular accident)

Addiction/withdrawal

Altered brain chemistry

Anxiety about tobacco's health effects

Hair

Odor and discoloration

Mouth & Throat

Cancers of lips, mouth, throat, larynx, and pharynx

Sore throat

Impaired sense of taste

Halitosis (bad breath)

Teeth

Periodontal (gum) disease; gingivitis; periodontitis

Loose teeth, tooth loss

Root-surface caries, plaque

Discoloration and staining

Lungs

Lung, bronchus, and tracheal cancer

Chronic obstructive pulmonary disease (COPD); emphysema

Chronic bronchitis

Respiratory infection; influenza; pneumonia; tuberculosis

Shortness of breath; asthma

Chronic cough; excessive sputum production

Liver

Liver cancer

Kidneys & Bladder

Kidney and bladder cancer

Skin

Psoriasis

Loss of skin tone; wrinkling; premature aging

Female Reproduction

Cervical cancer

Premature ovarian failure; early menopause

Reduced fertility

Painful menstruation

Wounds & Surgery

Impaired wound healing

Poor postsurgical recovery

Burns from cigarettes and from fires caused by cigarettes

Immune System

Impaired resistance to infection

Legs & Feet

Peripheral vascular disease; cold feet; leg pain; gangrene

Deep vein thrombosis (DVT)

!

Smoking ***increases the risk of tuberculosis*** and is responsible for approximately 20% of global TB incidence.

Smokers with HIV are nearly twice as likely to develop respiratory infections, resulting in poorer health outcomes.

Smoking 25 or more cigarettes a day was found to ***double the risk of type 2 diabetes*** in males in the US.

Risk Factors

Tobacco is the only risk factor shared by all of the four leading noncommunicable diseases.

	Tobacco Use	Unhealthy Diets	Lack of Physical Activity	Harmful Use of Alcohol
CARDIOVASCULAR	☑	☑	☑	☑
DIABETES	☑	☑	☑	☑
CANCER	☑	☑	☑	☑
CHRONIC RESPIRATORY	☑	☐	☐	☐

Health Risks of Smoking During Pregnancy

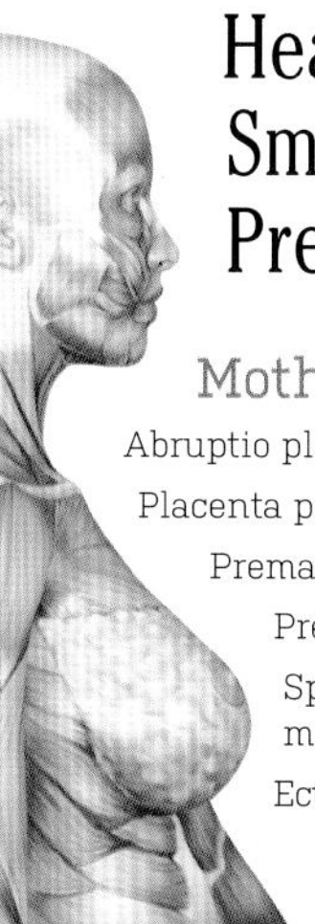

Mother

Abruptio placentae

Placenta previa

Premature rupture of membranes

Premature birth

Spontaneous abortion/ miscarriage

Ectopic pregnancy

Fetuses, Infants, Children

Stunted gestational development

Stillbirth

Sudden Infant Death Syndrome (SIDS)

Reduced lung function and impaired lung development

Asthma exacerbation

Acute lower respiratory infection; bronchitis; pneumonia

Respiratory irritation; cough; phlegm; wheeze

Childhood cancers

Oral cleft

RESEARCH SAYS:

"...even limited secondhand smoke exposure delivers enough nicotine to the brain to alter its function."

Nora Volkow, Director, National Institute on Drug Abuse, US, 2011

Harm Caused by Secondhand Smoke

ADULTS

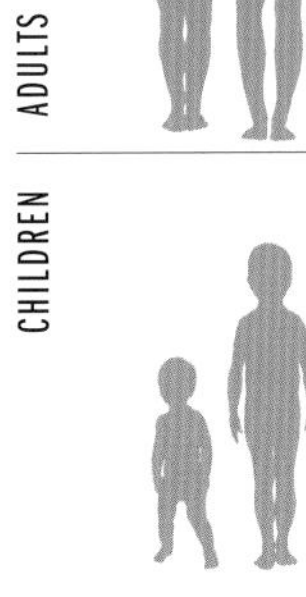

SUFFICIENT EVIDENCE
Coronary artery disease; Lung cancer

SUGGESTIVE EVIDENCE
Stroke; Nasal sinus cancer; Breast cancer; Carotid arterial wall thickening; Chronic obstructive pulmonary disease; Pre-term delivery

CHILDREN

SUFFICIENT EVIDENCE
Middle-ear disease; Respiratory symptoms (cough, wheeze, phlegm, breathlessness); Impaired lung function; Sudden Infant Death Syndrome (SIDS); Lower respiratory illness (including infections), Low birth weight

SUGGESTIVE EVIDENCE
Brain tumors; Lymphoma; Leukemia; Asthma

! Preteens who do not smoke but are exposed to secondhand smoke can experience symptoms of nicotine dependence.

THE INDUSTRY WAS TOLD:

"What the smoker does to himself may be his business, but what the smoker does to the nonsmoker is quite a different matter. [...] This we see as the most dangerous development to the viability of the tobacco industry that has yet occurred."

Roper Organization, US, 1978

Secondhand smoke, or "forced smoking," kills even those people who have consciously chosen not to smoke. Secondhand smoke, also known as environmental tobacco smoke, is a mixture of sidestream smoke from the burning tip of a cigarette, cigar, or pipe, and mainstream smoke, which smokers exhale. Sidestream smoke is the major component of secondhand smoke, and it contains higher concentrations of carcinogens than mainstream smoke.

There is no safe level of exposure to secondhand smoke. Globally, about 40% of children and a third of nonsmoking adults were exposed to secondhand smoke in 2004. The Western Pacific region has the highest rate of secondhand smoke exposure, with more than 50% of men, women, and children exposed to secondhand smoke in 2004.

AN ESTIMATED 600,000 INDIVIDUALS DIE ANNUALLY FROM EXPOSURE TO SECONDHAND SMOKE, AND THE MAJORITY OF SECONDHAND SMOKE DEATHS ARE AMONG WOMEN AND CHILDREN. Breathing secondhand smoke causes immediate harm to the cardiovascular and respiratory systems. Long-term exposure to secondhand smoke can even cause lung cancer. Expectant mothers, fetuses, and infants exposed to secondhand smoke are at particularly high risk of adverse health consequences. Sudden Infant Death Syndrome (SIDS), respiratory issues, and behavioral and learning problems can result when infants and children are exposed to secondhand smoke.

Exposure to secondhand smoke remains one of the world's most critical environmental health hazards, and is more harmful than all other indoor-air contaminants. The fact that nonsmokers have been forced to inhale other people's smoke has led to unprecedented citizen mobilization and the demand for tobacco control measures, including clean indoor-air laws, tax increases, restrictions on sales to minors, and advertising, promotion, and sponsorship bans.

United States of America
Bahamas
Mexico
Mexico City
Cuba
Haiti
Port Au Prince
Dominican Rep.
Jamaica
Belize
Honduras
Tegucigalpa
Guatemala
El Salvador
Nicaragua
Centro Managua
Costa Rica
Panama
St. Kitts & Nevis
Antigua & Barbuda
Dominica
St. Lucia
St. Vincent & the Grenadines
Barbados
Grenada
Trinidad & Tobago
Venezuela
Guyana
Suriname
Colombia
Bogotá
Ecuador
Quito
Peru
Bolivia
La Paz
Brazil
Sao Paulo
Paraguay
Chile
Metropolitana Santiago
Uruguay
Argentina

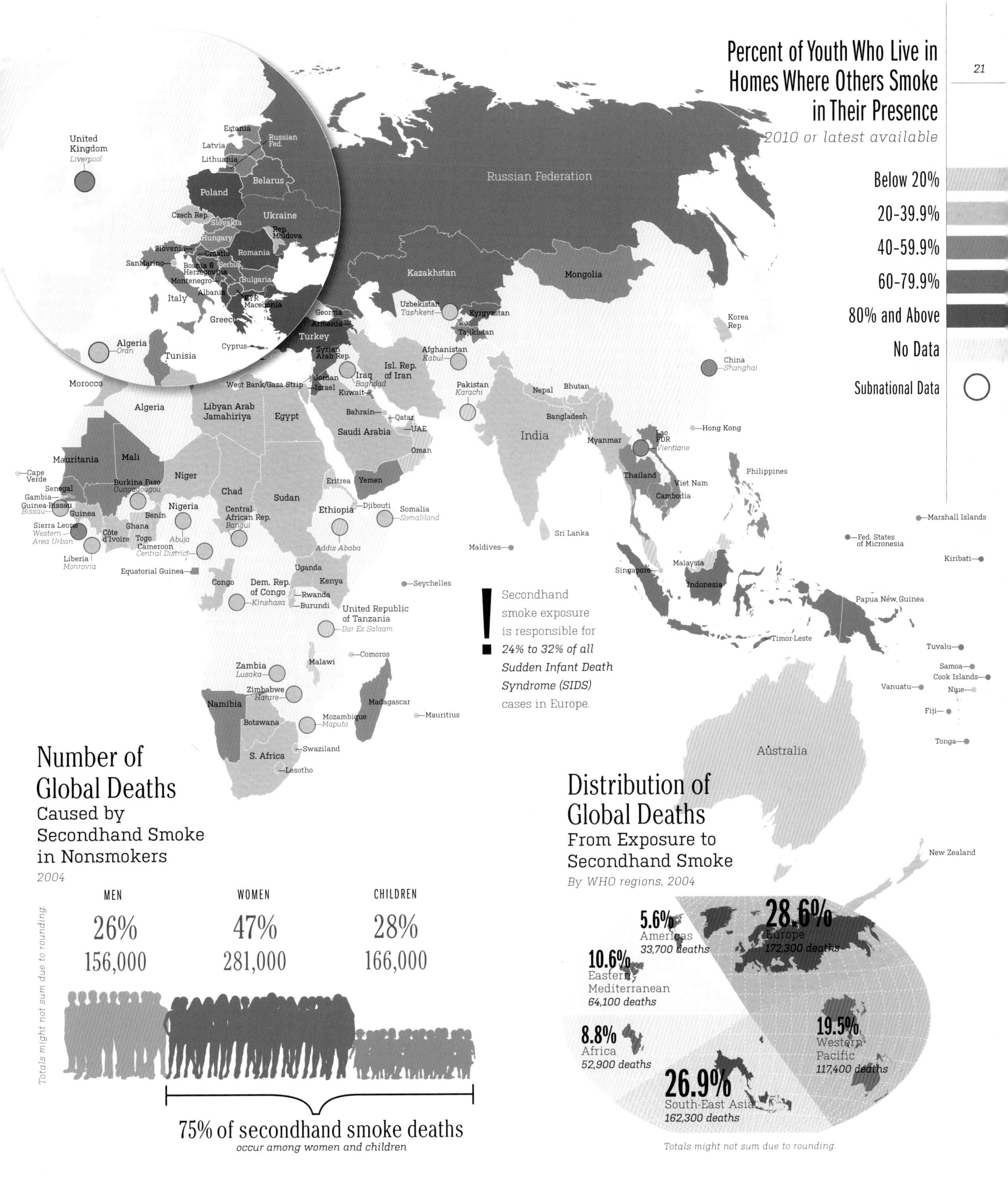
Percent of Youth Who Live in Homes Where Others Smoke in Their Presence
2010 or latest available
Below 20%
20-39.9%
40-59.9%
60-79.9%
80% and Above
No Data
Subnational Data
United Kingdom
Liverpool
Estonia
Latvia
Lithuania
Russian Fed.
Belarus
Poland
Czech Rep.
Slovakia
Ukraine
Rep. Moldova
Hungary
Slovenia
Croatia
Romania
SanMarino
Bosnia & Herzegovina
Serbia
Montenegro
Bulgaria
Albania
Italy
FYR Macedonia
Greece
Georgia
Armenia
Turkey
Cyprus
Algeria
Oran
Tunisia
Morocco
Russian Federation
Kazakhstan
Mongolia
Uzbekistan
Tashkent
Kyrgyzstan
Tajikistan
Korea Rep
China
Shanghai
Syrian Arab Rep.
Iraq
Baghdad
Isl. Rep. of Iran
Afghanistan
Kabul
Jordan
Israel
West Bank/Gaza Strip
Kuwait
Pakistan
Karachi
Nepal
Bhutan
Bahrain
Qatar
UAE
Saudi Arabia
Oman
Bangladesh
India
Myanmar
Lao PDR
Vientiane
Hong Kong
Algeria
Libyan Arab Jamahiriya
Egypt
Mauritania
Mali
Niger
Chad
Sudan
Eritrea
Yemen
Thailand
Viet Nam
Cambodia
Philippines
Cape Verde
Senegal
Gambia
Guinea-Bissau
Bissau
Guinea
Burkina Faso
Ouagadougou
Nigeria
Abuja
Benin
Central African Rep.
Bangui
Ethiopia
Addis Ababa
Djibouti
Somalia
Somaliland
Sierra Leone
Western Area Urban
Côte d'Ivoire
Ghana
Togo
Cameroon
Central District
Liberia
Monrovia
Equatorial Guinea
Maldives
Sri Lanka
Marshall Islands
Fed. States of Micronesia
Kiribati
Singapore
Malaysia
Indonesia
Papua New Guinea
Uganda
Kenya
Congo
Dem. Rep. of Congo
Kinshasa
Rwanda
Burundi
Seychelles
United Republic of Tanzania
Dar Es Salaam
Timor-Leste
Comoros
Malawi
Zambia
Lusaka
Zimbabwe
Harare
Namibia
Botswana
Madagascar
Mozambique
Maputo
Mauritius
Swaziland
S. Africa
Lesotho
Tuvalu
Samoa
Cook Islands
Vanuatu
Niue
Fiji
Tonga
Australia
New Zealand
!
Secondhand smoke exposure is responsible for 24% to 32% of all Sudden Infant Death Syndrome (SIDS) cases in Europe.
Number of Global Deaths
Caused by Secondhand Smoke in Nonsmokers
2004
MEN
26%
156,000
WOMEN
47%
281,000
CHILDREN
28%
166,000
Totals might not sum due to rounding.
75% of secondhand smoke deaths
occur among women and children
Distribution of Global Deaths
From Exposure to Secondhand Smoke
By WHO regions, 2004
5.6%
Americas
33,700 deaths
28.6%
Europe
172,300 deaths
10.6%
Eastern Mediterranean
64,100 deaths
8.8%
Africa
52,900 deaths
19.5%
Western Pacific
117,400 deaths
26.9%
South-East Asia
162,300 deaths
Totals might not sum due to rounding.

RESEARCH SAYS:

"Nobody should cry because of lower consumption of a product that kills half the people who use it."

Danny McGoldrick, Campaign for Tobacco-Free Kids, US, 2007

SINCE THE FIRST EDITION OF *THE TOBACCO ATLAS* A DECADE AGO,

MORE THAN 43 Trillion CIGARETTES HAVE BEEN SMOKED.

1 BUTT = 10 BILLION CIGARETTES

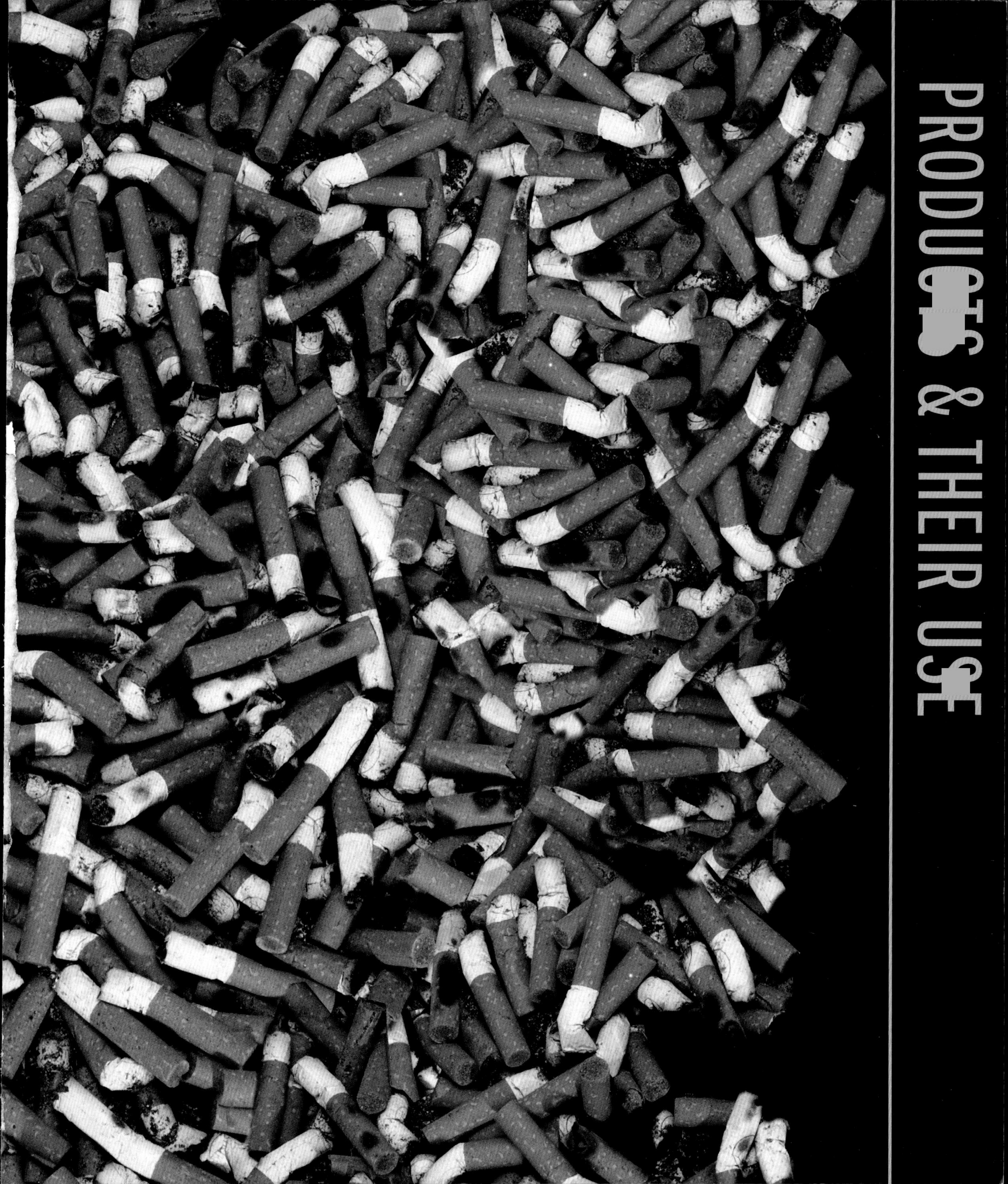
PRODUCTS & THEIR USE

GOVERNMENT SAYS:

"A jihad is needed against tobacco to tell that consumption of tobacco is dangerous. The whole nation needs to come together against it."

Ghulam Nabi Azad, Union Minister of Health & Family Welfare, India, 2010

Tobacco is used in many different ways around the world, but the global predominance is the use of MANUFACTURED CIGARETTES, WHICH ACCOUNT FOR 96% OF TOTAL WORLDWIDE SALES, and hence involves big business rather than small, local, rural enterprises.

The next largest components are the smoking of bidis in South-East Asia, the chewing of tobacco in India, the smoking of kreteks in Indonesia, and the use of moist snuff, which originated in Sweden but is now becoming global.

New forms of tobacco (and of its component nicotine) are constantly being invented, while older forms historically localized to specific regions of the world (such as the hookah and bidi) are becoming global. For instance, kreteks and moist snuff are currently being marketed to youth in many countries. These regional forms of tobacco sometimes gain footholds in new countries based on their exotic cachet, but to date they have not displaced manufactured cigarettes for a significant market share. Instead, they frequently serve as a gateway to addiction, luring youth and other fad smokers into lifelong dependence on nicotine.

New forms of tobacco may not be covered by existing tobacco control legislation and are thus a challenge to countries seeking to reduce the epidemic (especially to reduce youth uptake).

! Despite the introduction of many new forms of tobacco, ***there is still no safe way of using tobacco—whether inhaled, sniffed, sucked, or chewed;*** whether some of the harmful ingredients are reduced; or whether it is mixed with other ingredients.

SMOKING TOBACCO

Tobacco smoking is the act of burning dried or cured leaves of the tobacco plant and inhaling the smoke. Combustion uses heat to create new chemicals that are not found in unburned tobacco, such as tobacco-specific nitrosamines (TSNAs) and benzopyrene, and allows them to be absorbed through the lungs.

Manufactured cigarettes are the most commonly consumed tobacco products worldwide. They consist of shredded or reconstituted tobacco, processed with hundreds of chemicals and various flavors such as menthol, and rolled into a paper-wrapped cylinder. Usually tipped with a cellulose acetate filter, they are lit at one end and inhaled through the other.
Most prevalent: Worldwide

Kreteks are clove-flavored cigarettes. They may also contain a wide range of exotic flavorings and eugenol, which has an anesthetic effect, allowing for deeper and more harmful smoke inhalation.
Most prevalent: Indonesia

Roll-your-own (RYO) cigarettes are hand-filled by the smoker from fine-cut loose tobacco and a cigarette paper. RYO cigarette smokers are exposed to high concentrations of tobacco particulates, tar, nicotine, and TSNAs, and are at increased risk for developing cancers of the mouth, pharynx, larynx, lungs, and esophagus.
Most prevalent: Europe and New Zealand

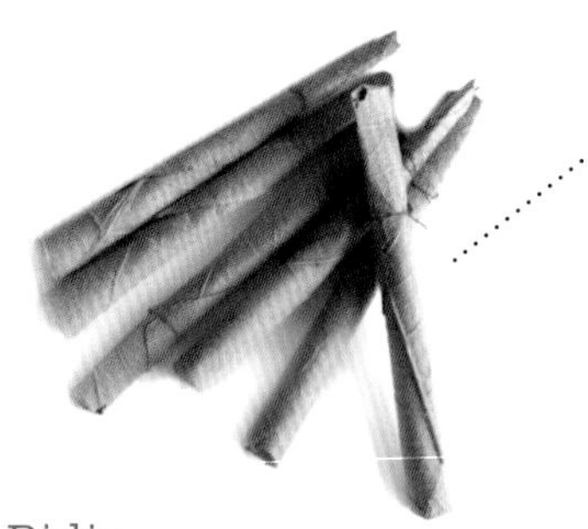

Bidis consist of a small amount of crushed tobacco, hand-wrapped in dried temburni or tendu leaves, and tied with string. Despite their small size, bidis tend to deliver more tar and carbon monoxide than manufactured cigarettes because users must puff harder to keep them lit.
Most prevalent: South Asia (and are the most heavily consumed smoked tobacco products in India)

Pipes are made of briar, slate, clay, or other substances. Tobacco is placed in the bowl, and the smoke is inhaled through the stem. In South-East Asia, clay pipes known as sulpa, chillum, and hookli are widely used.
Most prevalent: Worldwide

Sticks are made from sun-cured tobacco and wrapped in cigarette paper—for example, hand-rolled brus.
Most prevalent: Papua New Guinea

SMOKELESS TOBACCO

Smokeless tobacco is usually consumed orally or nasally, without burning or combustion. Smokeless tobacco increases the risk of cancer and leads to nicotine addiction similar to that produced by cigarette smoking. There are different types of smokeless tobacco: chewing tobacco, snuff, and dissolvables.

Chewing tobacco is an oral smokeless tobacco product that is placed in the mouth, cheek, or inner lip and sucked or chewed. It is sometimes referred to as "spit tobacco" because of the tendency by users to spit out the built-up tobacco juices and saliva.
Most prevalent: Worldwide

There are many varieties of chewing tobacco, including plug, loose-leaf, chimo, toombak, gutkha, and twist. Pan masala or betel quid consists of tobacco, areca nuts *(Areca catechu)*, slaked lime (calcium hydroxide), sweeteners, and flavoring agents wrapped in a betel leaf *(Piper betle)*. There are many varieties of pan masala, including kaddipudi, hogesoppu, gundi, kadapam, zarda, pattiwala, kiwam, and mishri.
Most prevalent: India

Moist snuff consists of ground tobacco held in the mouth between the cheek and the gum. Manufacturers are increasingly packaging moist snuff into small paper or cloth packets to make the product more convenient. Moist snuff products are known as snus, khaini, shammaah, nass, or naswa. Tobacco pastes or powders are similarly used, placed on the gums or teeth. Fine tobacco powder mixtures are usually inhaled and absorbed through the nasal passages.
Most prevalent: Scandinavia and US but becoming worldwide; banned in several countries

Cigars are made of air-cured and fermented tobaccos rolled in tobacco-leaf wrappers. The long aging and fermentation process produces high concentrations of carcinogenic compounds that are released upon combustion. The concentrations of toxins and irritants in cigars are higher than in cigarettes. Cigars come in many shapes and sizes, from cigarette-size cigarillos to double coronas, cheroots, stumpen, chuttas, and dhumtis. In reverse chutta and dhumti smoking, the ignited end is placed inside the mouth.
Most prevalent: Worldwide

Dry snuff is powdered tobacco that is inhaled through the nose or taken orally. Once widespread, particularly in Europe, the use of dry snuff is in decline.
Most prevalent: Europe

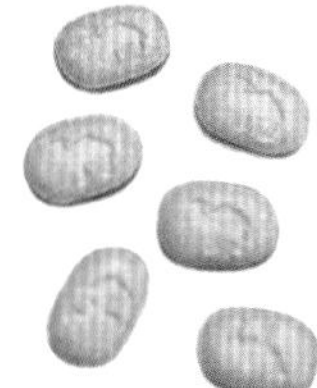

Dissolvable smokeless tobacco products dissolve in the mouth without expectoration; they contain tobacco and numerous added constituents whose purpose is to deliver nicotine to the user via oral mucosal absorption. They are often extensions of well-known cigarette brands, such as Camel Sticks, Strips, and Orbs; Marlboro Sticks; products by Star Scientific (Ariva, Stonewall); and Zerostyle Mint by Japan Tobacco. These newest oral smokeless tobacco products are developed for use by smokers in any situation where they cannot or choose not to smoke.
Most prevalent: High-income nations

Water pipes, also known as shisha, hookah, narghile, or hubble-bubble, operate by water filtration and indirect heat. Flavored tobacco is burned in a smoking bowl covered with foil and coal. The smoke is cooled by filtration through a basin of water and consumed through a hose and mouthpiece.
Most prevalent: North Africa, the Mediterranean region, and parts of Asia, but now spreading around the world

RESEARCH SAYS:

"Nicotine is a highly addictive drug, and to make it look like a piece of candy is recklessly playing with the health of children."

Gregory Connolly, Harvard University, US, 2010

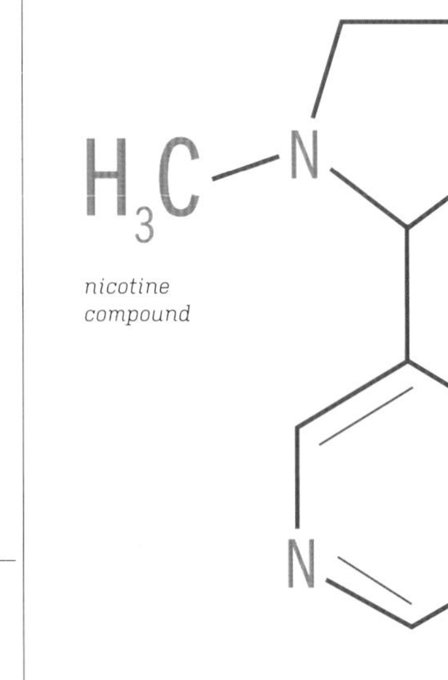

nicotine compound

THE INDUSTRY MUST SAY:

"We told Congress under oath that we believed nicotine is not addictive. We told you that smoking is not an addiction and all it takes to quit is willpower. Here's the truth: Smoking is very addictive. And it's not easy to quit. We manipulated cigarettes to make them more addictive."

One of the US Department of Justice's Proposed Corrective Statements for Cigarette Companies, 2011

With the exception of oral tobacco products, tobacco is typically consumed through combustion, in which tobacco leaves are burned at high temperatures and the resulting smoke is inhaled. Combustion is the most efficient method of delivering nicotine to the brain.

TOBACCO COMPANIES UNDERSTAND THE IMPORTANCE OF NICOTINE AND WANT TO CONTINUE TO BE THE PROVIDERS OF CHOICE FOR NICOTINE PRODUCTS, but they also understand the dangers created by the combustion of tobacco products, most notably that customers routinely die from their use. Therefore, tobacco companies are creating new products to keep individuals addicted to nicotine while reducing toxic exposures caused by combustion. Such products include noncombustible cigarettes (e.g., Eclipse, Premier) and oral tobacco (e.g., lozenges, strips, snus, orbs), some of which are dissolvable. There is an urgent need for research and regulation of these products.

Beginning in the 1970s, pharmaceutical companies began providing nicotine replacement therapy (NRT) to ease nicotine withdrawal symptoms.

Less harmful & heavily regulated

PHARMACEUTICAL COMPANIES

Pharmaceutical companies sell ***nicotine replacement therapy*** to assist with smoking cessation. These products are heavily regulated and companies are required to demonstrate that they are safe and effective.

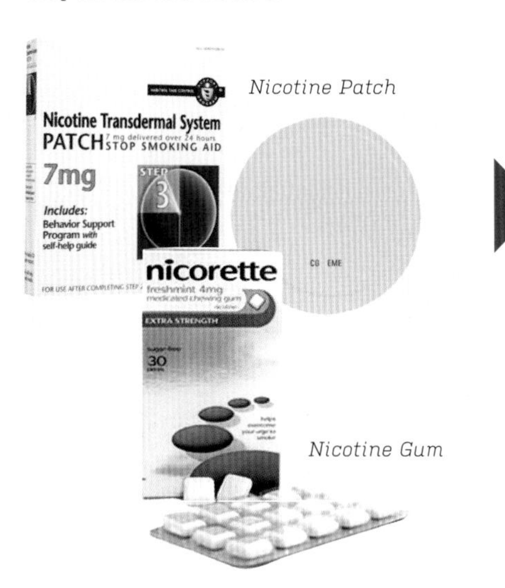

Nicotine Patch

Nicotine Gum

ENTREPRENEURS

Entrepreneurs create products to bypass tobacco bans while maintaining nicotine addiction. Examples of products include ***nicotine water, lollipops***, and ***electronic cigarettes.***

Nicotine Lollipop

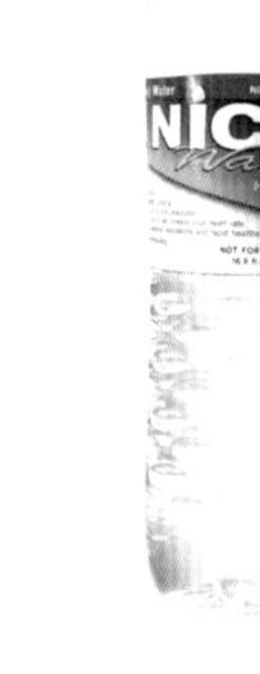

Nicotine Water

SIDE EFFECTS AND CONTINUUM OF HARM:

These products are generally safe when used as directed and are ***heavily regulated.*** Minor side effects include stomach irritation, rash, etc.

SIDE EFFECTS AND CONTINUUM OF HARM:

These products are ***unregulated***, and the side effects and dangers are unknown. Although e-cigarettes are marketed as a "safe" alternative to smoking, laboratory analyses found carcinogens and toxic chemicals in these products.

Because these products are considered pharmaceuticals, they must undergo rigorous approval to assure their safety and efficacy. NRT doubles smoking quit rates and is currently available through patches, gum, lozenges, and inhalers.

Entrepreneurs have created many novel nicotine delivery products, such as nicotine water, wafers, candy, inhalers, and electronic cigarettes. These products provide nicotine in an innovative yet unregulated manner, and the potential risks are largely unknown.

The arrival of novel nicotine delivery products in the mass market creates a new avenue for individuals to initiate or maintain nicotine addiction, which could result in increased addiction, fewer cessation attempts, increased use of multiple products, and addiction to higher levels of nicotine. However, these products could also potentially play a role in the cessation of combusted tobacco products.

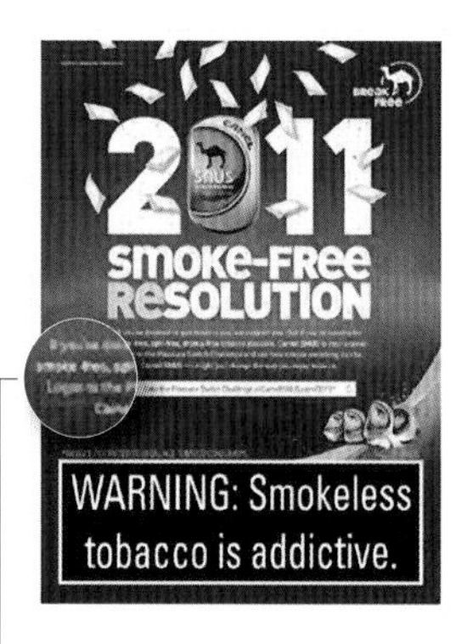

"If you've decided to quit tobacco use, we support you. But if you're looking for smoke-free, spit-free, drama-free tobacco pleasure, Camel Snus is your answer."

"Snus is less dangerous than cigarettes, for sure, but it is very hard to find anything more dangerous than cigarettes. There is no natural law that says 30 percent of the population should be nicotine addicts."

Goran Pershagen, Karolinska Institute, Sweden, 2007

CONTINUUM OF HARM ········ *More harmful & unregulated*

TOBACCO COMPANIES

! Tobacco companies are becoming more interested in nicotine delivery technology ***in an effort to capitalize on the $3.6 billion global market*** for smoking cessation aids.

Tobacco companies have launched nontraditional products, such as ***snus, orbs,*** and ***lozenges*** in high-income countries to ensure consumers maintain their tobacco addiction. They are also purchasing patents for alternative nicotine delivery systems, such as aerosol technology. Tobacco companies continue to provide traditional combustible cigarettes to consumers, especially those in low- and middle-income countries.

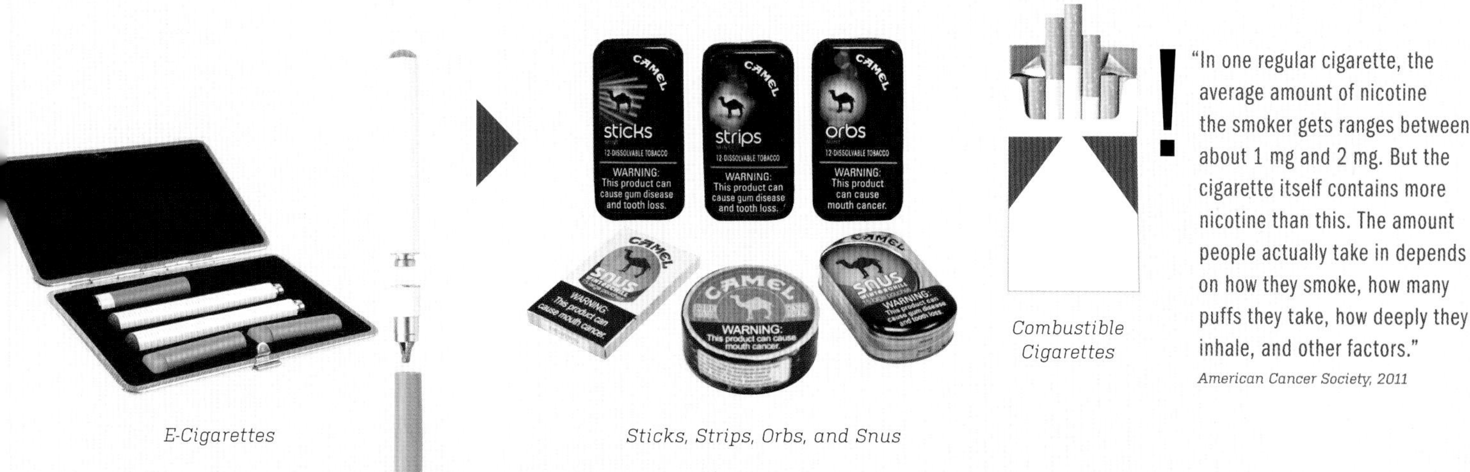

E-Cigarettes

Sticks, Strips, Orbs, and Snus

Combustible Cigarettes

! "In one regular cigarette, the average amount of nicotine the smoker gets ranges between about 1 mg and 2 mg. But the cigarette itself contains more nicotine than this. The amount people actually take in depends on how they smoke, how many puffs they take, how deeply they inhale, and other factors."

American Cancer Society, 2011

SIDE EFFECTS AND CONTINUUM OF HARM:

Combustible cigarettes result in significant morbidity and mortality. This is the most dangerous and harmful way to absorb nicotine, and the products are ***unregulated***. Smokeless tobacco products are known to be addictive and harmful. While less is known about newer products, they likely have some level of harm associated with their use.

RESEARCH SAYS:

> "For each 1,000 tons of tobacco produced, about 1,000 people will eventually die."
>
> *World Health Organization, Regional Office for the Eastern Mediterranean, undated*

NEARLY 20% OF THE WORLD'S ADULT POPULATION SMOKES CIGARETTES. Smokers consumed nearly 5.9 trillion cigarettes in 2009, representing a 13% increase in cigarette consumption in the past decade.

Cigarette consumption historically has been highest in high-income countries, but because of targeted marketing, increased social acceptability, continued economic development, and population increases, consumption is expected to increase in low- and middle-income countries. Cigarette consumption in Western Europe dropped by 26% between 1990 and 2009 but increased in the Middle East and Africa by 57% during the same period. This change has occurred as people in high-income countries increasingly understand the dangers of smoking and governments continue to implement tobacco control policy and legislation. Globally, the increase in cigarette consumption in low- and middle-income countries is significant enough to offset the decrease in high-income countries.

Cigarette consumption is responsible for a significant disease burden. As consumption rates continue to increase in low- and middle-income countries, these countries will experience a disproportionate amount of tobacco-related illness and death—particularly China, as Chinese men smoke a third of the world's cigarettes. If the smoking prevalence among Chinese women increases, global consumption of cigarettes will skyrocket, and the country's economy and health-care systems will be overwhelmed.

While global smoking prevalence is flat or decreasing, the total number of smokers worldwide continues to increase simply due to population growth. While almost 6 trillion cigarettes are consumed annually, the pattern of nicotine consumption may shift in the future as people seek alternative nicotine delivery systems (see Chapter 5 – *Nicotine Delivery Systems*). TOBACCO AND NICOTINE ADDICTION MUST BE TREATED COMMENSURATE WITH THE HARM CAUSED. The World Health Organization's Framework Convention on Tobacco Control (WHO FCTC) has outlined how best to reduce tobacco use, and the time has come to act on this information.

THE INDUSTRY SAYS:

> "We believe we can increase the consumption of kretek elsewhere.... We assured ourselves that they are not more or less dangerous than conventional cigarettes."
>
> *Louis Camilleri, CEO, Altria, US, 2005*

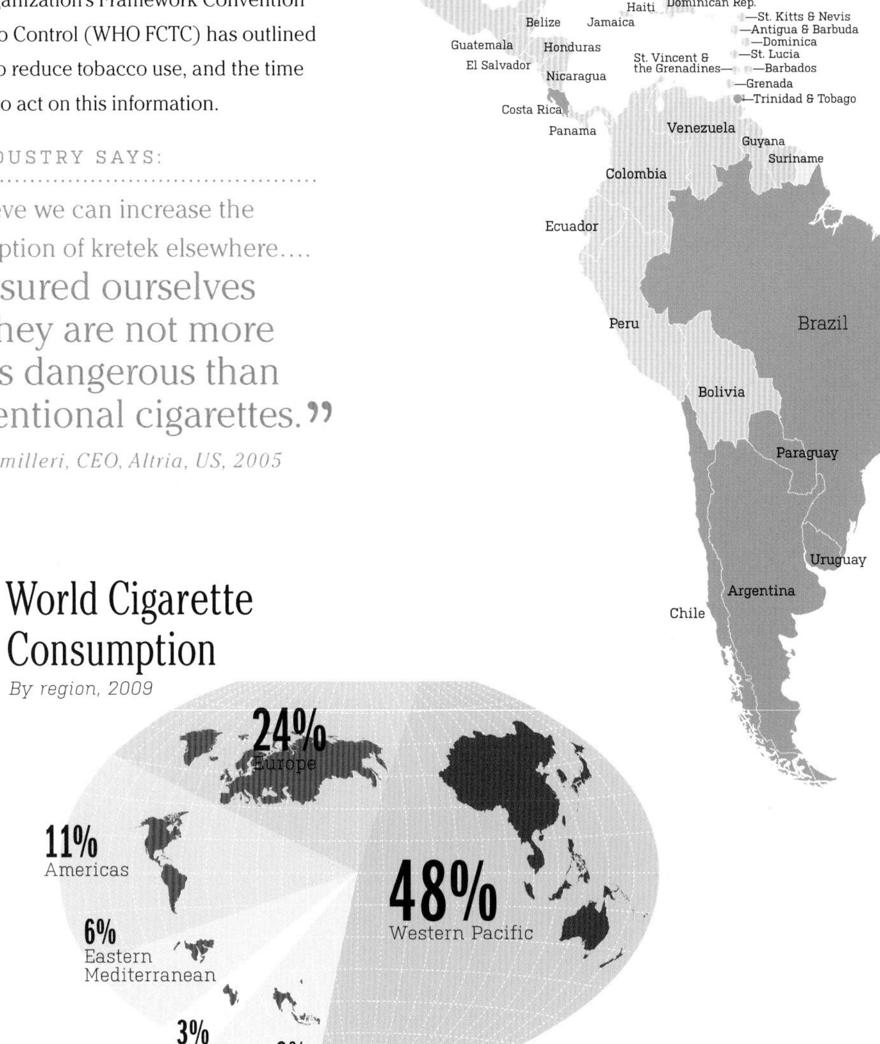

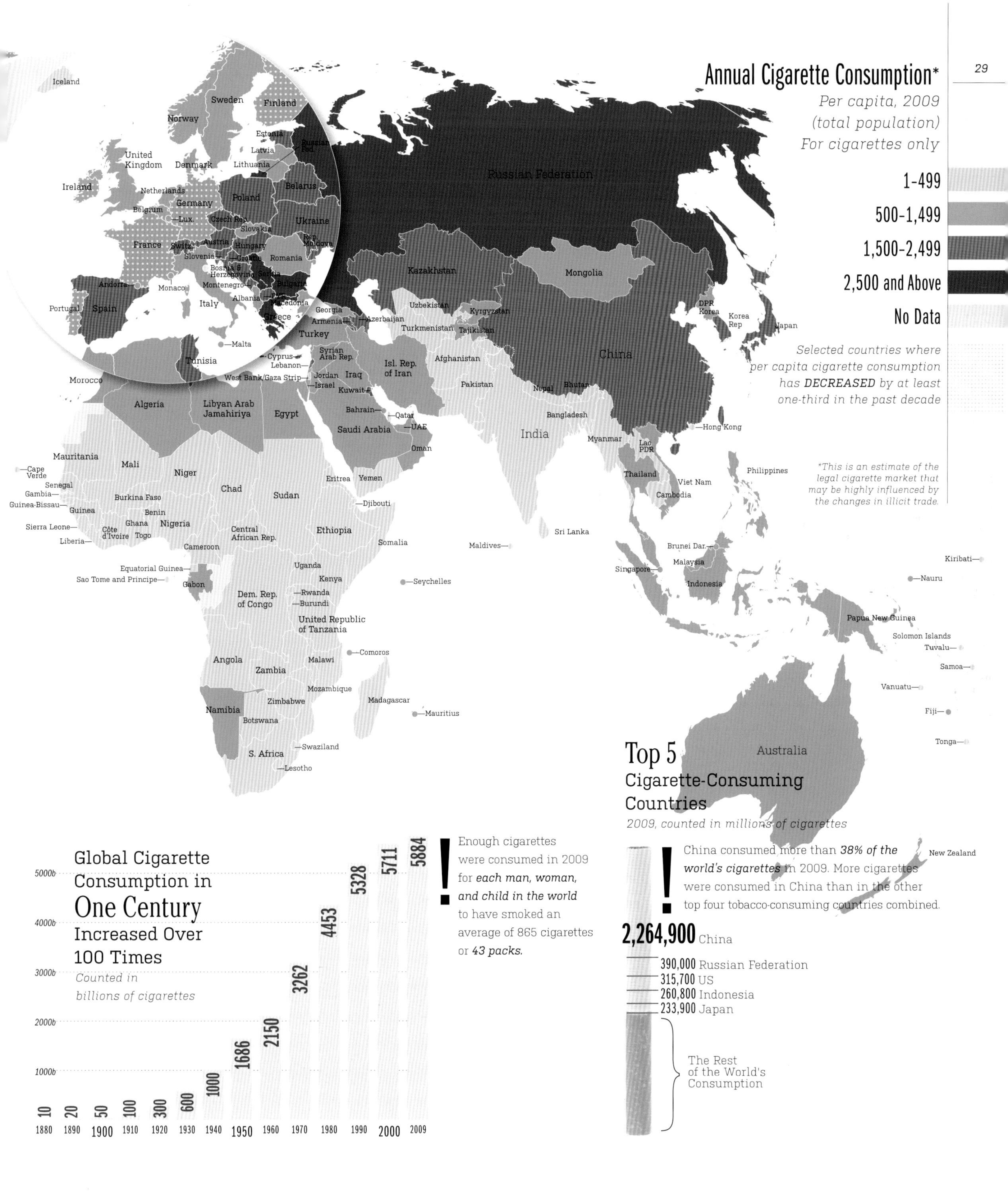
Annual Cigarette Consumption*
Per capita, 2009
(total population)
For cigarettes only
1-499
500-1,499
1,500-2,499
2,500 and Above
No Data
Selected countries where per capita cigarette consumption has DECREASED by at least one-third in the past decade
*This is an estimate of the legal cigarette market that may be highly influenced by the changes in illicit trade.
Iceland
Sweden
Finland
Norway
Estonia
Latvia
Lithuania
Russian Fed.
United Kingdom
Denmark
Ireland
Netherlands
Germany
Poland
Belarus
Belgium
Lux.
Czech Rep.
Slovakia
Ukraine
France
Switz.
Austria
Hungary
Rep. Moldova
Slovenia
Croatia
Romania
Bosnia & Herzegovina
Serbia
Bulgaria
Andorra
Monaco
Montenegro
Albania
Macedonia
Portugal
Spain
Italy
Greece
Malta
Tunisia
Morocco
Russian Federation
Kazakhstan
Mongolia
Uzbekistan
Kyrgyzstan
Georgia
Armenia
Azerbaijan
Turkmenistan
Tajikistan
Turkey
DPR Korea
Korea Rep
Japan
Cyprus
Lebanon
Syrian Arab Rep.
Isl. Rep. of Iran
Afghanistan
China
West Bank/Gaza Strip
Jordan
Iraq
Israel
Kuwait
Pakistan
Nepal
Bhutan
Algeria
Libyan Arab Jamahiriya
Egypt
Bahrain
Qatar
UAE
Saudi Arabia
Bangladesh
India
Myanmar
Hong Kong
Lao PDR
Oman
Mauritania
Mali
Niger
Cape Verde
Senegal
Gambia
Guinea-Bissau
Guinea
Chad
Sudan
Eritrea
Yemen
Thailand
Philippines
Viet Nam
Cambodia
Burkina Faso
Benin
Djibouti
Sierra Leone
Côte d'Ivoire
Ghana
Togo
Nigeria
Central African Rep.
Ethiopia
Liberia
Cameroon
Somalia
Maldives
Sri Lanka
Brunei Dar.
Malaysia
Singapore
Indonesia
Kiribati
Nauru
Equatorial Guinea
Sao Tome and Principe
Gabon
Uganda
Kenya
Seychelles
Dem. Rep. of Congo
Rwanda
Burundi
United Republic of Tanzania
Papua New Guinea
Solomon Islands
Tuvalu
Comoros
Angola
Zambia
Malawi
Samoa
Vanuatu
Mozambique
Zimbabwe
Madagascar
Namibia
Botswana
Mauritius
Fiji
Tonga
Swaziland
S. Africa
Lesotho
Australia
New Zealand
Global Cigarette Consumption in One Century Increased Over 100 Times
Counted in billions of cigarettes
5000b
4000b
3000b
2000b
1000b
10 1880
20 1890
50 1900
100 1910
300 1920
600 1930
1000 1940
1686 1950
2150 1960
3262 1970
4453 1980
5328 1990
5711 2000
5884 2009
!
Enough cigarettes were consumed in 2009 for each man, woman, and child in the world to have smoked an average of 865 cigarettes or 43 packs.
Top 5 Cigarette-Consuming Countries
2009, counted in millions of cigarettes
!
China consumed more than 38% of the world's cigarettes in 2009. More cigarettes were consumed in China than in the other top four tobacco-consuming countries combined.
2,264,900 China
390,000 Russian Federation
315,700 US
260,800 Indonesia
233,900 Japan
The Rest of the World's Consumption

"When I began smoking, about 80 percent of men were smokers. The advertising phrase was, 'You're healthy when a cigarette tastes so good.'"

Masanobu Mizuno, plaintiff in a suit against Japan Tobacco, Japan, 2009

About 800 million adult men worldwide smoke cigarettes. **ALMOST 20% OF THE WORLD'S ADULT MALE SMOKERS LIVE IN HIGH-INCOME COUNTRIES, WHILE OVER 80% ARE IN LOW- AND MIDDLE-INCOME COUNTRIES.**

The global tobacco epidemic can be segmented into four stages in which men typically precede women. Stage 1 represents the very beginning of the epidemic when the prevalence of smoking has begun to rise but there is as yet no appreciable smoking attributed mortality. In Stage 2 smoking prevalence increases rapidly but smoking attributed deaths still account for a small proportion (less than 5%) of all deaths. In Stage 3 smoking prevalence is stable or decreasing but smoking attributed mortality increases to a maximum of 20%- 50% of all deaths in middle age (35-69 years). In stage 4 smoking prevalence (and eventually smoking-attributed mortality) decrease towards lower limits that are not yet defined. While countries may have similar prevalence rates, each country's location on the curve is important. Countries on the upslope of the trajectory are in the early stages of the epidemic and experience different challenges than those countries on the downslope.

Tobacco marketing associates male smoking with masculinity, happiness, wealth, virility, and power. In reality, smoking kills nearly 4 million men annually and leads to infertility, health disparities, illness, and premature death. Overall, smoking prevalence rates are declining, but the number of smokers is increasing due to general population growth. Even the most successful tobacco control programs can only desire to cap the number of new tobacco users. People are increasingly using innovative and alternative products, such as oral tobacco, electronic cigarettes, and nicotine replacement therapy, to obtain nicotine. As we continue to monitor smoking rates throughout the world, we must become increasingly cognizant of these alternative manners of maintaining nicotine addiction (see Chapter 5 – *Nicotine Delivery Systems*).

THE INDUSTRY SAYS:

"I'm no cowboy and I don't ride horseback, but I like to think I have the freedom the Marlboro man exemplifies. He's the man who doesn't punch a clock. He's not computerized. He's a free spirit."

George Weissman, Former President and CEO, Philip Morris USA, 1978

! Among the 14 countries where 50% or more of men smoke, ***all but one country (Greece) are classified as low- or middle-income.***

Male Smoking Prevalence and Deaths Over a Century

Weighted average of smoking prevalence, 2010

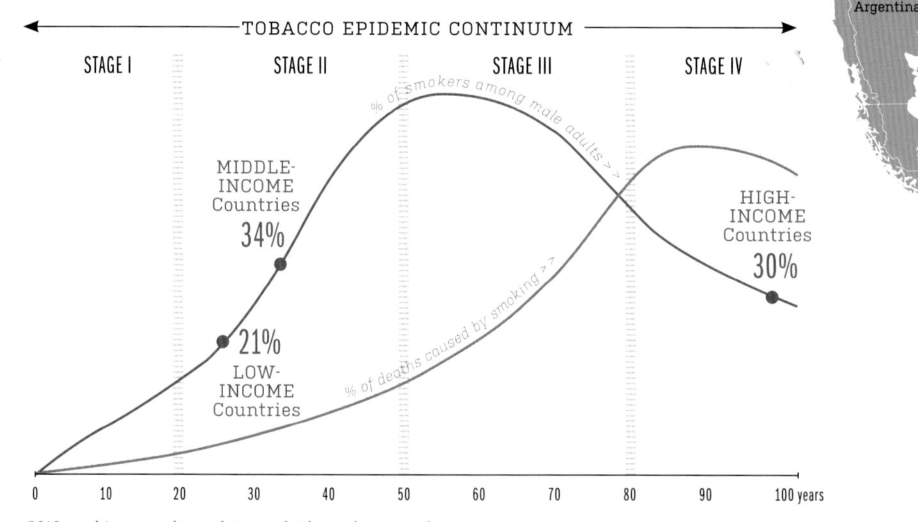

2010 smoking prevalence data overlaid on tobacco epidemic continuum.

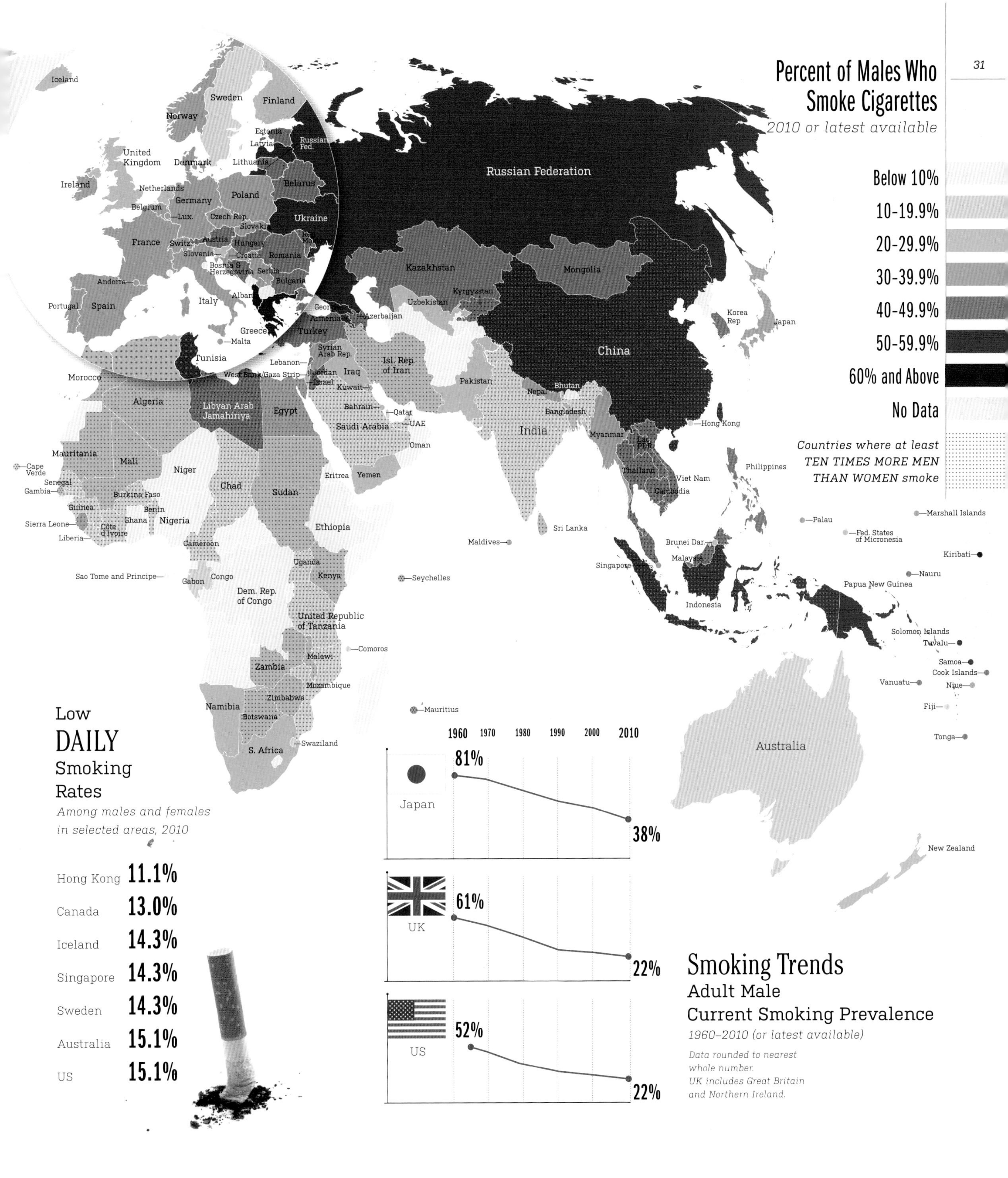
Percent of Males Who
Smoke Cigarettes
2010 or latest available
Below 10%
10-19.9%
20-29.9%
30-39.9%
40-49.9%
50-59.9%
60% and Above
No Data
Countries where at least
TEN TIMES MORE MEN
THAN WOMEN smoke
Iceland
Sweden
Finland
Norway
Estonia
Latvia
Russian Fed.
United Kingdom
Denmark
Lithuania
Ireland
Netherlands
Belarus
Germany
Poland
Belgium
Lux.
Czech Rep.
Ukraine
Slovakia
France
Switz.
Austria
Hungary
Slovenia
Croatia
Romania
Bosnia & Herzegovina
Serbia
Bulgaria
Andorra
Italy
Alban
Portugal
Spain
Greece
Malta
Tunisia
Morocco
Russian Federation
Kazakhstan
Mongolia
Uzbekistan
Kyrgyzstan
Georgia
Armenia
Azerbaijan
Turkey
Korea Rep
Japan
China
Syrian Arab Rep.
Lebanon
Isl. Rep. of Iran
West Bank/Gaza Strip
Jordan
Iraq
Israel
Kuwait
Pakistan
Bhutan
Nepal
Bahrain
Qatar
UAE
Bangladesh
Saudi Arabia
India
Hong Kong
Algeria
Libyan Arab Jamahiriya
Egypt
Oman
Myanmar
Lao PDR
Mauritania
Mali
Niger
Cape Verde
Senegal
Gambia
Chad
Sudan
Eritrea
Yemen
Thailand
Viet Nam
Cambodia
Philippines
Burkina Faso
Guinea
Benin
Sierra Leone
Ghana
Nigeria
Côte d'Ivoire
Liberia
Ethiopia
Sri Lanka
Palau
Marshall Islands
Fed. States of Micronesia
Cameroon
Maldives
Brunei Dar.
Malaysia
Kiribati
Singapore
Nauru
Sao Tome and Principe
Gabon
Congo
Uganda
Kenya
Seychelles
Papua New Guinea
Dem. Rep. of Congo
Indonesia
United Republic of Tanzania
Solomon Islands
Tuvalu
Comoros
Malawi
Samoa
Zambia
Cook Islands
Mozambique
Vanuatu
Niue
Zimbabwe
Namibia
Mauritius
Fiji
Botswana
Swaziland
S. Africa
Australia
Tonga
New Zealand
Low
DAILY
Smoking
Rates
Among males and females
in selected areas, 2010
Hong Kong 11.1%
Canada 13.0%
Iceland 14.3%
Singapore 14.3%
Sweden 14.3%
Australia 15.1%
US 15.1%
1960
1970
1980
1990
2000
2010
Japan
81%
38%
UK
61%
22%
US
52%
22%
Smoking Trends
Adult Male
Current Smoking Prevalence
1960–2010 (or latest available)
Data rounded to nearest whole number.
UK includes Great Britain and Northern Ireland.

HISTORY SAYS:

> “What Bernays had created [in the 1920s in the United States] was the idea that if a woman smoked it made her more powerful and independent. An idea that still persists today.”
>
> *Adam Curtis*, Century of the Self, *UK, 2002*

NEARLY 200 MILLION ADULT WOMEN WORLDWIDE SMOKE CIGARETTES. As observed among high-income countries in the 20th century, the first stage of the tobacco epidemic occurred as the rate of smoking among men increased and surpassed 50%. During the next stage, smoking rates decreased among men and increased among women. There is a concern that this pattern may occur in the future in low- and middle-income countries as well. In 2010, half of the world's female smokers were in high-income countries and the remaining half in low- and middle-income countries.

Tobacco companies market directly to women and create an association between smoking and gender equality. This is happening today in many low- and middle-income countries where there are potential new smokers and sparse marketing restrictions, but this practice is not new for tobacco companies. ALMOST A CENTURY AGO, THE AMERICAN TOBACCO COMPANY PURPOSEFULLY LINKED SMOKING WITH WOMEN'S RIGHT TO VOTE, WITH CIGARETTES CALLED "TORCHES OF FREEDOM." This type of forced association between smoking and gender equality can be expected worldwide.

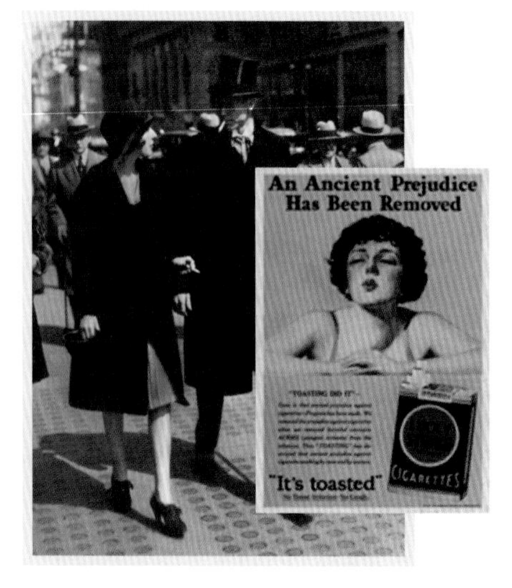

Women are the target of marketing campaigns, specifically ones promoting “light” or “low-tar” cigarettes. Women often choose these cigarettes because of a false assumption that the products are less harmful than full-flavor cigarettes. In reality, all cigarettes contain approximately the same amount of tar and nicotine, but smokers of “light” and “low-tar” cigarettes compensate (e.g., covering ventilation holes, sucking harder, etc.) to more efficiently extract nicotine from the cigarettes. This has resulted in no net benefit for women who continue to smoke and use these “lighter” products.

Smoking decreases fertility in women, combines with oral contraceptives to increase the risk of heart attacks and stroke, and results in poor health outcomes for fetuses and newborns. If women begin smoking at rates equivalent to men, the world will face a public health disaster of enormous proportions.

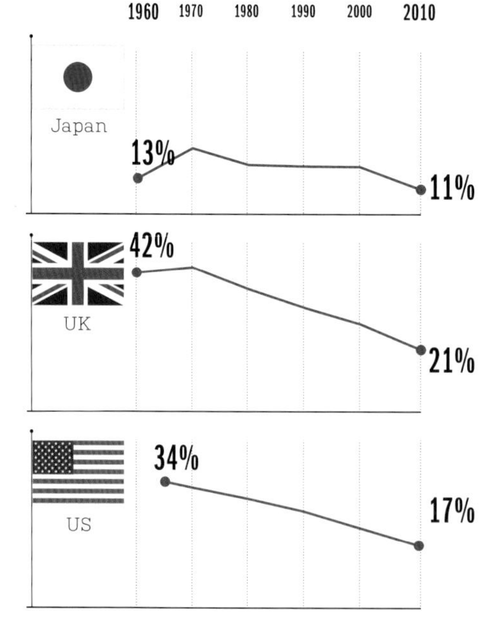

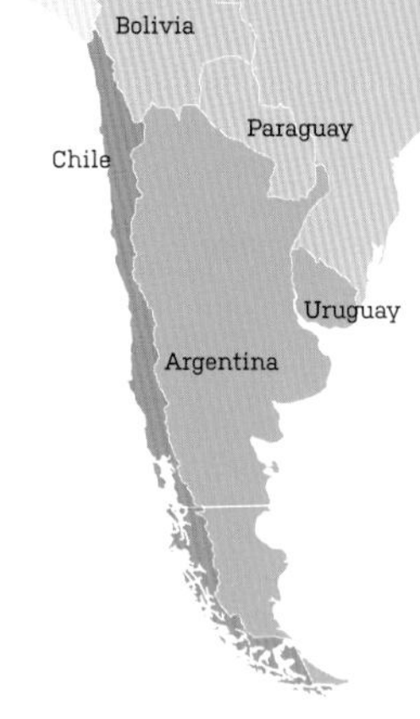

Smoking Trends
Adult Female Current Smoking Prevalence

1960–2010 (or latest available)

Data rounded to nearest whole number.
UK includes Great Britain and Northern Ireland.

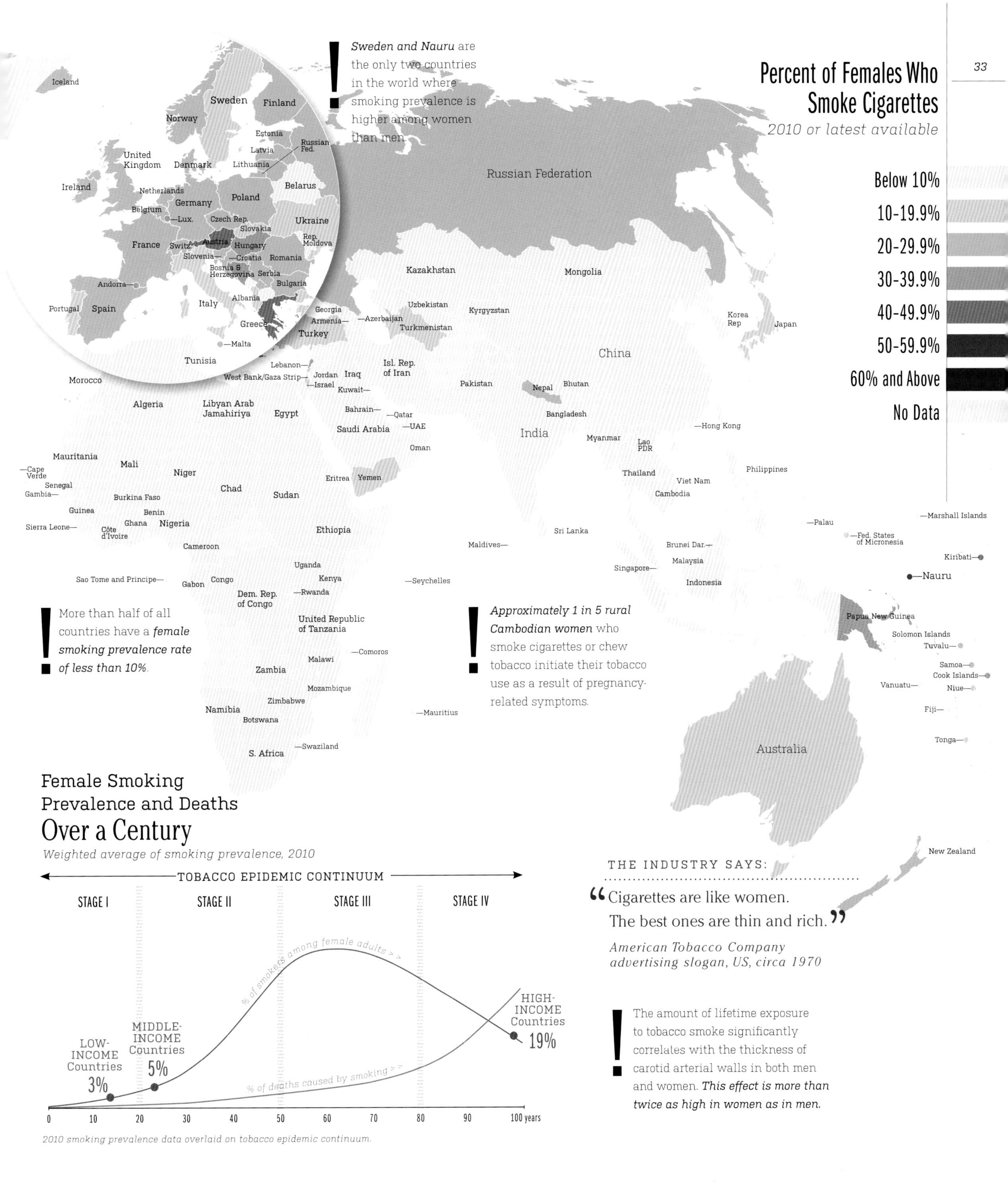

2010 smoking prevalence data overlaid on tobacco epidemic continuum.

RESEARCH SAYS:

“Kids who see others smoking are more likely to take up the habit because they don't perceive cigarettes as unhealthy.”

Simon Racicot, Concordia University, US, 2011

While there are large differences in smoking rates among adults by gender, smoking rates among boys and girls (ages 13–15) vary minimally in many regions of the world. Smoking rates between boys and girls differ by less than five percentage points in almost half of the world's countries. Tobacco companies view youth smoking as an opportunity to secure new smokers at a young age. **THE MAJORITY OF SMOKERS BEGIN SMOKING IN THEIR YOUTH.** For example, 83% of smokers in the US begin smoking before the age of 18. Even the tobacco industry understands the importance of youth smoking, and a 1984 R.J. Reynolds document stated that “younger adults are the only source of replacement smokers.”

Boys begin smoking during their youth in response to peer pressure, misconceptions that smoking is cool or enhances popularity, easy access to tobacco products, cigarette pricing, and tobacco marketing. Both marketing and pricing of cigarettes are proven to encourage youth initiation of smoking, because marketing makes smoking appealing to youth, and low pricing makes smoking affordable.

Smoking has an immediate harmful impact on boys' health, such as a reduction in stamina, and an increase in respiratory symptoms, mental health visits, and school absenteeism. Smoking endangers health, and the longer an individual smokes, the more severe the repercussions. Youth smokers are entering into an addiction that shortens their life span and increases the likelihood they will die early from diseases caused by smoking.

THE INDUSTRY SAYS:

“It is important to know as much as possible about teenage smoking patterns and attributes. Today's teenager is tomorrow's potential regular customer, and the overwhelming majority of smokers first begin to smoke while still in their teens.... The smoking patterns of teenagers are particularly important to Philip Morris.”

Philip Morris USA, 1981

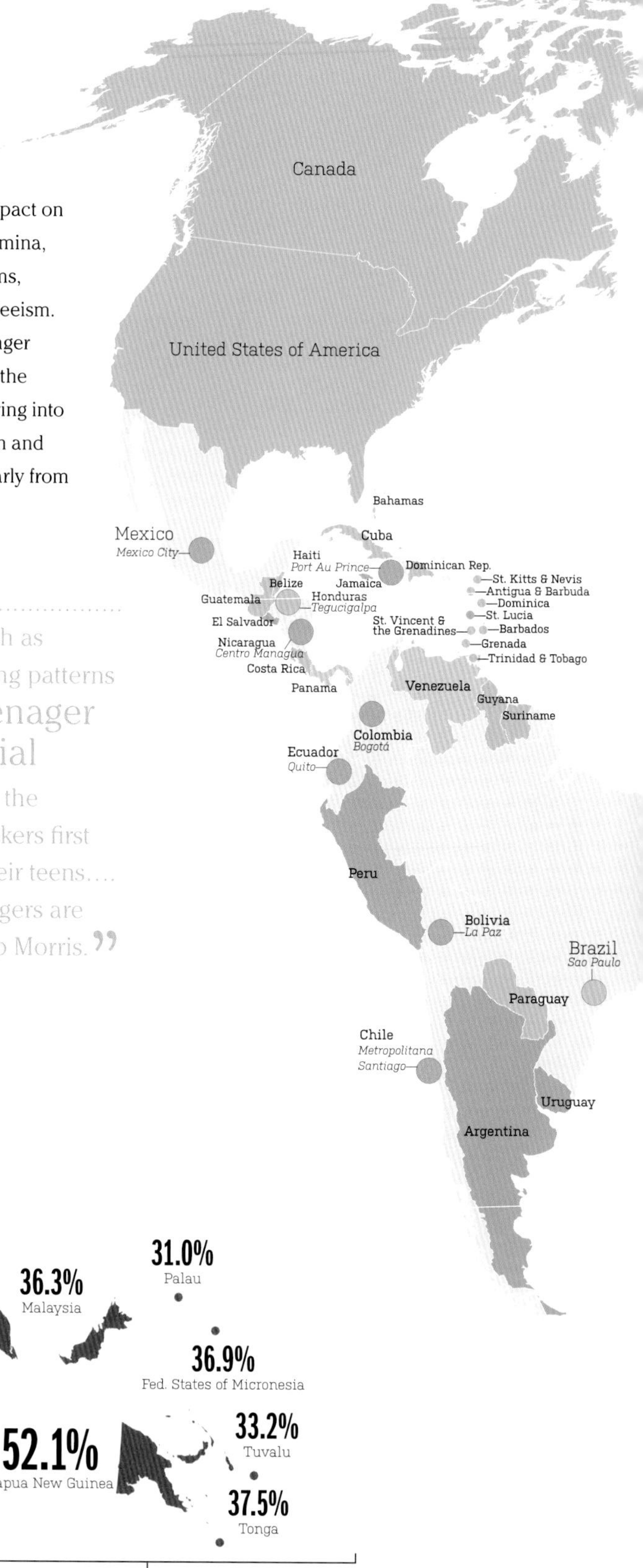

Countries With the Highest Smoking Rates Among Boys

Ages 13–15, 2011 or latest available

Africa	Madagascar	30.7%
Europe	Lithuania	33.8%
Europe	Latvia	36.3%
Europe	Belarus	31.2%
South-East Asia	Timor-Leste	50.6%
Western Pacific	Malaysia	36.3%
Western Pacific	Palau	31.0%
Western Pacific	Fed. States of Micronesia	36.9%
Western Pacific	Papua New Guinea	52.1%
Western Pacific	Tuvalu	33.2%
Western Pacific	Tonga	37.5%

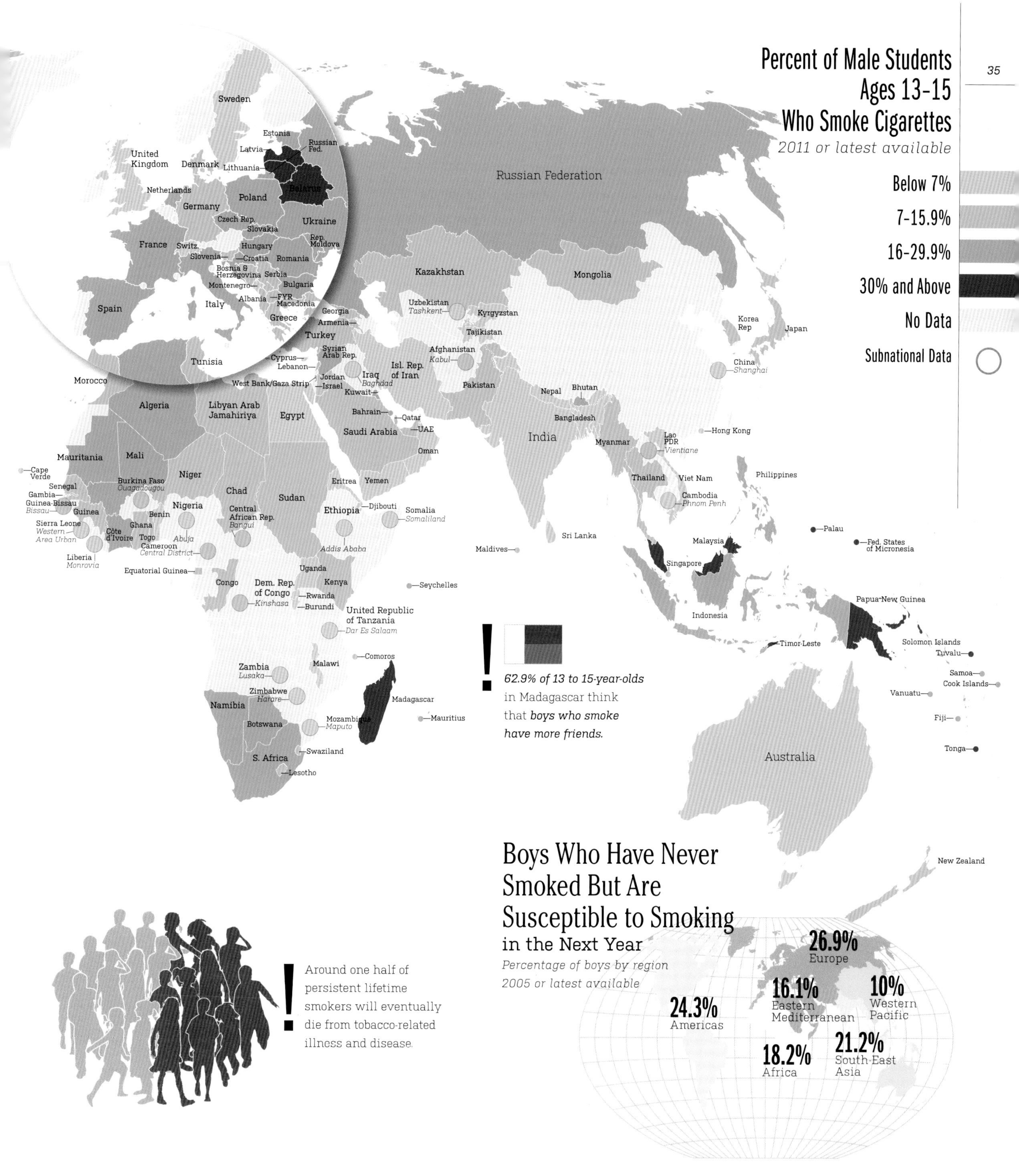

Percent of Male Students Ages 13-15 Who Smoke Cigarettes
2011 or latest available
Below 7%
7-15.9%
16-29.9%
30% and Above
No Data
Subnational Data
Sweden
Estonia
Latvia
Russian Fed.
United Kingdom
Denmark
Lithuania
Belarus
Netherlands
Poland
Germany
Czech Rep.
Slovakia
Ukraine
France
Switz.
Hungary
Rep. Moldova
Slovenia
Croatia
Romania
Bosnia & Herzegovina
Serbia
Montenegro
Bulgaria
Albania
FYR Macedonia
Spain
Italy
Greece
Georgia
Armenia
Turkey
Tunisia
Cyprus
Lebanon
Syrian Arab Rep.
Morocco
West Bank/Gaza Strip
Jordan
Israel
Iraq
Baghdad
Isl. Rep. of Iran
Kuwait
Bahrain
Qatar
UAE
Saudi Arabia
Oman
Algeria
Libyan Arab Jamahiriya
Egypt
Russian Federation
Kazakhstan
Mongolia
Uzbekistan
Tashkent
Kyrgyzstan
Tajikistan
Afghanistan
Kabul
Pakistan
Nepal
Bhutan
Bangladesh
India
Myanmar
Korea Rep
Japan
China
Shanghai
Hong Kong
Lao PDR
Vientiane
Thailand
Viet Nam
Cambodia
Phnom Penh
Philippines
Mauritania
Mali
Cape Verde
Senegal
Gambia
Guinea-Bissau
Bissau
Guinea
Sierra Leone
Western Area Urban
Liberia
Monrovia
Burkina Faso
Ouagadougou
Niger
Chad
Nigeria
Abuja
Benin
Ghana
Côte d'Ivoire
Togo
Cameroon
Central District
Equatorial Guinea
Central African Rep.
Bangui
Sudan
Eritrea
Yemen
Djibouti
Ethiopia
Addis Ababa
Somalia
Somaliland
Uganda
Kenya
Congo
Dem. Rep. of Congo
Kinshasa
Rwanda
Burundi
United Republic of Tanzania
Dar Es Salaam
Seychelles
Comoros
Malawi
Zambia
Lusaka
Zimbabwe
Harare
Namibia
Botswana
Mozambique
Maputo
Madagascar
Mauritius
Swaziland
S. Africa
Lesotho
Maldives
Sri Lanka
Malaysia
Singapore
Indonesia
Palau
Fed. States of Micronesia
Papua New Guinea
Timor-Leste
Solomon Islands
Tuvalu
Samoa
Cook Islands
Vanuatu
Fiji
Tonga
Australia
New Zealand
62.9% of 13 to 15-year-olds in Madagascar think that boys who smoke have more friends.
Boys Who Have Never Smoked But Are Susceptible to Smoking in the Next Year
Percentage of boys by region
2005 or latest available
26.9% Europe
24.3% Americas
16.1% Eastern Mediterranean
10% Western Pacific
18.2% Africa
21.2% South-East Asia
Around one half of persistent lifetime smokers will eventually die from tobacco-related illness and disease.

RESEARCH SAYS:

> “There is an important public-health message here that we need to get to teenage girls: Smoking is not going to help you lose weight.”
>
> *Louise Pilote, McGill University, Canada, 2006*

As with boys, most female smokers initiate the habit before reaching adulthood. Girls begin smoking during their youth in response to peer pressure, misconceptions that smoking is cool or enhances popularity, easy access to tobacco products, and tobacco marketing. Both marketing and pricing of cigarettes encourage youth initiation of smoking. Marketing makes smoking appealing to youth, and low pricing makes smoking affordable.

Some girls initiate smoking or continue to smoke due to the belief that smoking will assist with weight loss. This is especially common in cultures where women are subjected to unrealistic body-image goals. The tobacco industry has promoted the adoption of this belief, and a 1982 R.J. Reynolds document stated that “[a] brand which contains a natural appetite suppressant (in tobacco or tipping) will be perceived as controlling weight.”

Among today's adults, more men consistently smoke than women. In fact, there are at least 49 countries in which ten times more men than women smoke. The same is not the case for today's teenagers. **IN MOST OF THE WORLD, THE DIFFERENCE IN SMOKING RATES BETWEEN GIRLS AND BOYS IS SMALL.** In fact, more girls smoke than boys in at least 25 countries. The similarity of today's boys' and girls' smoking rates suggests that, in the future, today's teenage girls may be more likely to smoke than today's adult women. If this pattern continues in the future, the consequences will be deadly.

RESEARCH SAYS:

> “...if the movie stars smoke, especially in romance films, they are effectively encouraging young girls to smoke.”
>
> *John Pierce et al., University of California, San Diego, US, 2005*

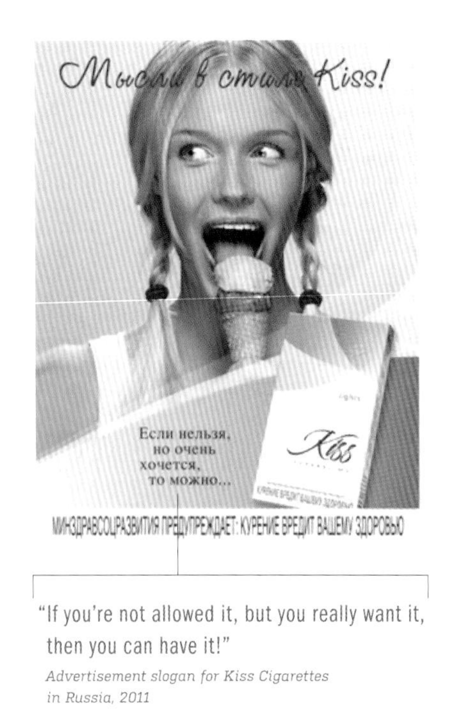

“If you're not allowed it, but you really want it, then you can have it!”

Advertisement slogan for Kiss Cigarettes in Russia, 2011

Places Where Substantially

More Girls Than Boys Smoke Cigarettes

Ages 13–15, 2010 or latest available

Boys | Girls

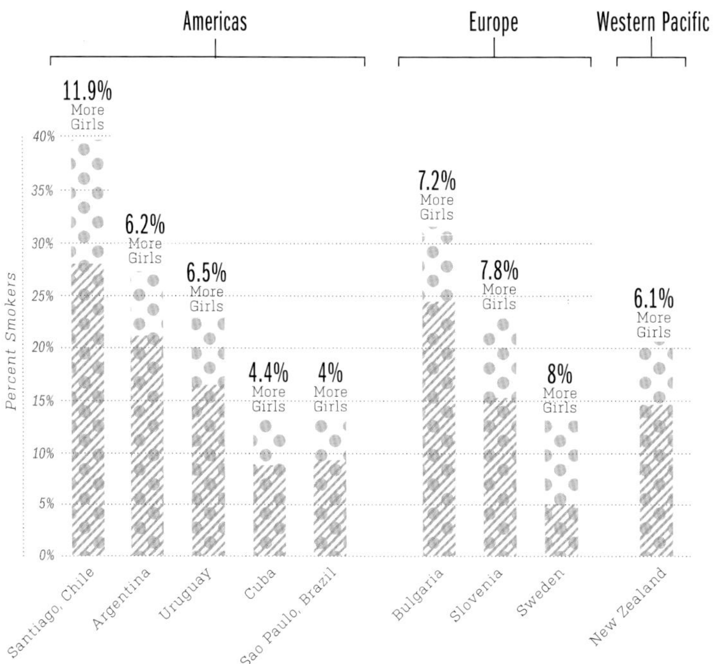

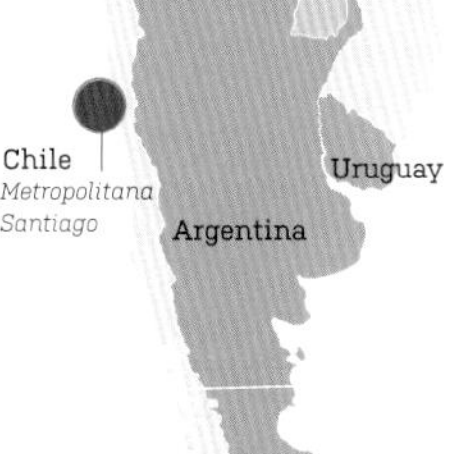

Percent of Female Students Ages 13-15 Who Smoke Cigarettes

2011 or latest available

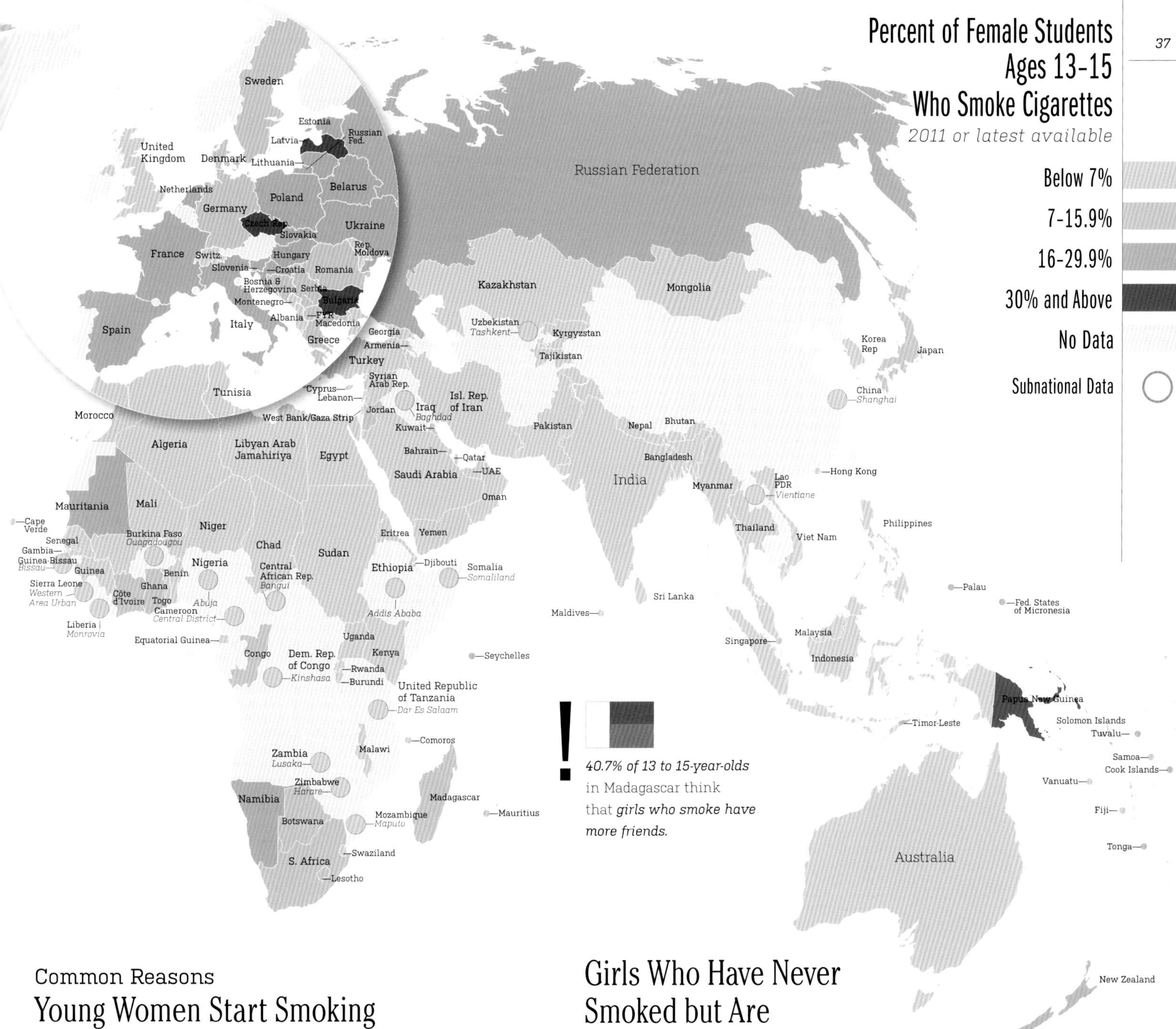

! *40.7% of 13 to 15-year-olds* in Madagascar think that *girls who smoke have more friends.*

Common Reasons
Young Women Start Smoking

- Association with others *(parents and friends)* who smoke.
- Concern with *weight, body image, or social acceptance.*
- Interest in *rebelling or stating individuality.*
- Reaction to positive images of smoking in *magazines, movies, and youth culture.*
- Influence from cigarette *marketing campaigns* targeting women.

Girls Who Have Never Smoked but Are Susceptible to Smoking
in the Next Year

Percentage of girls by region
2005 or latest available

33.0% Europe

25.6% Americas

10.9% Eastern Mediterranean

7.1% Western Pacific

17.4% Africa

10.7% South-East Asia

CONSUMER SAYS:

"*Beta ek gutka khane ka itna shauk hai to ek kaam kar. Ek dost aur banna. Kaandha deney ke kaam aayega.*
Son, if you are so fond of eating gutka [chewing tobacco], make sure you make a friend so that you have someone to help carry your coffin."

Title track from Bollywood movie, Wanted, *India, 2009*

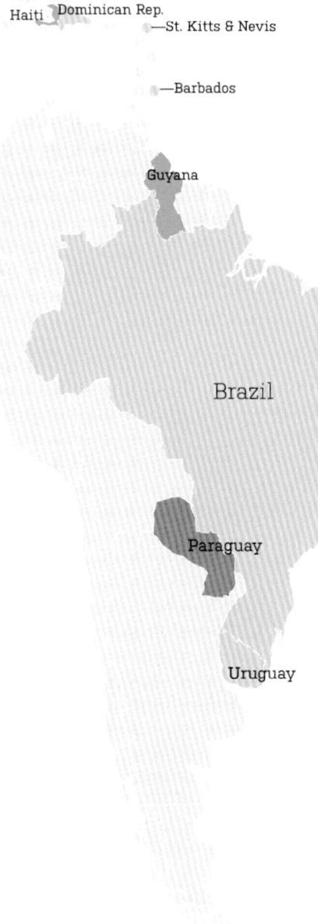

Smokeless tobacco accounts for a significant and growing portion of global tobacco use, especially in South Asia. Over 25 distinct types of smokeless tobacco products are used worldwide, including both commercialized and local or homegrown products, used orally and nasally. Some products combine tobacco with substantial amounts of chemical additives and other plant material that may confer additional risk to the user. Moreover, smokeless tobacco products contain many of the toxins and carcinogens found in cigarettes, and thus result in many of the same diseases caused by smoking. In addition, smokeless tobacco use increases periodontal disease, tooth loss, and precancerous mouth lesions.

Despite the harm from smokeless tobacco use to both individuals and society at large, these products are not sufficiently regulated in many countries. The landscape of smokeless tobacco manufacturing and marketing is rapidly evolving. **THE LARGEST AMERICAN, BRITISH, AND JAPANESE CIGARETTE COMPANIES HAVE ENTERED THE SMOKELESS TOBACCO MARKET AND ARE BRANDING THEIR SMOKELESS PRODUCTS AS AN EXTENSION OF CIGARETTE BRANDS, A COMPLEMENT TO BE USED IN SMOKE-FREE ENVIRONMENTS.** Understanding this "dual-use" consumption pattern will be essential to developing an appropriate regulatory structure for smokeless tobacco.

Global patterns of smokeless tobacco use vary widely. The import and sale of smokeless tobacco products are banned in 40 countries and areas. In some countries, like Finland and Egypt, men use smokeless tobacco products in much greater numbers than women because such products are perceived as masculine; in countries like South Africa, Thailand, and Bangladesh, women use smokeless tobacco products more than men because they are seen as a discreet way to consume tobacco.

Research addressing smokeless tobacco is limited. Monitoring and surveillance systems are scarce, and significant research gaps exist in identifying ingredients, additives, and toxicities of smokeless tobacco products. Little is known about product pricing, substitution of smokeless tobacco for smoked tobacco, and youth susceptibility to smokeless tobacco use. Policies to control smokeless tobacco are underdeveloped. The integration of smokeless tobacco control measures into the wider framework of tobacco control can help to curb its use.

THE INDUSTRY SAYS:

"We adopted our core strategy for growth: and that was to expand the smokeless tobacco category by converting adult smokers to smokeless tobacco."

Daniel Butler, President, U.S. Smokeless Tobacco Company, 2008

Global Smokeless Tobacco Sales Volume

Measured in tonnes

447,924
tonnes

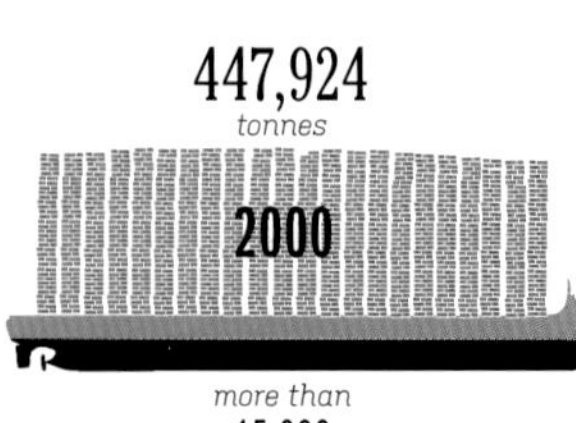

more than
15,000
shipping containers

574,164
tonnes

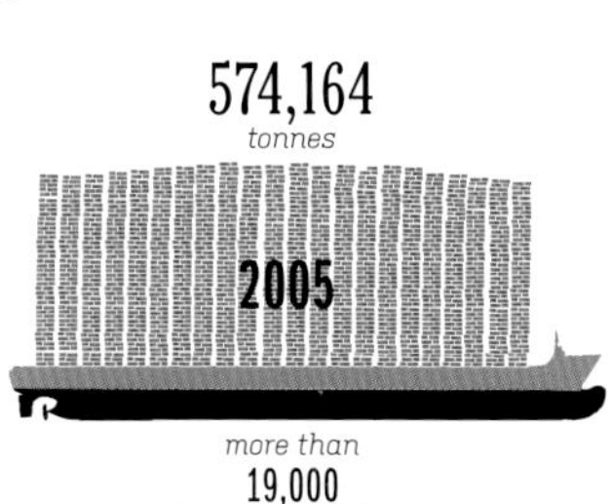

more than
19,000
shipping containers

710,211
tonnes

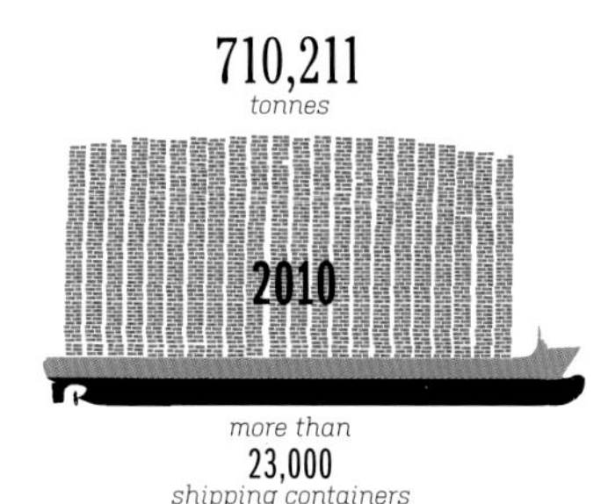

more than
23,000
shipping containers

749,424
tonnes

2015
forecast

more than
25,000
shipping containers

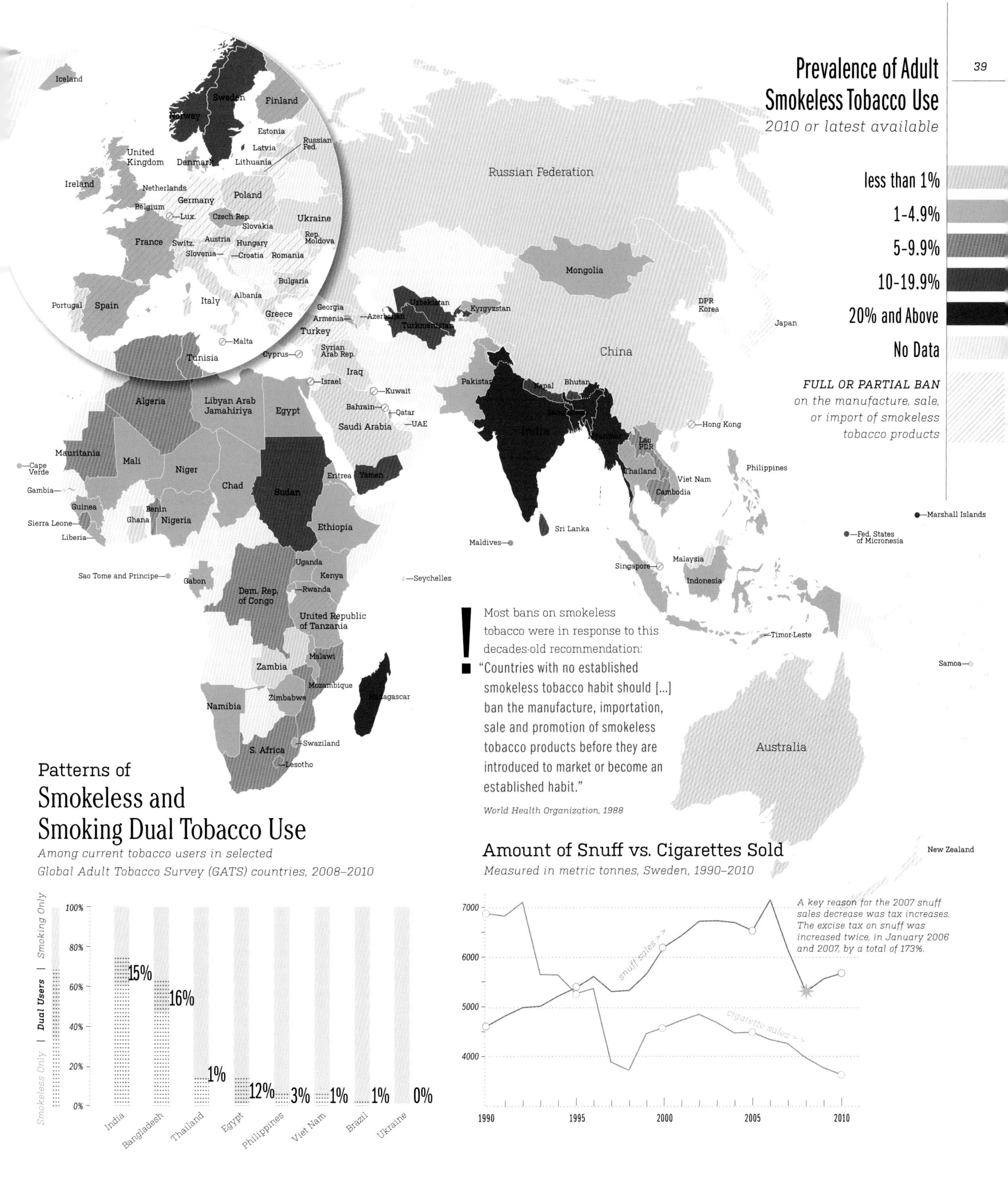
Prevalence of Adult Smokeless Tobacco Use
2010 or latest available
less than 1%
1-4.9%
5-9.9%
10-19.9%
20% and Above
No Data
FULL OR PARTIAL BAN
on the manufacture, sale, or import of smokeless tobacco products
Iceland
Sweden
Finland
Norway
Estonia
Russian Fed.
Latvia
United Kingdom
Denmark
Lithuania
Ireland
Netherlands
Poland
Germany
Belgium
Lux.
Czech Rep.
Ukraine
Slovakia
France
Switz.
Austria
Hungary
Rep. Moldova
Slovenia
Croatia
Romania
Bulgaria
Portugal
Spain
Italy
Albania
Greece
Georgia
Armenia
Azerbaijan
Turkey
Malta
Tunisia
Cyprus
Syrian Arab Rep.
Iraq
Israel
Kuwait
Bahrain
Qatar
UAE
Saudi Arabia
Russian Federation
Mongolia
Uzbekistan
Turkmenistan
Kyrgyzstan
DPR Korea
Japan
China
Pakistan
Nepal
Bhutan
India
Bangladesh
Myanmar
Hong Kong
Lao PDR
Thailand
Viet Nam
Cambodia
Philippines
Sri Lanka
Maldives
Marshall Islands
Fed. States of Micronesia
Malaysia
Singapore
Indonesia
Timor-Leste
Samoa
Australia
New Zealand
Algeria
Libyan Arab Jamahiriya
Egypt
Mauritania
Mali
Niger
Chad
Sudan
Eritrea
Yemen
Cape Verde
Gambia
Guinea
Benin
Ghana
Nigeria
Sierra Leone
Liberia
Ethiopia
Sao Tome and Principe
Gabon
Uganda
Kenya
Rwanda
Seychelles
Dem. Rep. of Congo
United Republic of Tanzania
Malawi
Zambia
Mozambique
Madagascar
Zimbabwe
Namibia
Swaziland
S. Africa
Lesotho
Most bans on smokeless tobacco were in response to this decades-old recommendation:
"Countries with no established smokeless tobacco habit should [...] ban the manufacture, importation, sale and promotion of smokeless tobacco products before they are introduced to market or become an established habit."
World Health Organization, 1988
Patterns of
Smokeless and Smoking Dual Tobacco Use
Among current tobacco users in selected Global Adult Tobacco Survey (GATS) countries, 2008–2010
Smokeless Only | Dual Users | Smoking Only
100%
80%
60%
40%
20%
0%
15%
16%
1%
12%
3%
1%
1%
0%
India
Bangladesh
Thailand
Egypt
Philippines
Viet Nam
Brazil
Ukraine
Amount of Snuff vs. Cigarettes Sold
Measured in metric tonnes, Sweden, 1990–2010
7000
6000
5000
4000
snuff sales >>
cigarette sales >>
A key reason for the 2007 snuff sales decrease was tax increases. The excise tax on snuff was increased twice, in January 2006 and 2007, by a total of 173%.
1990
1995
2000
2005
2010

RESEARCH SAYS:

“Doctors and other health-care workers are most effective in assisting patients to quit when they serve as role models by not smoking themselves. Their effectiveness increases further if they are visibly involved in local and national tobacco control activities.”

World Health Organization, 2011

While over 93% of medical students in Hong Kong believe that health professionals should receive training in smoking cessation counseling, ***only 38% of students have received formal training.***

Proportion of Countries Providing Cessation Support Services in the Offices of Health Professionals

2010

No data for 3.6% of countries

12.8%
Services available in most offices

45.6%
Services available in some offices

38.0%
Services not available

Canada

United States of America

Mexico

Cuba
Havana

Bahamas

Belize

Jamaica

Guatemala

—Barbados
—Grenada
—Trinidad & Tobago

Costa Rica

Panama

Guyana

Suriname

Peru
Costa Region

Bolivia

Brazil
Rio De Janiero

Paraguay
Asuncion

Chile

Uruguay

Argentina

Only 5% of medical students in Buenos Aires, Argentina, received formal training in smoking cessation counseling.

Worldwide, health professionals are respected and trusted as opinion leaders and trendsetters. They have the ability to affect social norms and have led the charge for smoking cessation in high-income countries. It is important that this also happens in low- and middle-income countries, since overall smoking rates are unlikely to decline until physician rates decrease.

All health professionals have the responsibility to advise patients about life-changing decisions and health matters, such as the importance of quitting smoking and how to quit. Even brief smoking cessation interventions are effective, and cessation support can double quit rates. But health professionals must be educated about how to conduct these conversations. Training and education build confidence among health professionals and increase their ability to discuss smoking cessation with patients, which in turn leads to more cessation success.

Health professionals who are smokers are less likely to advise their patients to quit smoking. The smoking status of health professionals varies throughout the world based on socio-demographic patterns and the stages of the tobacco epidemic.

THE MEDICAL STUDENTS OF TODAY ARE THE DOCTORS OF TOMORROW, AND IT IS IMPORTANT THAT THESE STUDENTS RECEIVE FORMAL SMOKING CESSATION TRAINING AS PART OF THEIR MEDICAL CURRICULUM. Unfortunately, this formal training does not always occur, and in many parts of the world, medical students smoke at rates equal to or higher than those of the general population.

In addition to educating health professionals about tobacco cessation, health facilities, such as hospitals, clinics, and doctors' offices, must adopt smoke-free policies to protect against secondhand smoke exposure. Smoke-free policies should also be adopted in medical schools. In some countries, smoking rates among medical students increase during their schooling, a circumstance that proper policies can help prevent.

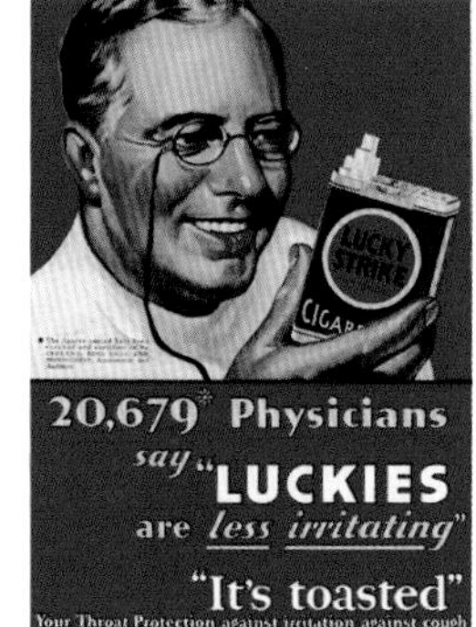

“20,679 physicians say ‘Luckies are less irritating.’”

American Tobacco Company, US, 1931

Smoking Prevalence Among Health Professions Students

2010 or latest available

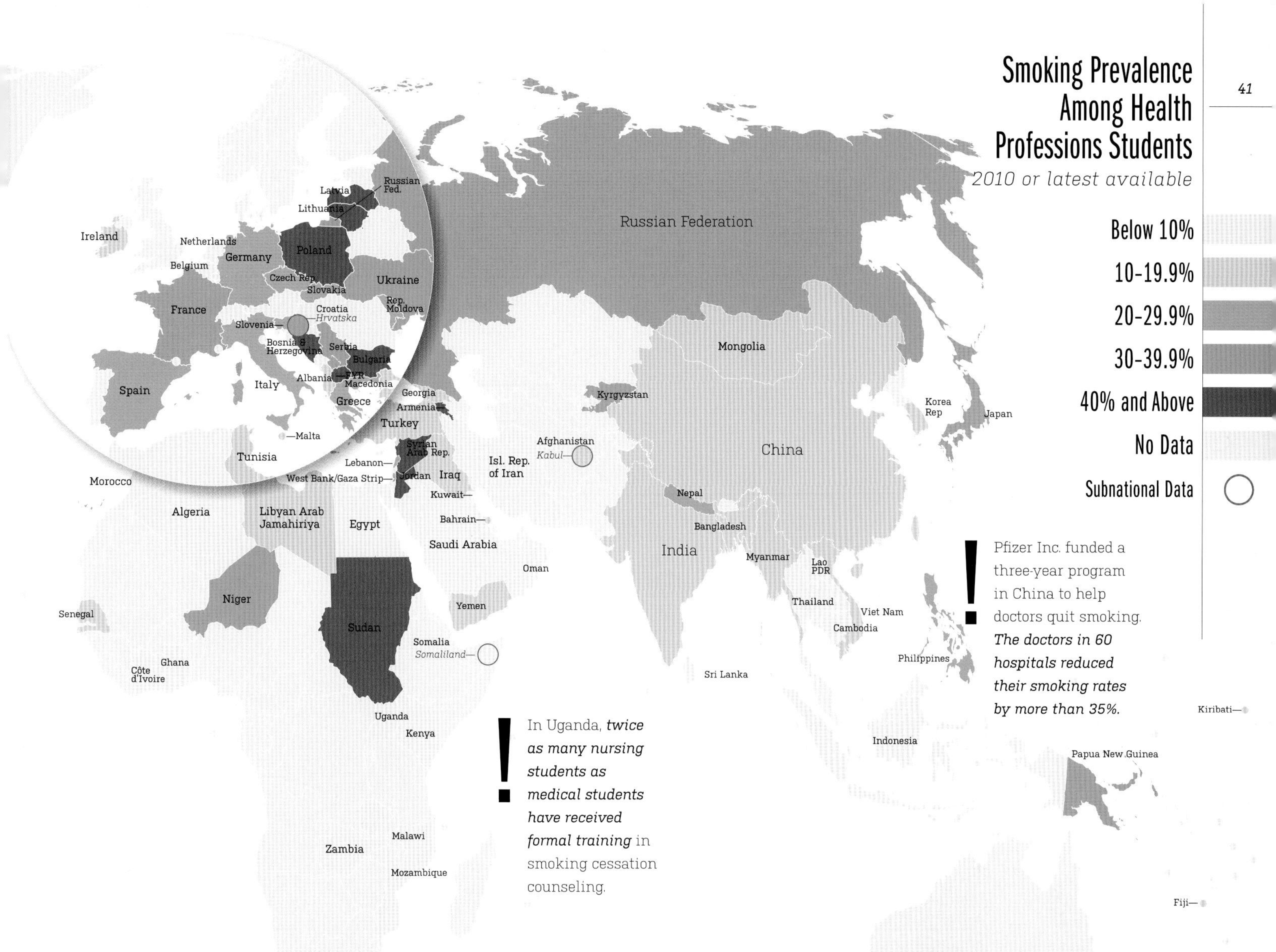

Pfizer Inc. funded a three-year program in China to help doctors quit smoking. *The doctors in 60 hospitals reduced their smoking rates by more than 35%.*

In Uganda, ***twice*** *as many nursing students as medical students have received formal training* in smoking cessation counseling.

Percent of Countries With Smoke-Free Health Facilities

2010 or latest available

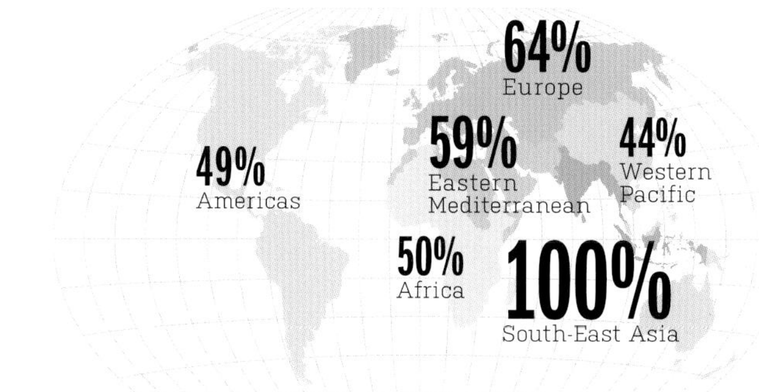

Even Brief Tobacco Cessation Interventions Are Effective

All health professionals should screen patients for tobacco use and follow the five steps below:

1. **ASK** about tobacco use
2. **ADVISE** to quit
3. **ASSESS** interest in quitting
4. **ASSIST** in quitting
5. **ARRANGE** follow-up

RESEARCH SAYS:

"Smokers often do not realize that they pay twice for cigarettes.
First with cash out of pocket,then later with their health or [their] lives."

AydaYurekli, World Bank, 2001

BETWEEN 2000 AND 2008, TOTAL COSTS IN China ATTRIBUTABLE TO TOBACCO USE MORE THAN Quadruple

2000
$7.2 BILLION

Values include direct and indirect costs. Direct costs include all health-care expenditures for treating smoking-related illnesses. Indirect costs largely include the value of lost productivity and cost of premature deaths caused by smoking-related illnesses. Measured in US dollars.

2008

$28.9 BILLION

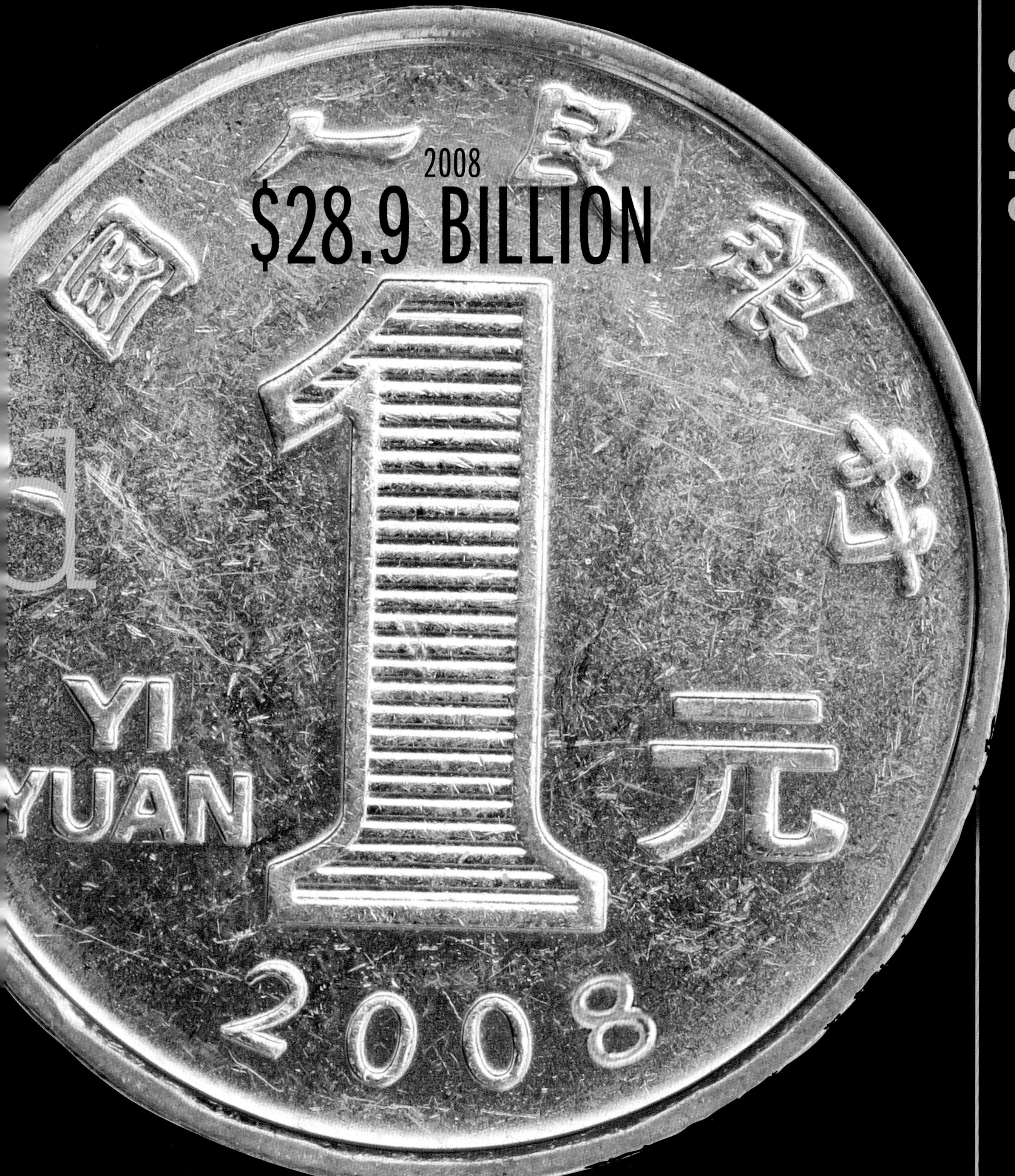

RESEARCH SAYS:

“The monetary value of the health damage from a single pack of cigarettes is $35 to an American smoker.”

Jonathan Gruber, Massachusetts Institute of Technology, Botond Köszegi, University of California, Berkeley, US, 2008

The Opportunity Costs of Smoking

Every society gives up the opportunity to buy something important when valuable resources are spent treating smoking-related illnesses.

Direct cost of tobacco use in USD — *How else could these resources be spent?*

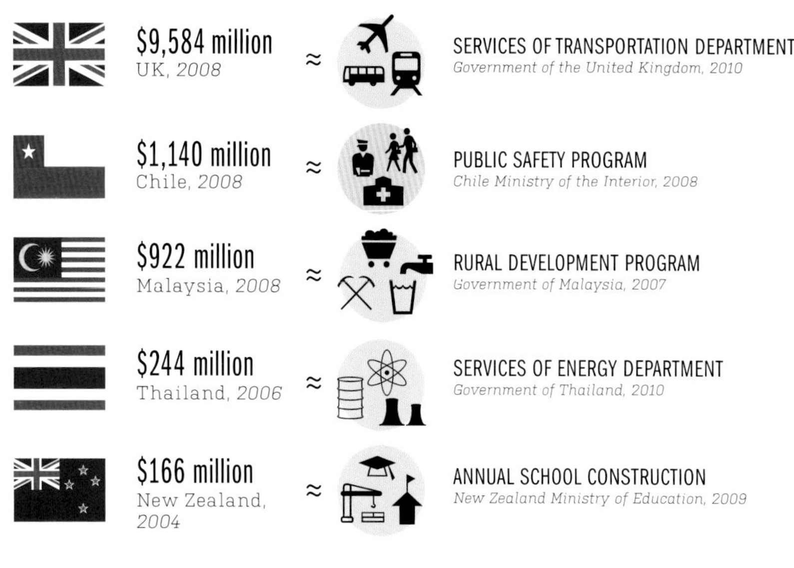

$2,803m Canada
$96,000m United States of America
$5,700m Mexico
$800m Guatemala
$21m Barbados
$71m Panama
$409m Venezuela
$185m Brazil
$1,140m Chile
$150m Uruguay
$2,200m Argentina

This map reflects estimates of both private and public direct medical costs of treating tobacco-related illnesses, which are only a portion of the total cost of tobacco to society. Indirect costs such as losses in labor productivity, cigarette butt littering, fire damage, environmental harm from destructive farming practices, and the intangible suffering of the victims and their families are not included. These losses further strengthen the argument that tobacco consumption has serious economic consequences.

Tobacco companies insist that their business is essential for global and local economies, ignoring the enormous resource drain that the use of tobacco products has on society as a whole.

THE BURDEN OF DEATH, DISEASE, AND DISABILITY CAUSED BY THE USE OF TOBACCO PRODUCTS MORE THAN OUTWEIGHS ANY ECONOMIC BENEFIT FROM THEIR MANUFACTURE AND SALE. The tobacco industry has even commissioned studies that claim early mortality from tobacco use eases the financial burden on public pension funds—an argument never advanced to combat prevention efforts against HIV/AIDS, tuberculosis, or diabetes. This grim conclusion is not only immoral, but also incorrect.

The direct cost of tobacco-related illnesses is determined by both the number of persons being treated and the cost of treatment. The number of patients depends on a country's population and stage in the tobacco epidemic, whereas cost of treatment depends on the country's health system. Estimates may also vary depending on the research method used. Tobacco-related health-care costs have only been calculated in a few nations, primarily due to limited or poor-quality data, dearth of research funding, and absence of research capacity. As health systems of low- and middle-income countries develop along with their economies, the medical costs of tobacco-related diseases will continue to grow, and so will the need to evaluate these costs.

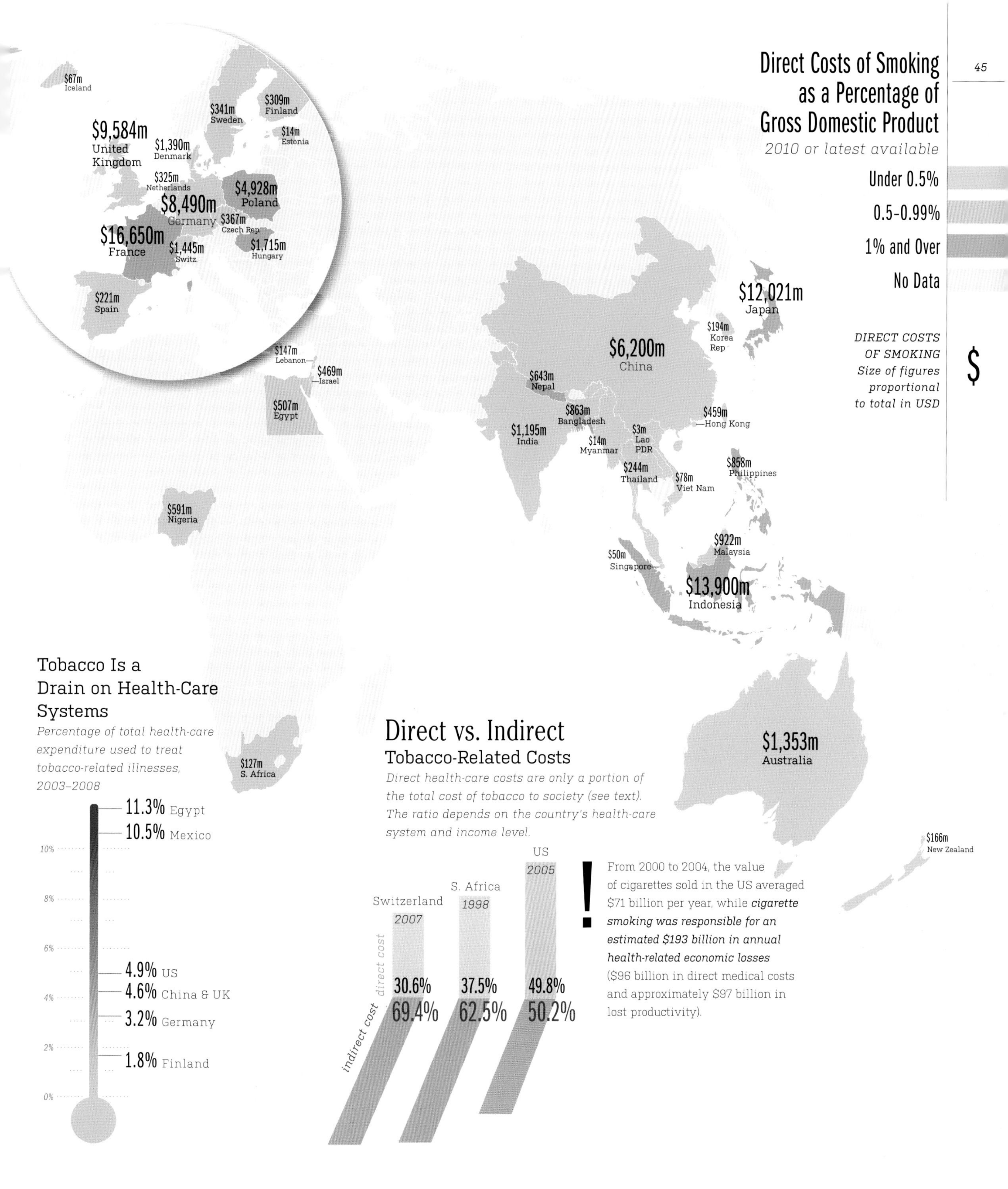

Direct Costs of Smoking as a Percentage of Gross Domestic Product
2010 or latest available
Under 0.5%
0.5-0.99%
1% and Over
No Data
DIRECT COSTS OF SMOKING
Size of figures proportional to total in USD
$
$67m Iceland
$9,584m United Kingdom
$1,390m Denmark
$341m Sweden
$309m Finland
$14m Estonia
$325m Netherlands
$8,490m Germany
$4,928m Poland
$367m Czech Rep.
$16,650m France
$1,445m Switz.
$1,715m Hungary
$221m Spain
$147m Lebanon
$469m Israel
$507m Egypt
$591m Nigeria
$127m S. Africa
$643m Nepal
$863m Bangladesh
$1,195m India
$14m Myanmar
$3m Lao PDR
$244m Thailand
$78m Viet Nam
$6,200m China
$194m Korea Rep
$12,021m Japan
$459m Hong Kong
$858m Philippines
$922m Malaysia
$50m Singapore
$13,900m Indonesia
$1,353m Australia
$166m New Zealand
Tobacco Is a Drain on Health-Care Systems
Percentage of total health-care expenditure used to treat tobacco-related illnesses, 2003–2008
11.3% Egypt
10.5% Mexico
4.9% US
4.6% China & UK
3.2% Germany
1.8% Finland
10%
8%
6%
4%
2%
0%
Direct vs. Indirect
Tobacco-Related Costs
Direct health-care costs are only a portion of the total cost of tobacco to society (see text). The ratio depends on the country's health-care system and income level.
Switzerland 2007
S. Africa 1998
US 2005
direct cost
indirect cost
30.6%
69.4%
37.5%
62.5%
49.8%
50.2%
!
From 2000 to 2004, the value of cigarettes sold in the US averaged $71 billion per year, while cigarette smoking was responsible for an estimated $193 billion in annual health-related economic losses ($96 billion in direct medical costs and approximately $97 billion in lost productivity).

CONSUMERS SAY:

"Eggs? Where will the money come from to buy them?"

Hasan, a rickshaw puller from Bangladesh who could feed each of his three children an egg a day if he bought eggs instead of tobacco, 2001

Money spent on tobacco often reduces resources available for basic necessities, such as nutrition, health care, and education. These opportunity costs impose a significant burden on tobacco users and their families, burying many of them in a vicious cycle of poverty that can span generations. **SPENDING ON TOBACCO PRODUCTS DIVERTS RESOURCES FROM ESSENTIAL GOODS AND SERVICES, INCLUDING EDUCATION, FOOD, CLOTHING, SHELTER, AND TRANSPORTATION.** Expenditures on tobacco inhibit progress toward UN Millennium Development Goals.

The retail price of a pack of cigarettes varies among and within nations. Cigarette prices are influenced by many factors, including the tobacco market structure (a monopoly, oligopoly, or competitive market) and tobacco tax system (the size and structure of the excise tax—see Chapter 29 – *Tobacco Taxes*). Significant price differentials may exist between so-called premium cigarette brands and economy brands, a result of a tobacco industry strategy to target specific segments of the population, or of the tax structure favoring ad-valorem over specific tax. Specific tax, established as a fixed amount of money collected by the government per cigarette, would result in more uniform cigarette prices, reducing the price gap between cheap and premium brands. This would encourage smokers to quit or lower consumption as opposed to simply switching to cheaper cigarette brands. Making the prices of all tobacco products more homogeneous would limit consumers' option to substitute other tobacco products to avoid price or tax increases. Therefore, efforts should be made to equalize taxes across different tobacco products.

!

In striving for greater profits, *the big tobacco firms have pushed the average price of cigarettes up in rich countries,* such as Britain — where 20 cigarettes now cost more than £6 a pack — *while hammering down the price paid to tobacco growers in poorer countries,* such as India and Malawi.

In Viet Nam, *smokers spent 3.6 times more on tobacco than on education, 2.5 times more than on clothing,* and *1.9 times more than on health care* in 2003.

Tobacco consumption *impoverished roughly 15 million people in India in 2004.*

Students in *Niger spent 40% of their income on cigarettes in 2003.*

Canada

United States of America

Mexico

Cuba

Haiti

Dominican Rep.

Belize

Jamaica

St. Kitts & Nevis

Antigua & Barbuda

Dominica

Guatemala

Honduras

St. Vincent & the Grenadines

St. Lucia

El Salvador

Nicaragua

Barbados

Grenada

Trinidad & Tobago

Costa Rica

Panama

Venezuela

Guyana

Suriname

Colombia

Ecuador

Peru

Brazil

Bolivia

Paraguay

Uruguay

Argentina

Chile

Price of Other Tobacco Products

Compared to Cigarettes

per 20 sticks/units in USD

Marlboro | Local Cigarette | Other Tobacco Product

$12.00 $10.00 $8.00 $6.00 $4.00 $2.00 $0

	Marlboro	Local Cigarette	Other Tobacco Product
Norway, 2009 — Snus	$11.88	$11.88	$7.54
Belgium, 2011 — Roll-Your-Own Cigarettes	$6.34	$5.85	$2.28
Indonesia, 2009 — Kreteks	$1.05	$1.30	$1.44
India, 2010 — Bidis	$1.96	$1.74	$0.10

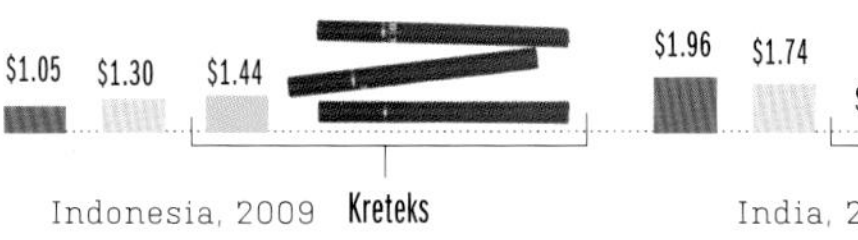

Cigarette Prices

Price in USD of 20 Marlboro cigarettes or equivalent international brand

2011 or latest available

More than $8.00

$4.00-$7.99

$2.00-$3.99

Less than $2.00

No Data

Countries where ***REAL*** *(inflation-adjusted)* ***PRICE*** *of Marlboro* ***DECREASED*** *between 2000 and 2011; data considered for 70 countries*

Iceland
Sweden
Finland
Norway
Estonia
Russian Fed.
Latvia
United Kingdom
Denmark
Lithuania
Ireland
Netherlands
Belarus
Germany
Poland
Belgium
Lux.
Czech Rep.
Ukraine
Slovakia
France
Switz.
Austria
Hungary
Rep. Moldova
Slovenia
Croatia
Romania
San Marino
Bosnia & Herzegovina
Serbia
Andorra
Monaco
Montenegro
Bulgaria
Albania
FYR Macedonia
Portugal
Spain
Italy
Georgia
Greece
Armenia
Azerbaijan
Turkey
Malta
Tunisia
Cyprus
Lebanon
Syrian Arab Rep.
Morocco
Jordan
Iraq
Isl. Rep. of Iran
Israel
Kuwait
Algeria
Libyan Arab Jamahiriya
Egypt
Bahrain
Qatar
Saudi Arabia
UAE
Oman
Russian Federation
Kazakhstan
Mongolia
Uzbekistan
Kyrgyzstan
Turkmenistan
Tajikistan
Korea Rep
Japan
Afghanistan
China
Pakistan
Nepal
Bangladesh
India
Hong Kong
Lao PDR
Mauritania
Mali
Niger
Cape Verde
Senegal
Gambia
Guinea-Bissau
Guinea
Chad
Sudan
Eritrea
Yemen
Burkina Faso
Djibouti
Benin
Sierra Leone
Côte D'Ivoire
Ghana
Nigeria
Togo
Liberia
Central African Rep.
Ethiopia
Cameroon
Somalia
Thailand
Viet Nam
Cambodia
Philippines
Palau
Marshall Islands
Sri Lanka
Fed. States of Micronesia
Maldives
Brunei Dar.
Malaysia
Kiribati
Singapore
Nauru
Uganda
Kenya
Seychelles
Sao Tome and Principe
Congo
Rwanda
Dem. Rep. of Congo
Burundi
Indonesia
United Republic of Tanzania
Papua New Guinea
Timor-Leste
Tuvalu
Angola
Zambia
Samoa
Cook Islands
Vanuatu
Niue
Mozambique
Zimbabwe
Madagascar
Fiji
Namibia
Botswana
Mauritius
Tonga
Swaziland
S. Africa
Australia
Lesotho
New Zealand

Price of Local Brand

as a Percent of Marlboro Prices

The greater the difference in cigarette prices, the easier for the smoker to switch to a cheaper brand (downtrade).

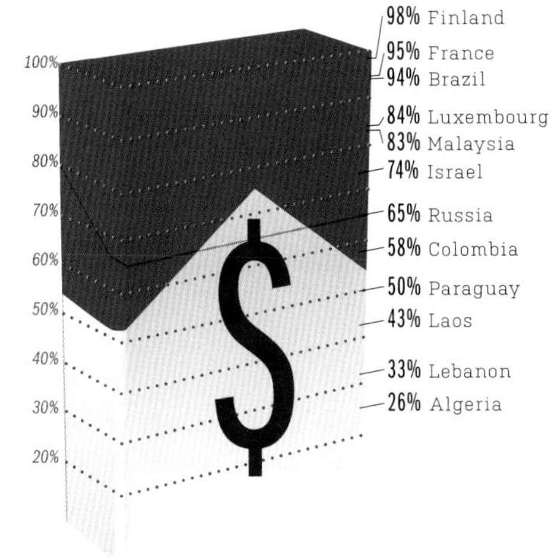

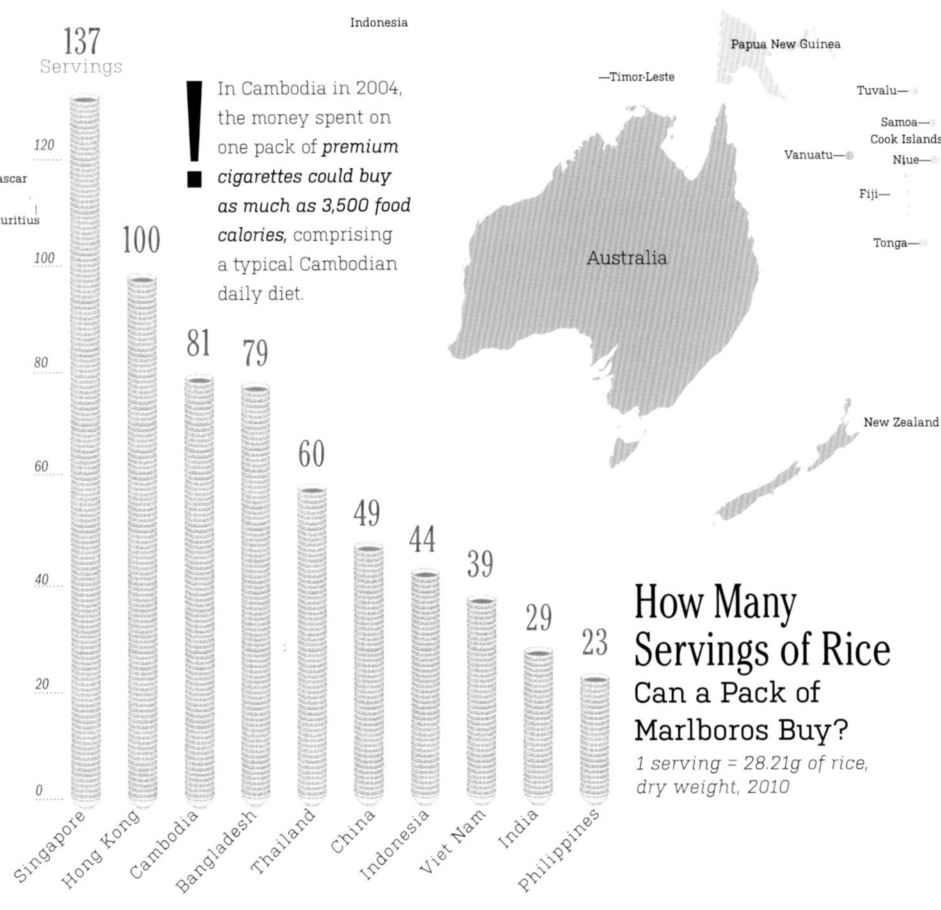

! In Cambodia in 2004, the money spent on one pack of ***premium cigarettes could buy as much as 3,500 food calories,*** comprising a typical Cambodian daily diet.

How Many Servings of Rice

Can a Pack of Marlboros Buy?

1 serving = 28.21g of rice, dry weight, 2010

“If real cigarette prices do not rise faster than consumer purchasing power, tobacco becomes relatively more affordable and consumption increases.”

World Health Organization, WHO Report on the Global Tobacco Epidemic, 2011

In recent decades, many low- and middle-income countries have achieved unprecedented economic growth. The economies of many countries in Asia, Eastern Europe, and South America have grown at annual rates of 6% or more. Rapid growth increases consumers' purchasing power, and people discover that many things, including cigarettes, become more affordable. Therefore, fast-growing countries face greater tobacco control challenges.

Consumers' decisions to buy cigarettes are influenced by their available income and the price of cigarettes. Economists call this combination "affordability," expressed as the percentage of a worker's income or duration of work time required to buy a product. The more income required to purchase cigarettes or the more one must work to earn enough money for cigarettes, the less affordable cigarettes are.

Despite cigarette prices being much higher in high-income countries, cigarettes are on average more affordable in those countries. For example, in 2009 THE MEDIAN EMPLOYED PERSON IN KENYA HAD TO WORK ALMOST AN HOUR TO BUY A PACK OF THE CHEAPEST CIGARETTES, WHILE THE CHEAPEST CIGARETTES COST JUST OVER 11 MINUTES OF LABOR FOR THE MEDIAN WORKER IN JAPAN. In low- and middle-income countries, cigarettes are generally becoming more affordable as economies develop, with the highest increase in affordability within the last decade being observed in China, Libya, and the Russian Federation.

The growth in average income significantly affects the affordability of cigarettes, and in that sense is bad for public health efforts to reduce consumption by making tobacco products less affordable. But tobacco control policymakers cannot argue against economic growth. The best way to make cigarettes less affordable is to increase tobacco taxes and prices (see Chapter 29 – *Tobacco Taxes*). To the extent that tobacco control is a priority for government and policymakers, tobacco taxes and prices should be adjusted to reduce affordability.

Minutes of Labor
Required to Purchase a Pack of Cigarettes
At median wage in 2009

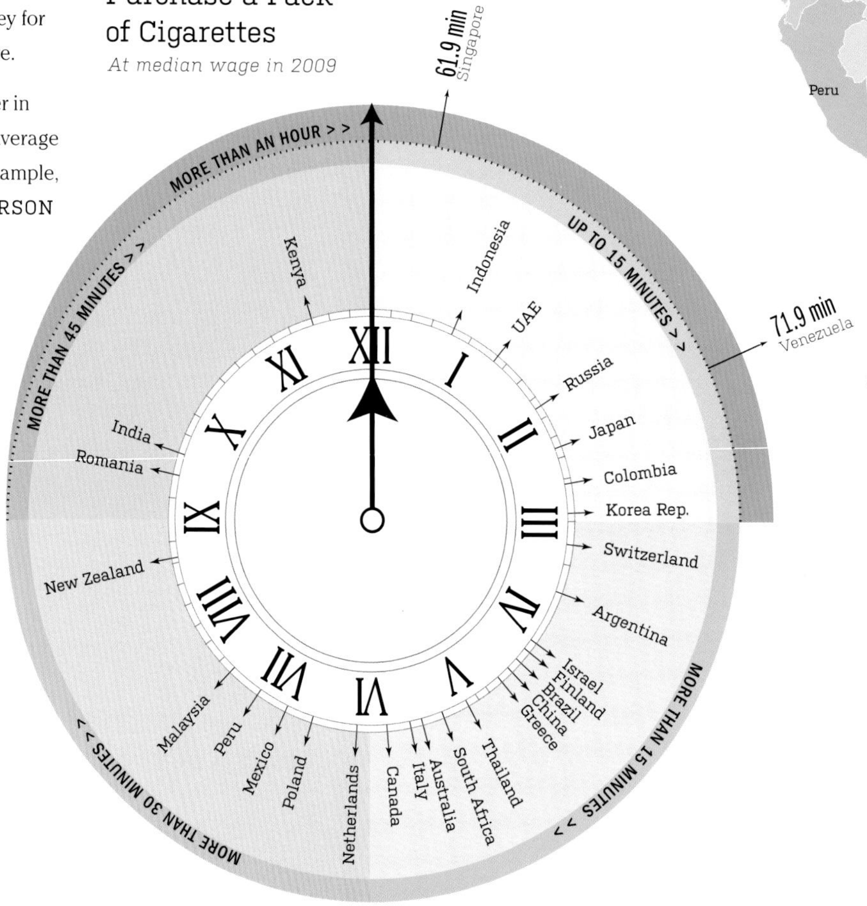

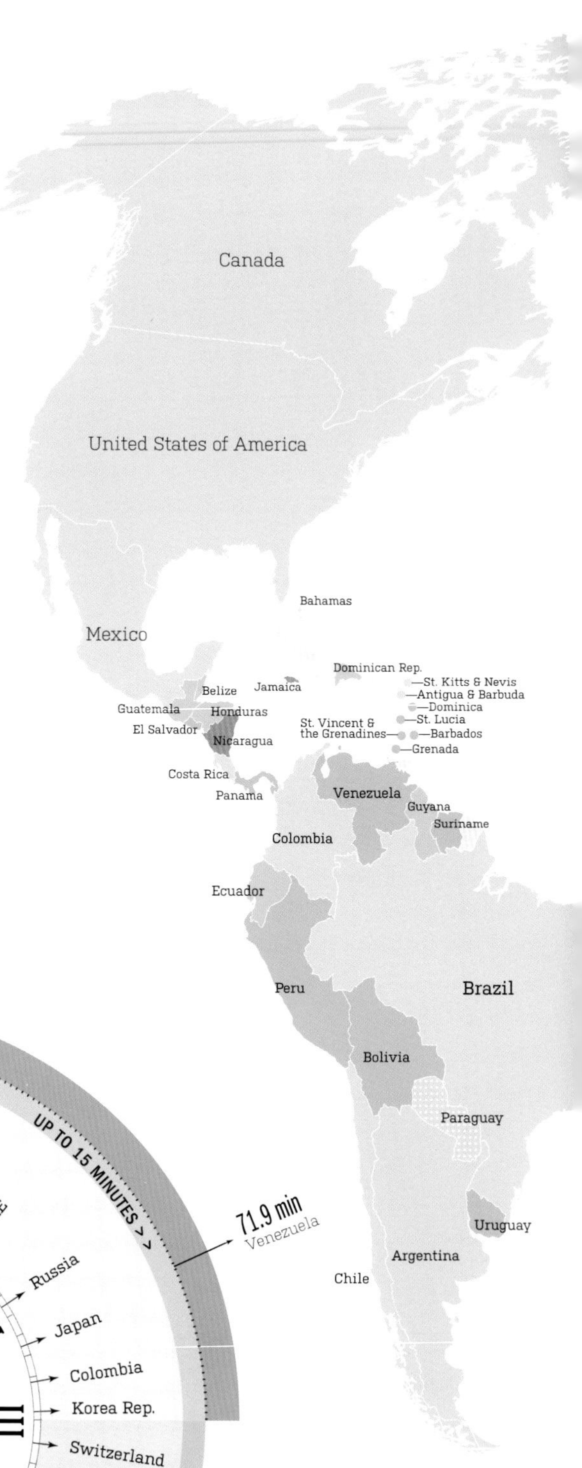

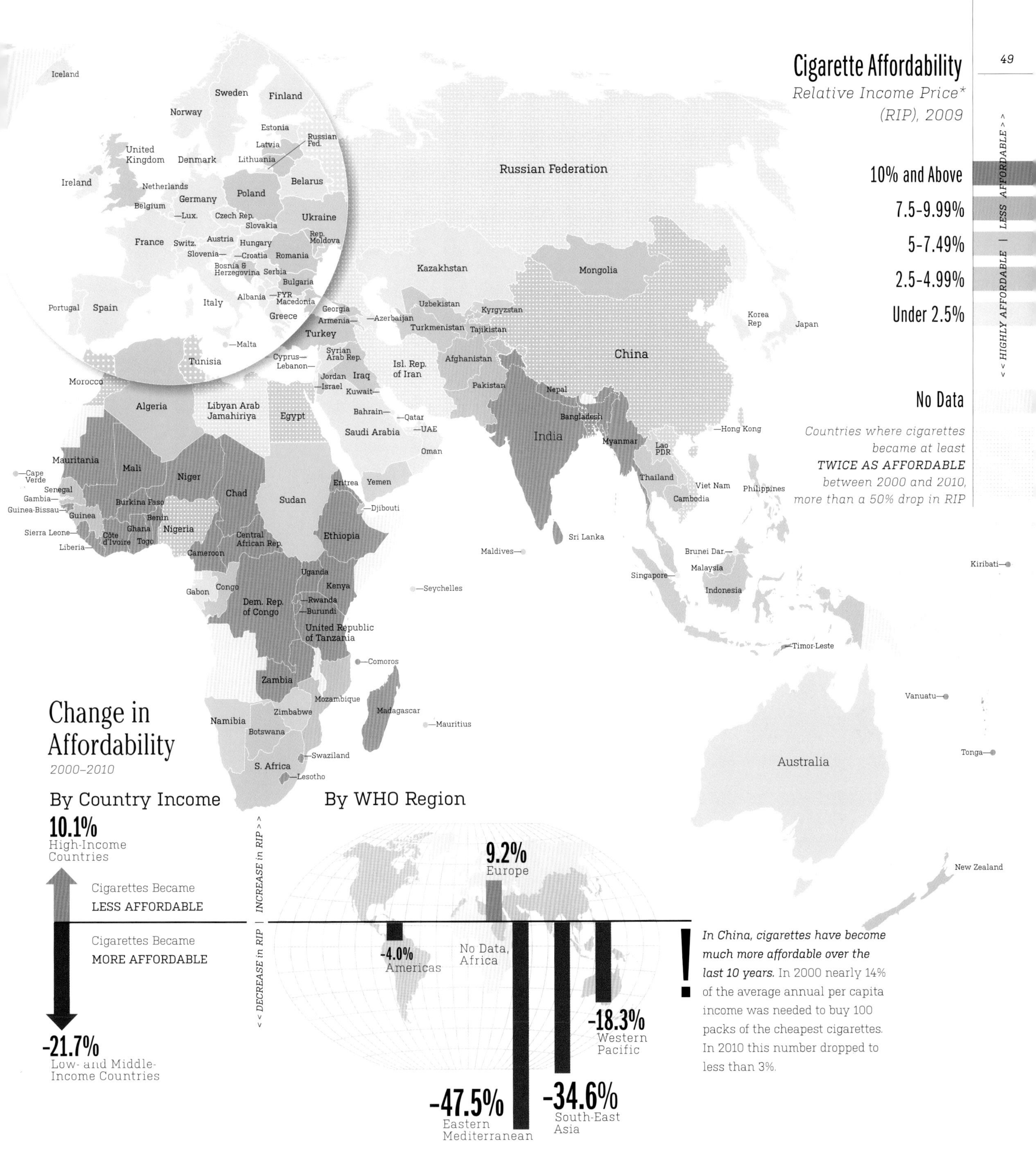

*Relative Income Price (RIP) = Percentage of annual per capita income, measured by per capita GDP, needed to purchase 100 packs of cheapest cigarettes.

RESEARCH SAYS:

"Tobacco use is unlike other threats to global health. Infectious diseases do not employ multinational public relations firms. There are no front groups to promote the spread of cholera. Mosquitoes have no lobbyists."

WHO Zeltner Report, 2000

BETWEEN 2000 AND 2010,

WORLD CIGARETTE PRODUCTION INCREASED BY 12%.

TODAY, CIGARETTE COMPANIES PRODUCE NEARLY

6 Trillion

CIGARETTES PER YEAR.

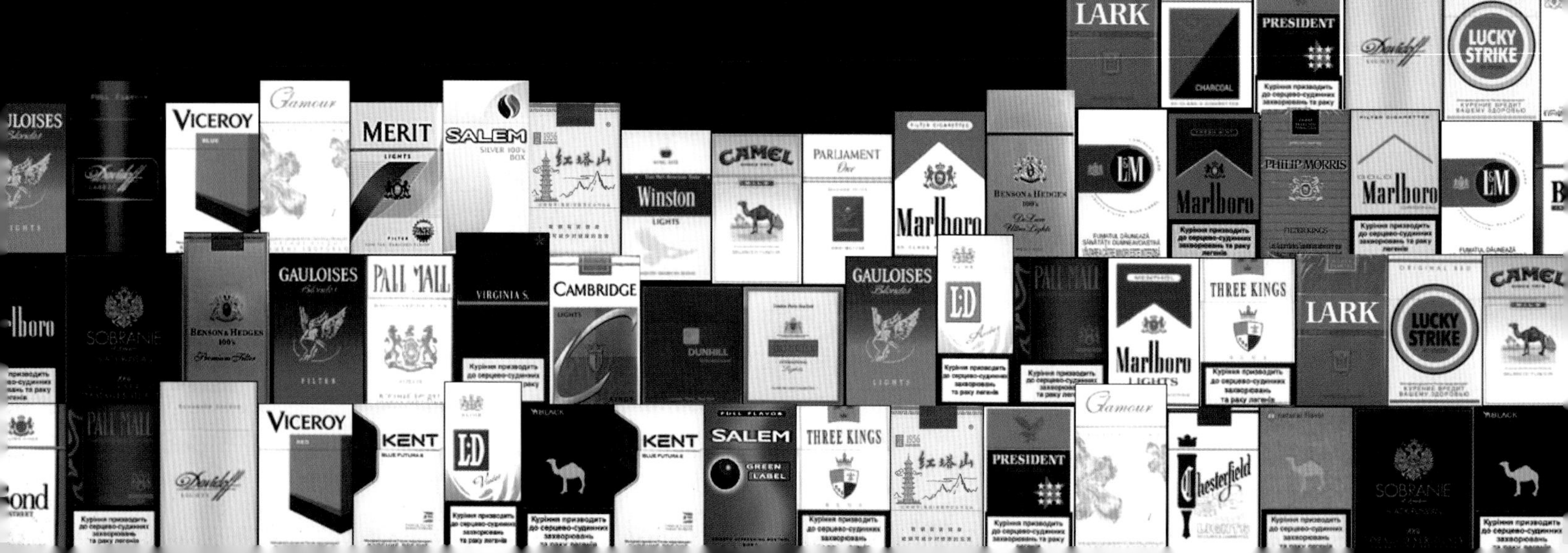

TOBACCO INDUSTRY

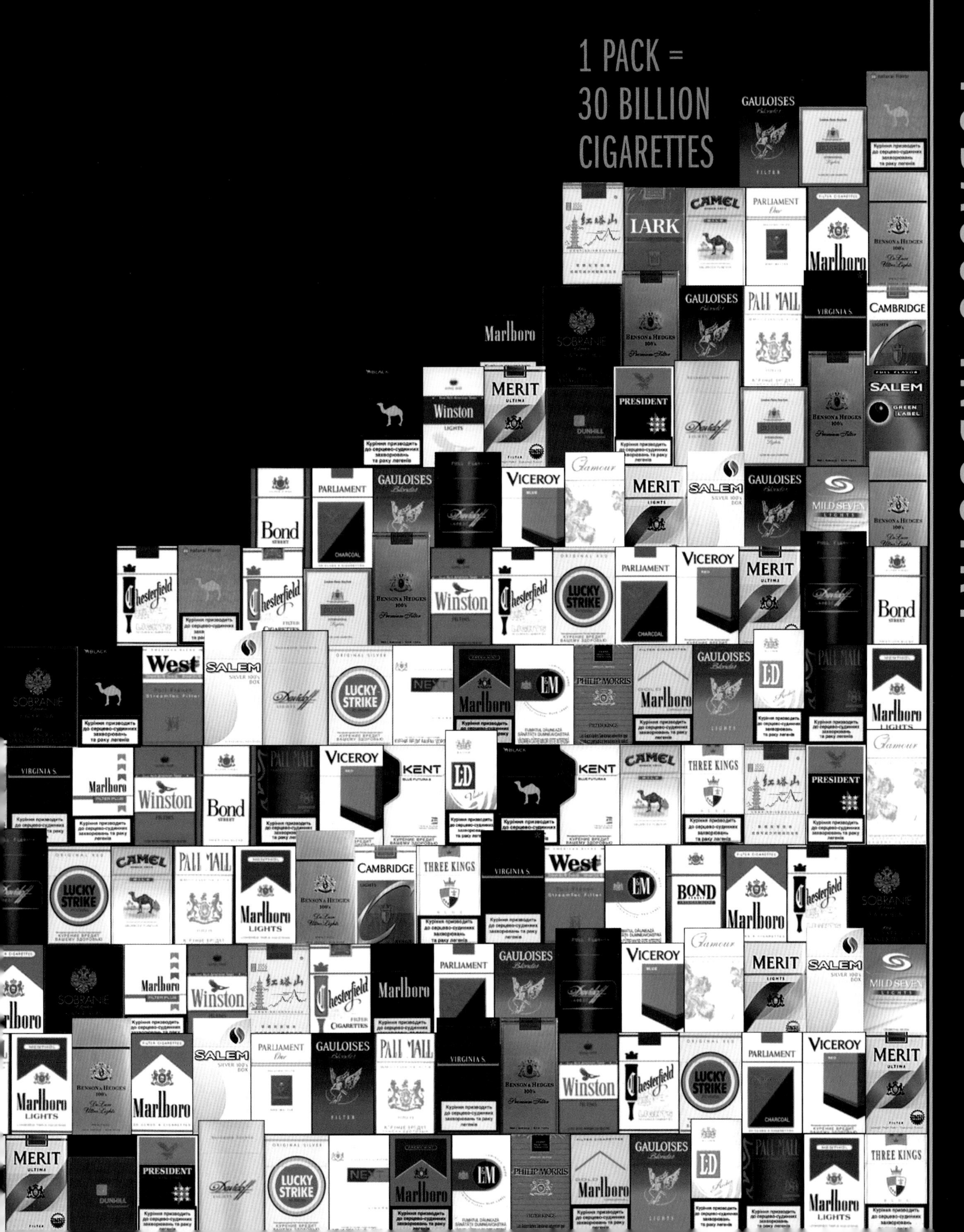

ADVOCATES SAY:

> “...they cheated the farmers. Tobacco farmers have families, they run businesses, they work real hard on the land.... I think they are the innocent people in this.”
>
> *Harvey Strosberg, Lawyer, Canada, 2010*

Tobacco is known to be grown in at least 124 countries, occupying 3.8 million hectares of agricultural land. There are only 5 countries in which tobacco is not grown, and it is unknown whether or not tobacco is grown in the remaining countries of the world. World tobacco production peaked in 1997 at over 9 million tonnes and has since declined by almost a quarter to 7.1 million tonnes in 2009.

Tobacco is primarily grown in low- and middle-income countries, where it is a contributor to undernourishment, because the land is used to grow tobacco rather than food. IN 2009, SIX OF THE TOP TEN TOBACCO-PRODUCING COUNTRIES HAD UNDERNOURISHMENT RATES BETWEEN 5% AND 27%. In 2008 in Malawi, a top tobacco-producing country with 27% undernourishment, each hectare of land devoted to tobacco produced 1 tonne of tobacco leaf; a hectare of land growing potatoes produced 14.6 tonnes in the same year.

Tobacco farming negatively affects the environment. Deforestation results from wood being needed for the curing process and for hanging leaves to dry. Each year, 20,000 hectares of forests are cleared to cure tobacco. Tobacco leaches the soil of many nutrients, so fertilizers and pesticides are heavily used in tobacco production. These chemicals endanger workers and create runoff that pollutes the environment.

No matter where tobacco farmers work, these individuals experience illnesses through their exposure to pesticides (which cause neurological damage) and nicotine (which results in green tobacco sickness). In addition to health impacts, many tobacco farmers are trapped in a cycle of poverty, as they are required to purchase high-cost equipment and infrastructure with little profit remaining. In 2003, tobacco farmers in the US received less than 1% of consumer spending on tobacco.

The WHO FCTC calls for financial and technical assistance to tobacco growers in countries dependent on tobacco agriculture. Although shifting from growing tobacco to growing economically and environmentally viable alternatives, such as food, addresses the issue of malnutrition, few countries have implemented such measures.

Trend in Tobacco Production

Production quantity in million metric tonnes for selected countries, 1965–2009

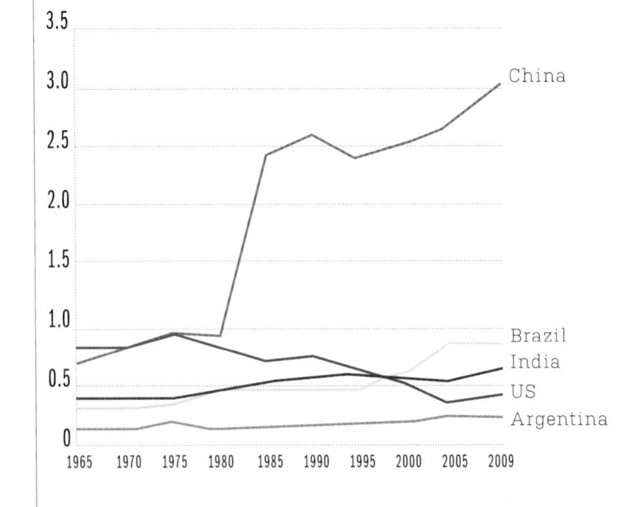

Leading Producers of Tobacco Leaf

Production quantity in metric tonnes

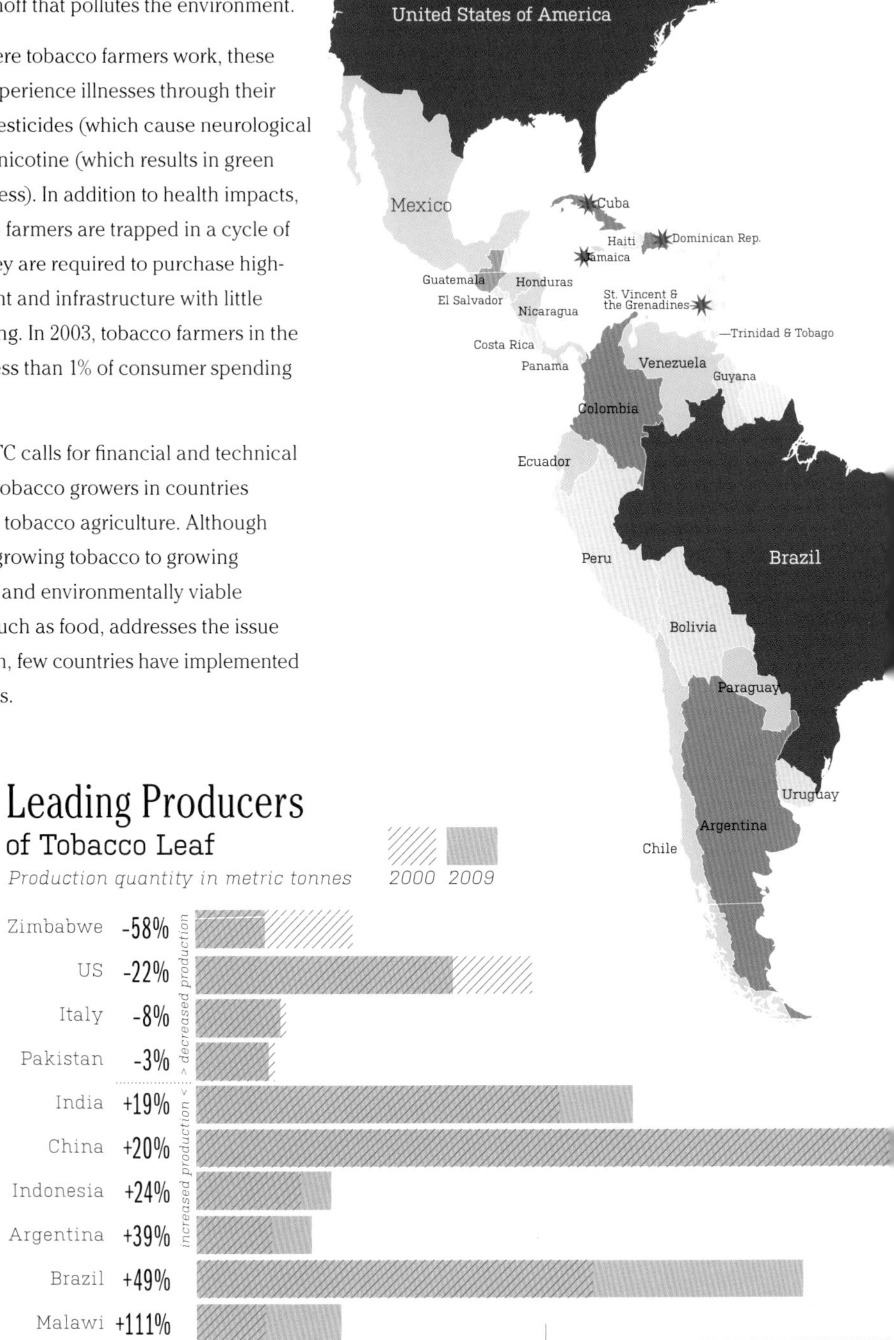

Land Devoted to Growing Tobacco

Area in hectares, 2009

One hectare = 2.47 acres

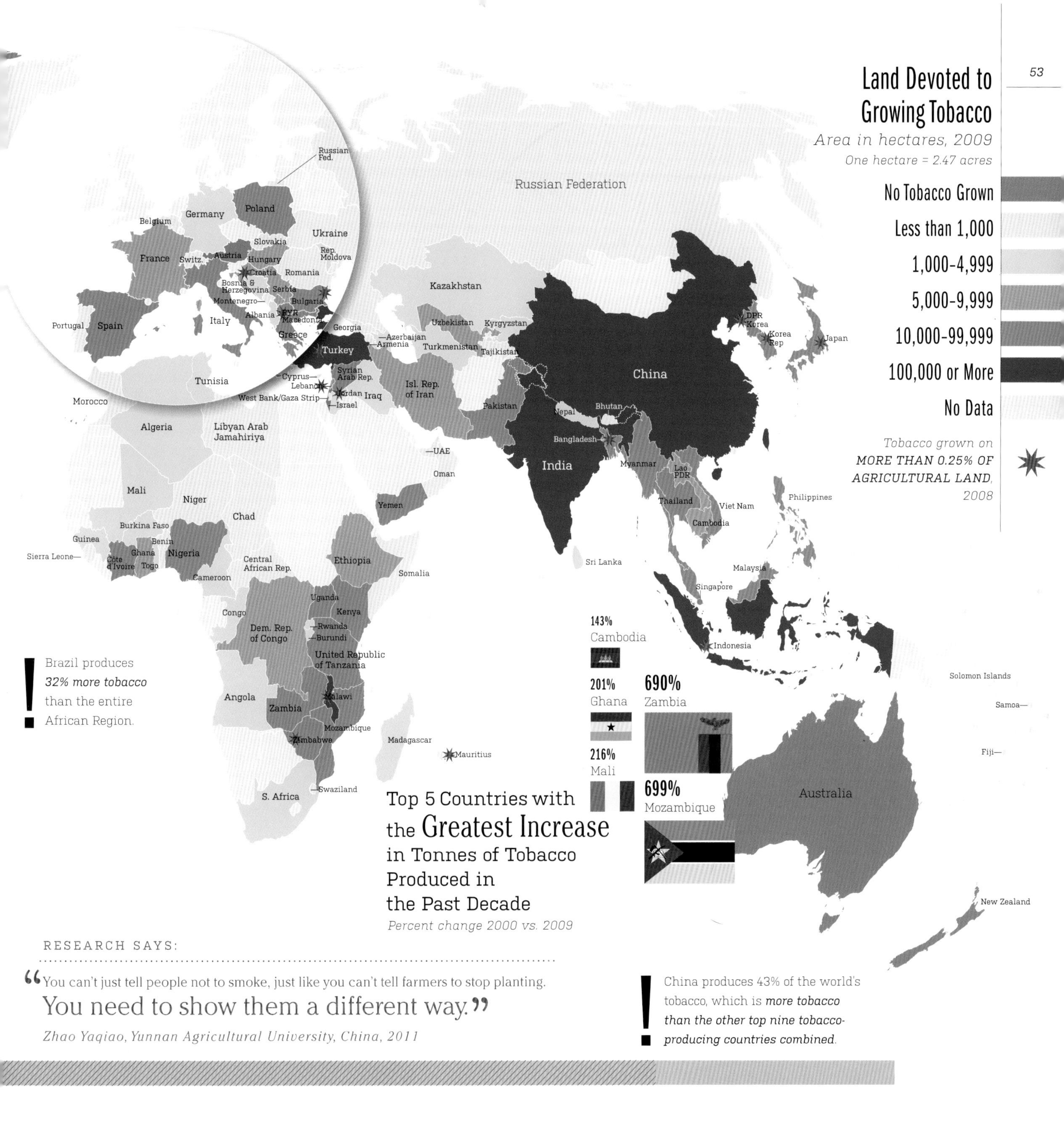

Top 5 Countries with the Greatest Increase in Tonnes of Tobacco Produced in the Past Decade

Percent change 2000 vs. 2009

143% Cambodia

201% Ghana

216% Mali

690% Zambia

699% Mozambique

! Brazil produces *32% more tobacco* than the entire African Region.

RESEARCH SAYS:

“You can't just tell people not to smoke, just like you can't tell farmers to stop planting. You need to show them a different way.”

Zhao Yaqiao, Yunnan Agricultural University, China, 2011

! China produces 43% of the world's tobacco, which is *more tobacco than the other top nine tobacco-producing countries combined.*

1,500,000 | 2,000,000 | 2,500,000 | 3,000,000

RESEARCH SAYS:

"Cigarettes are being extruded – and therefore smoked – at a rate of more than 300 million miles per year, which is about 34,000 miles per hour, 24 hours a day."

Robert Proctor, Stanford University, US, 2011

There are well over 500 cigarette factories spread around the globe, each responsible for thousands of premature deaths and massive, avoidable costs to society. THESE FACTORIES COLLECTIVELY PRODUCE NEARLY 6 TRILLION CIGARETTES EVERY YEAR, ROUGHLY 12% MORE THAN A DECADE AGO. In 2010, cigarettes were produced in the majority of countries worldwide, and about a million cigarettes were manufactured every five seconds. That year, 41% of the world's cigarettes were produced in China, followed by Russia (7%), the US (6%), Germany (4%), and Indonesia (3%).

Where are these cigarettes manufactured, wrapped, and boxed for shipment? Cigarette factories are located in every corner of the world, concentrated in Europe and China, and new ones are still being built. These factories are often hidden from sight behind high walls, given vague titles like "manufacturing facility" or "production center," and serviced by unmarked trucks. That is not true in China, however, where smoking is much more socially acceptable than in other countries; factories are highly visible and prominently featured in their communities.

With advances in satellite imaging technology, projects such as Stanford University's Cigarette Citadels now make it possible to locate hundreds of these factories online. For instance, Internet users can view one of the world's largest cigarette factories in Bergen op Zoom, near the Hague, Netherlands. This facility, built by Philip Morris in the 1980s, currently manufactures about 96 billion cigarettes annually, with most exported to other European countries and Japan. About 90,000 people could die prematurely every year as a result of consuming cigarettes manufactured in this single facility.

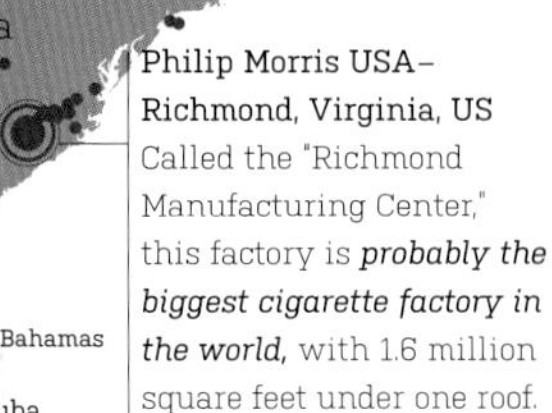

Philip Morris USA–Richmond, Virginia, US
Called the "Richmond Manufacturing Center," this factory is ***probably the biggest cigarette factory in the world,*** with 1.6 million square feet under one roof.

Souza Cruz BAT–Uberlândia, Brazil
This factory works 24 hours a day, 7 days a week to produce ***49 billion cigarettes annually.***

Who Is Getting the Money Spent on a Cigarette?

Distribution of value of a premium cigarette, 2009–2010

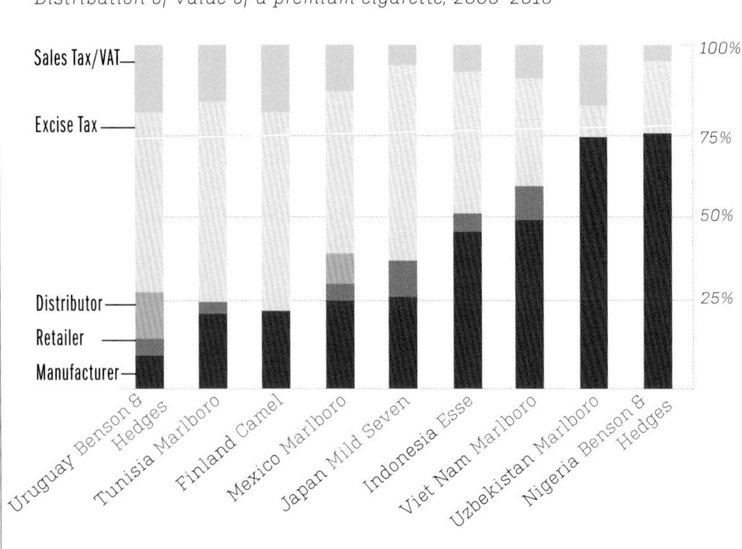

Cigarettes Dominate, but Are Not the Only Tobacco Product of the Tobacco Industry

Value of global tobacco industry production measured at retail sales price (all taxes included) in 2010, in billions, USD

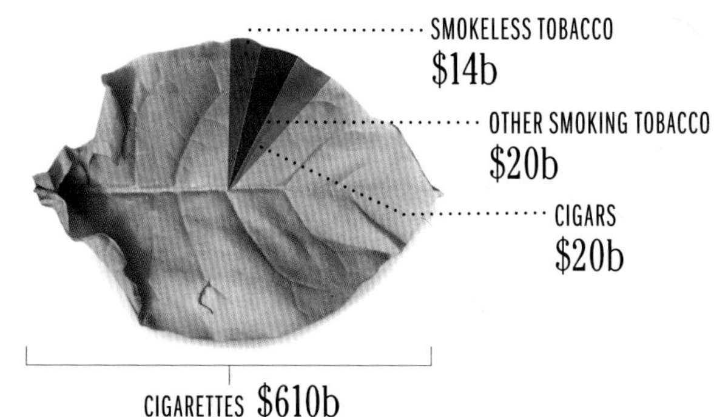

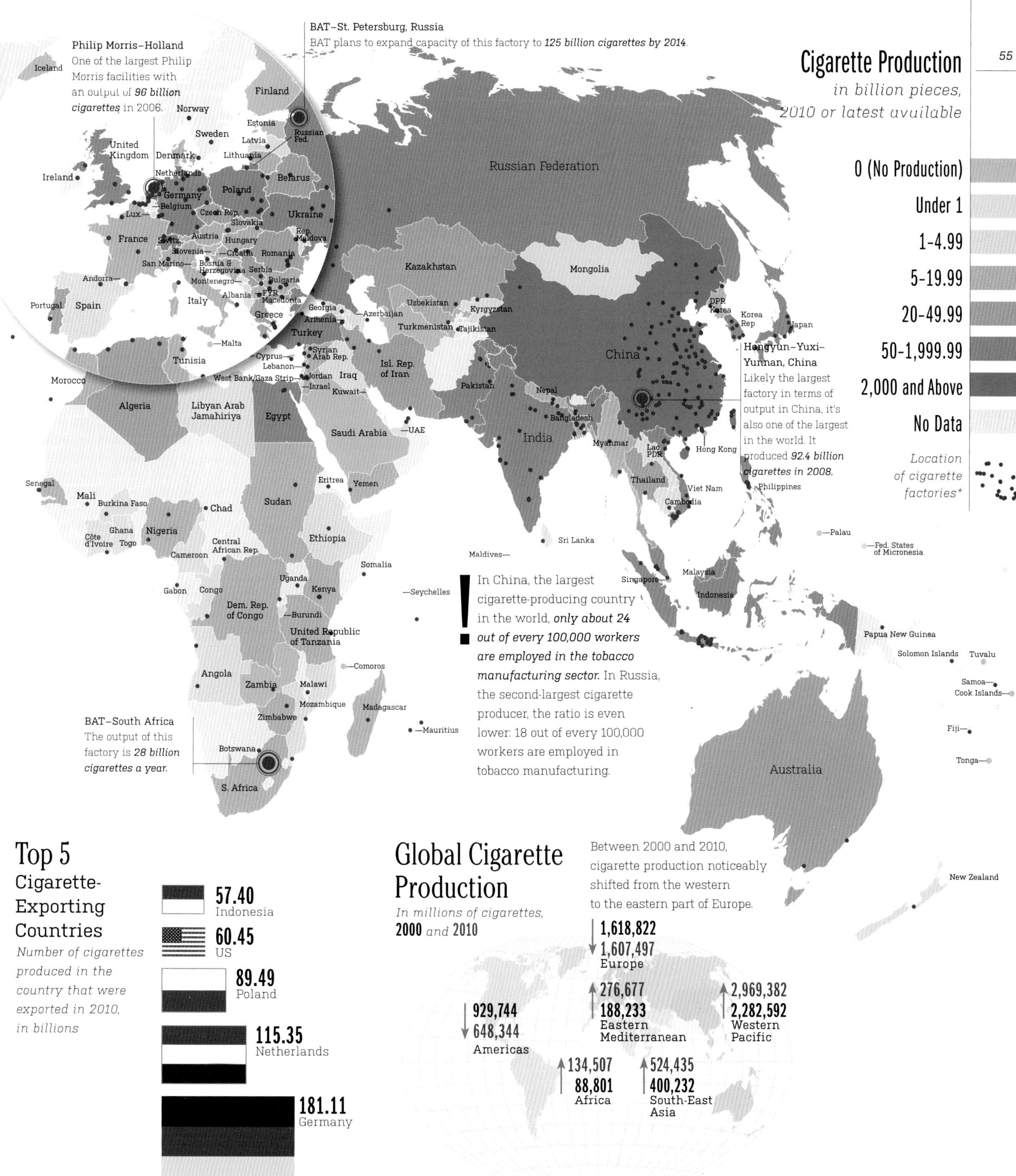

Cigarette Production
in billion pieces, 2010 or latest available
0 (No Production)
Under 1
1-4.99
5-19.99
20-49.99
50-1,999.99
2,000 and Above
No Data
Location of cigarette factories*
Philip Morris–Holland
One of the largest Philip Morris facilities with an output of 96 billion cigarettes in 2006.
BAT–St. Petersburg, Russia
BAT plans to expand capacity of this factory to 125 billion cigarettes by 2014.
Hongyun–Yuxi–Yunnan, China
Likely the largest factory in terms of output in China, it's also one of the largest in the world. It produced 92.4 billion cigarettes in 2008.
BAT–South Africa
The output of this factory is 28 billion cigarettes a year.
In China, the largest cigarette-producing country in the world, only about 24 out of every 100,000 workers are employed in the tobacco manufacturing sector. In Russia, the second-largest cigarette producer, the ratio is even lower: 18 out of every 100,000 workers are employed in tobacco manufacturing.
Iceland
Finland
Norway
Sweden
Estonia
Latvia
Lithuania
Russian Fed.
United Kingdom
Denmark
Ireland
Netherlands
Belarus
Poland
Germany
Belgium
Lux.
Czech Rep.
Ukraine
Slovakia
Rep. Moldova
France
Switz.
Austria
Hungary
Slovenia
Croatia
Romania
San Marino
Bosnia & Herzegovina
Serbia
Andorra
Montenegro
Bulgaria
Albania
FYR Macedonia
Italy
Portugal
Spain
Greece
Georgia
Armenia
Azerbaijan
Turkey
Malta
Tunisia
Cyprus
Syrian Arab Rep.
Lebanon
West Bank/Gaza Strip
Jordan
Israel
Iraq
Kuwait
Isl. Rep. of Iran
Morocco
Algeria
Libyan Arab Jamahiriya
Egypt
Saudi Arabia
UAE
Russian Federation
Kazakhstan
Mongolia
Uzbekistan
Kyrgyzstan
Turkmenistan
Tajikistan
China
DPR Korea
Korea Rep
Japan
Pakistan
Nepal
Bangladesh
India
Myanmar
Lao PDR
Hong Kong
Thailand
Viet Nam
Cambodia
Philippines
Sri Lanka
Maldives
Palau
Fed. States of Micronesia
Singapore
Malaysia
Indonesia
Papua New Guinea
Solomon Islands
Tuvalu
Samoa
Cook Islands
Fiji
Tonga
Australia
New Zealand
Senegal
Mali
Burkina Faso
Chad
Sudan
Eritrea
Yemen
Côte d'Ivoire
Ghana
Togo
Nigeria
Central African Rep.
Cameroon
Ethiopia
Somalia
Gabon
Congo
Uganda
Kenya
Seychelles
Dem. Rep. of Congo
Burundi
United Republic of Tanzania
Comoros
Angola
Zambia
Malawi
Mozambique
Madagascar
Zimbabwe
Mauritius
Botswana
S. Africa
Top 5 Cigarette-Exporting Countries
Number of cigarettes produced in the country that were exported in 2010, in billions
57.40 Indonesia
60.45 US
89.49 Poland
115.35 Netherlands
181.11 Germany
Global Cigarette Production
In millions of cigarettes, 2000 and 2010
Between 2000 and 2010, cigarette production noticeably shifted from the western to the eastern part of Europe.
1,618,822
1,607,497
Europe
929,744
648,344
Americas
276,677
188,233
Eastern Mediterranean
2,969,382
2,282,592
Western Pacific
134,507
88,801
Africa
524,435
400,232
South-East Asia
*http://tobaccoresearch.stanford.edu

RESEARCH SAYS:

> “These companies remain some of the most profitable in the world. This is thanks in part to their endless inventive ways of undermining and circumventing regulation.”
>
> *Anna Gilmore, University of Bath, UK, 2011*

In recent years, publicly traded tobacco companies have consolidated through privatization and mergers. Today there are five major private tobacco companies: Philip Morris International, Altria/Philip Morris USA, Japan Tobacco International, British American Tobacco, and Imperial Tobacco. In addition to these corporations, there are sixteen state-owned tobacco companies that are the leading cigarette manufacturers in specific countries. CHINA NATIONAL TOBACCO CORPORATION IS THE LARGEST STATE-OWNED TOBACCO COMPANY, PRODUCING MORE CIGARETTES THAN ANY OTHER COMPANY IN THE WORLD. In 2008 CNTC manufactured 2.1 trillion of the 5.9 trillion cigarettes produced worldwide.

As the tobacco market has consolidated under a few major companies, the direction of these companies is beginning to change. Traditionally, company buyouts took place in order to consolidate and expand cigarette market share. Now tobacco companies are branching out into other areas of tobacco products and technology. In recent years, the major tobacco companies have purchased corporations that produce oral tobacco, such as snus. In 2011 Philip Morris International bought patent rights to a technology that delivers nicotine-infused aerosol. In the same year, British American Tobacco established Nicoventures, a separate company dedicated to creating alternative nicotine products that offer the same experience expected from cigarettes without some of the risks of smoking.

Estimates of revenues from the global tobacco industry vary widely but are likely approaching half a trillion dollars annually. Although tobacco is ultimately a financial burden on the governments and health-care systems of countries, it is also a source of government revenue, through tobacco taxes and additional profit for those countries with state-owned tobacco companies. Each year the tobacco industry in China contributes over 7% of the central government's total revenue. If Big Tobacco were a country, it would have a gross domestic product (GDP) similar to that of Poland and Sweden.

THE INDUSTRY SAYS:

> “Altria Group has outperformed the S&P 500 every year since 2000 and has increased its dividend 44 times in the last 42 years. Its scale, balance sheet strength and improved operational focus make the company a compelling consumer products investment opportunity, and enable the company to have large-scale economic impact.”
>
> *Altria website, US, 2011*

Global Cigarette Market Share

Percent of total number of cigarettes produced, 2000 and 2008

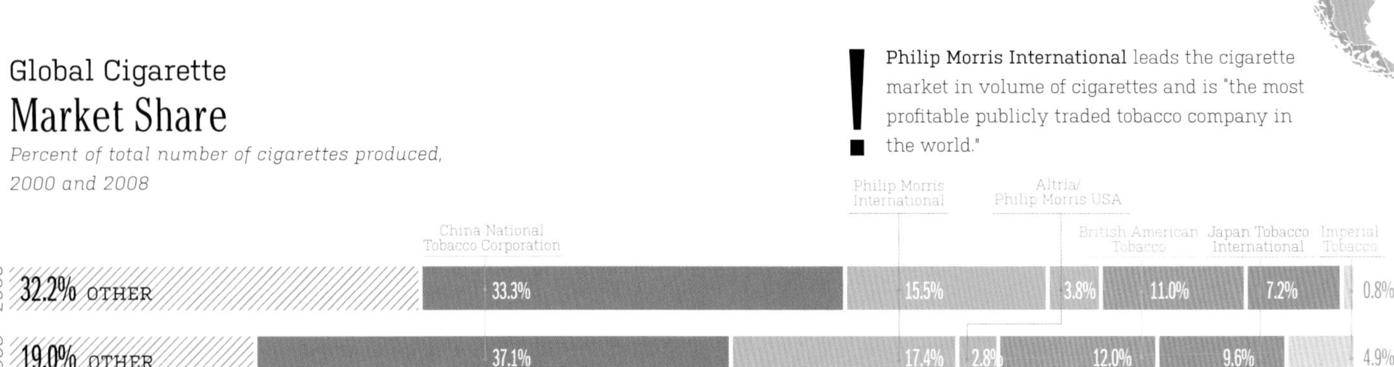

Totals might not sum due to rounding.

! **Philip Morris International** leads the cigarette market in volume of cigarettes and is "the most profitable publicly traded tobacco company in the world."

Canada
United States of America
Philip Morris International New York, NY
Altria Group/Philip Morris USA Richmond, VA
Mexico
Cuba
Dominican Rep.
Jamaica
Guatemala
Honduras
El Salvador
Nicaragua
Costa Rica
Panama
Trinidad & Tobago
Venezuela
Colombia
Ecuador
Peru
Brazil
Bolivia
Paraguay
Uruguay
Argentina
Chile

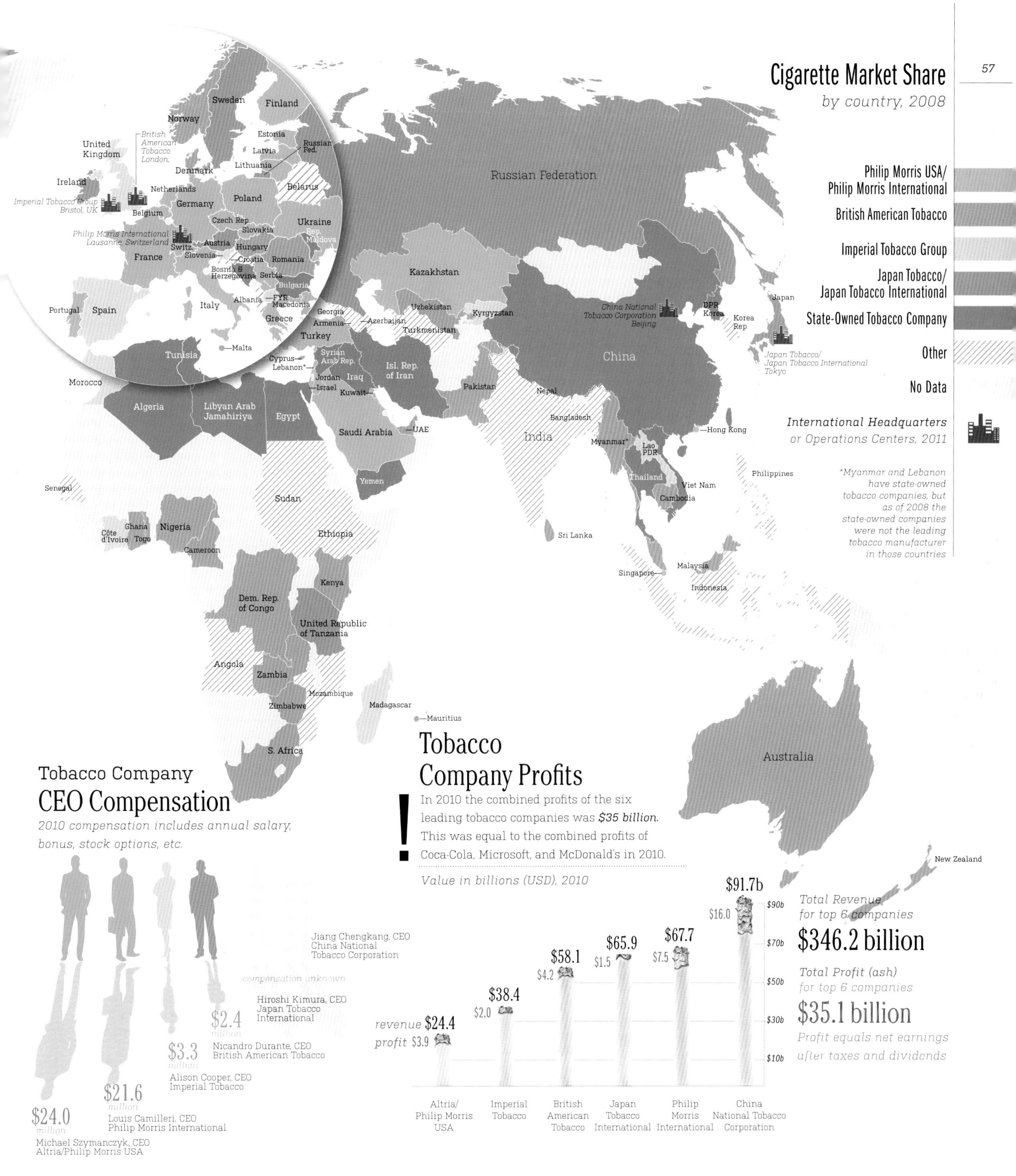

Cigarette Market Share
by country, 2008
Philip Morris USA/
Philip Morris International
British American Tobacco
Imperial Tobacco Group
Japan Tobacco/
Japan Tobacco International
State-Owned Tobacco Company
Other
No Data
International Headquarters
or Operations Centers, 2011
*Myanmar and Lebanon have state-owned tobacco companies, but as of 2008 the state-owned companies were not the leading tobacco manufacturer in those countries
British American Tobacco London,
Imperial Tobacco Group Bristol, UK
Philip Morris International Lausanne, Switzerland
China National Tobacco Corporation Beijing
Japan Tobacco/ Japan Tobacco International Tokyo
Sweden
Finland
Norway
Estonia
United Kingdom
Latvia
Russian Fed.
Lithuania
Ireland
Denmark
Netherlands
Belarus
Germany
Poland
Belgium
Czech Rep.
Slovakia
Ukraine
Rep. Moldova
Austria
Switz.
Hungary
France
Slovenia
Croatia
Romania
Bosnia & Herzegovina
Serbia
Bulgaria
Albania
FYR Macedonia
Portugal
Spain
Italy
Greece
Georgia
Armenia
Azerbaijan
Turkey
Malta
Tunisia
Cyprus
Lebanon*
Syrian Arab Rep.
Morocco
Jordan
Iraq
Isl. Rep. of Iran
Israel
Kuwait
Algeria
Libyan Arab Jamahiriya
Egypt
Saudi Arabia
UAE
Yemen
Senegal
Sudan
Côte d'Ivoire
Ghana
Togo
Nigeria
Cameroon
Ethiopia
Kenya
Dem. Rep. of Congo
United Republic of Tanzania
Angola
Zambia
Mozambique
Zimbabwe
Madagascar
Mauritius
S. Africa
Russian Federation
Kazakhstan
Uzbekistan
Kyrgyzstan
Turkmenistan
Pakistan
Nepal
India
Bangladesh
Sri Lanka
China
DPR Korea
Korea Rep
Japan
Myanmar*
Lao PDR
Thailand
Hong Kong
Viet Nam
Cambodia
Philippines
Malaysia
Singapore
Indonesia
Australia
New Zealand
Tobacco Company
CEO Compensation
2010 compensation includes annual salary, bonus, stock options, etc.
Jiang Chengkang, CEO China National Tobacco Corporation
compensation unknown
$2.4 million
Hiroshi Kimura, CEO Japan Tobacco International
$3.3 million
Nicandro Durante, CEO British American Tobacco
Alison Cooper, CEO Imperial Tobacco
$21.6 million
Louis Camilleri, CEO Philip Morris International
$24.0 million
Michael Szymanczyk, CEO Altria/Philip Morris USA
Tobacco
Company Profits
!
In 2010 the combined profits of the six leading tobacco companies was $35 billion. This was equal to the combined profits of Coca-Cola, Microsoft, and McDonald's in 2010.
Value in billions (USD), 2010
revenue $24.4
profit $3.9
$38.4
$2.0
$58.1
$4.2
$65.9
$1.5
$67.7
$7.5
$91.7b
$16.0
$90b
$70b
$50b
$30b
$10b
Altria/ Philip Morris USA
Imperial Tobacco
British American Tobacco
Japan Tobacco International
Philip Morris International
China National Tobacco Corporation
Total Revenue for top 6 companies
$346.2 billion
Total Profit (ash) for top 6 companies
$35.1 billion
Profit equals net earnings after taxes and dividends

RESEARCH SAYS:

“Smuggling of cigarettes gives opportunities for organized crime networks to survive and may increase the general level of corruption in a country.”

WHO, Western Pacific Regional Office, 2000

Cigarette Prices and Illicit Cigarette Trade in the UK

Contrary to tobacco industry claims, the increase in retail price has not led to any corresponding increase in illicit trade.

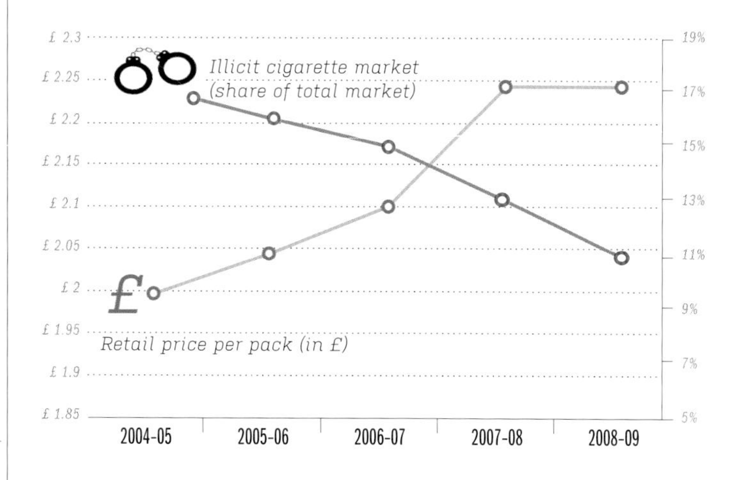

! If illicit trade were eliminated, governments worldwide would gain at least ***$31.3 billion a year in tax revenue,*** and from 2030 onward, ***more than 164,000 premature deaths would be avoided annually due to higher average cigarette prices.***

The share of the illicit cigarette trade in the global cigarette market (estimated at 9–11%) has remained relatively stable since 2000, even though some countries have managed to reduce the penetration of illicit cigarettes within their markets (e.g., UK). On average, this percentage is significantly higher in low- and middle-income countries than in high-income countries.

Illicit trade in tobacco products has serious health, economic, and social implications. Circumventing tobacco taxes undermines tax and price policies, which are among the most effective mechanisms to control tobacco use, as well as other tobacco control measures, such as youth access laws or mandatory health-warning labels. Tobacco smuggling can also lead to higher levels of corruption. Illicit cigarette trade is highly profitable for the transnational tobacco companies, allowing them to circumvent tobacco taxation. In Canada, the industry was found guilty of organizing illicit trade and paid billions of dollars in penalties.

The illicit tobacco trade is addressed by Article 15 of the WHO Framework Convention on Tobacco Control (WHO FCTC). Parties to the Convention are negotiating a protocol that builds upon the original treaty and aims to strengthen international cooperation in fighting the illicit tobacco trade. Despite the irreconcilable conflicts of interest between the tobacco industry and the public health community, the industry is seeking to enter WHO FCTC illicit trade protocol negotiations and national-level illicit trade control activities. In many parts of the world, the tobacco industry works closely with governments to combat illicit trade. This collaboration involves many risks and conflicts with Article 5.3 of the WHO FCTC.

THE TOBACCO INDUSTRY HAS CONSISTENTLY ARGUED THAT TOBACCO TAX INCREASES CREATE MORE ILLICIT TRADE. HOWEVER, NO RESEARCH EVIDENCE SUPPORTS THIS CLAIM. On the contrary, evidence shows that factors other than tax and price are more important determinants of illicit tobacco trade, and that illicit trade is generally lesser where cigarette prices are higher. Policies that can decrease illicit trade include licensing all participants in the tobacco business, introducing enhanced tax stamps and higher trafficking penalties, and tracking tobacco product packages.

Canada
United States of America
Mexico
Bahamas
Dominican Rep.
Belize
Jamaica
Guatemala
El Salvador
Nicaragua
Barbados
Trinidad & Tobago
Costa Rica
Panama
Venezuela
Guyana
Colombia
Ecuador
Peru
Brazil
Bolivia
Paraguay
Uruguay
Argentina
Chile

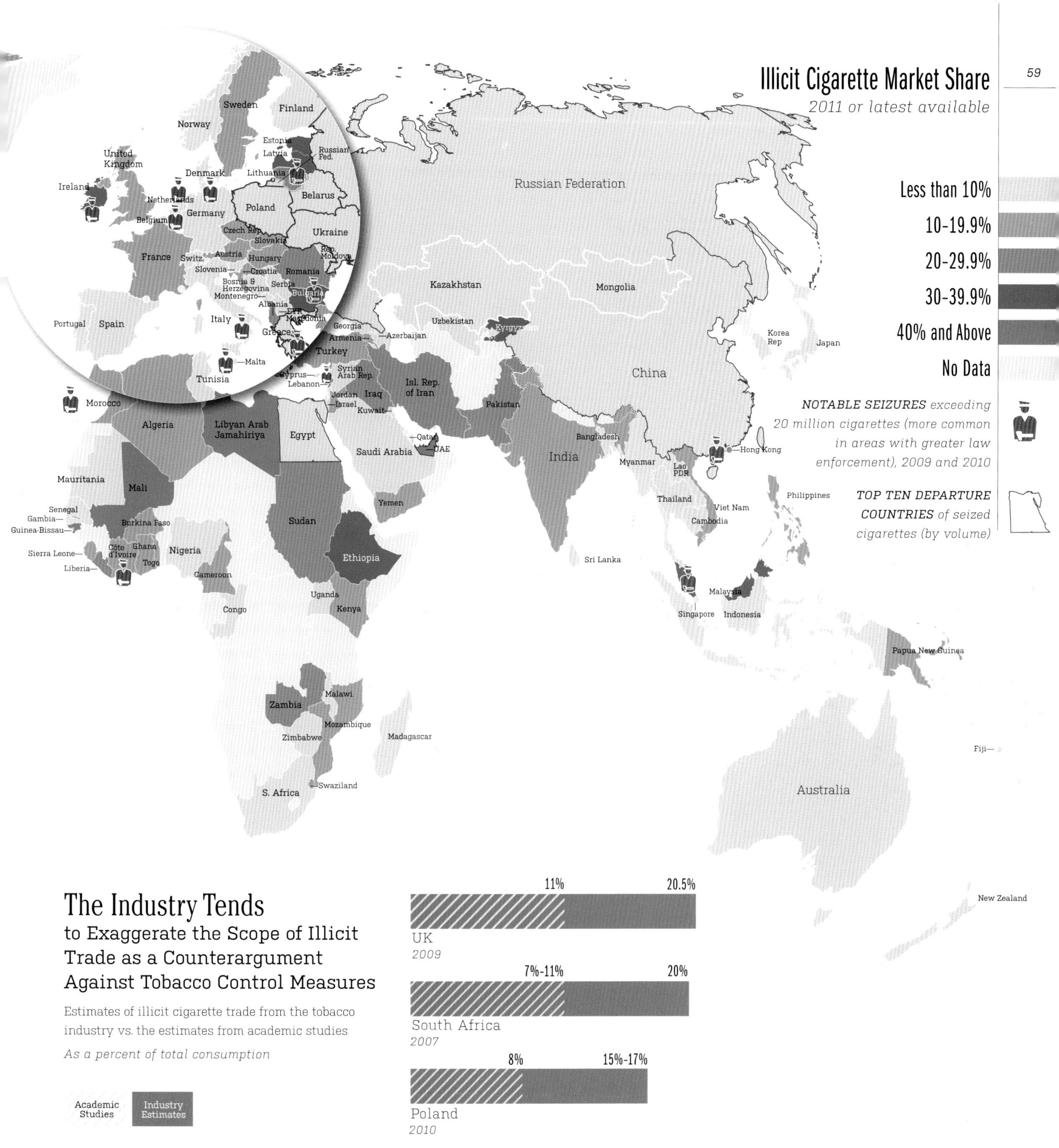

Illicit Cigarette Market Share
2011 or latest available
Less than 10%
10-19.9%
20-29.9%
30-39.9%
40% and Above
No Data
NOTABLE SEIZURES exceeding 20 million cigarettes (more common in areas with greater law enforcement), 2009 and 2010
TOP TEN DEPARTURE COUNTRIES of seized cigarettes (by volume)
Sweden
Finland
Norway
Estonia
Latvia
Russian Fed.
United Kingdom
Denmark
Lithuania
Ireland
Netherlands
Belarus
Poland
Germany
Belgium
Czech Rep.
Ukraine
Slovakia
France
Switz.
Austria
Hungary
Rep. Moldova
Slovenia
Croatia
Romania
Bosnia & Herzegovina
Serbia
Montenegro
Bulgaria
Albania
FYR Macedonia
Portugal
Spain
Italy
Greece
Georgia
Armenia
Azerbaijan
Turkey
Malta
Tunisia
Cyprus
Lebanon
Syrian Arab Rep.
Isl. Rep. of Iran
Jordan
Iraq
Israel
Kuwait
Morocco
Algeria
Libyan Arab Jamahiriya
Egypt
Qatar
UAE
Saudi Arabia
Russian Federation
Kazakhstan
Mongolia
Uzbekistan
Kyrgyzstan
China
Korea Rep
Japan
Pakistan
India
Bangladesh
Myanmar
Lao PDR
Hong Kong
Thailand
Viet Nam
Cambodia
Philippines
Sri Lanka
Malaysia
Singapore
Indonesia
Papua New Guinea
Mauritania
Mali
Senegal
Gambia
Guinea-Bissau
Burkina Faso
Sierra Leone
Liberia
Côte d'Ivoire
Ghana
Togo
Nigeria
Cameroon
Sudan
Ethiopia
Yemen
Uganda
Kenya
Congo
Malawi
Zambia
Mozambique
Zimbabwe
Madagascar
Swaziland
S. Africa
Australia
Fiji
New Zealand
The Industry Tends
to Exaggerate the Scope of Illicit Trade as a Counterargument Against Tobacco Control Measures
Estimates of illicit cigarette trade from the tobacco industry vs. the estimates from academic studies
As a percent of total consumption
Academic Studies
Industry Estimates
11%
20.5%
UK
2009
7%-11%
20%
South Africa
2007
8%
15%-17%
Poland
2010

INDUSTRY SAYS:

“If you can market a product that kills people, you can sell anything.”

Chris Reiter, R.J. Reynolds Campaign Program Manager, US, 2003

Cigarette Marketing Expenditures

2008, in millions (USD)

% of Costs

83% PRICE DISCOUNTS, COUPONS, RETAIL-VALUE-ADDED $8,263.7m

1% DIRECT MAIL $89.9m

1% SPECIALTY ITEM DISTRIBUTION $101.0m (Branded and Non-Branded)

2% POINT OF SALE $163.7m

2% PUBLIC ENTERTAINMENT $154.7m (Adult Only)

2% ALL OTHERS $236.8m (plus Magazine/Outdoor, Sampling Distribution, Company Website)

9% PROMOTIONAL ALLOWANCES $931.2m (Retailers, Wholesalers, Others)

TOTAL $9,941 million

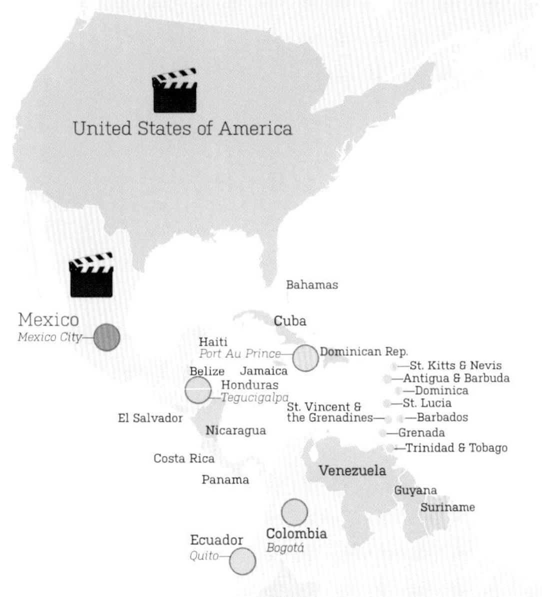

THE TOBACCO INDUSTRY CLAIMS THAT IT DOES NOT MARKET TO CHILDREN AND THAT THE PURPOSE OF ITS ADVERTISING IS ONLY TO ENCOURAGE ADULT SMOKERS TO SWITCH BRANDS. US Federal Judge Gladys Kessler found this argument baseless, and concluded that tobacco advertising contributes to youth smoking. Despite increasing restrictions on marketing and advertising, tobacco companies continue to spend billions of dollars annually to maintain brand loyalty among current smokers, to influence young people to use tobacco, and to keep smokers addicted.

In 2008, $9.9 billion was spent on cigarette advertising and promotion in the US alone, and an additional $548 million was spent on smokeless tobacco marketing. This equated to more than $34 being spent on tobacco marketing for every man, woman, and child in the US that year.

Mass media tobacco advertising is banned in many countries, but tobacco companies are utilizing other marketing techniques to attract and retain smokers. In some countries these methods include advertisements at the point of sale, promotional allowances paid to retailers to facilitate product placement, promotions such as “buy one, get one free,” and price discounts. Price discounts include the costs that cigarette companies incur when they pay cigarette retailers and wholesalers to reduce the overall price of cigarettes. In the US in 2008, price discounts, coupons, and retail-value-added promotions accounted for 83% of all tobacco marketing expenditures.

In addition to these techniques, tobacco companies are actively engaged in brand-stretching and other strategies to avoid regulation and marketing bans. They also utilize the Internet and other new media. The Internet allows participation and engagement unlike any other form of media, and has great potential for tobacco advertising. Additional attention must be paid to the use of the Internet in cigarette marketing, particularly social media sites.

Continued implementation of the WHO FCTC and its provisions will increase comprehensive tobacco advertising, marketing, promotion, and sponsorship bans throughout the world.

! *British American Tobacco and Philip Morris researched the Chinese culture of gift giving* and subsequently marketed cigarettes to strengthen the image of their brands while promoting the acceptability of cigarettes as a present and the social norm of giving gifts.

Percent of Youth Who Have Something With a Tobacco Logo on It

(T-Shirt, pen, backpack, etc.)
2010 or latest available

Under 10%
10-14.9%
15-19.9%
20-24.9%
Above 25%
No Data
Subnational Data

Selected countries where portrayal of ***SMOKING IN MOVIES HAS BEEN LINKED TO YOUTH SMOKING*** *in the past decade*

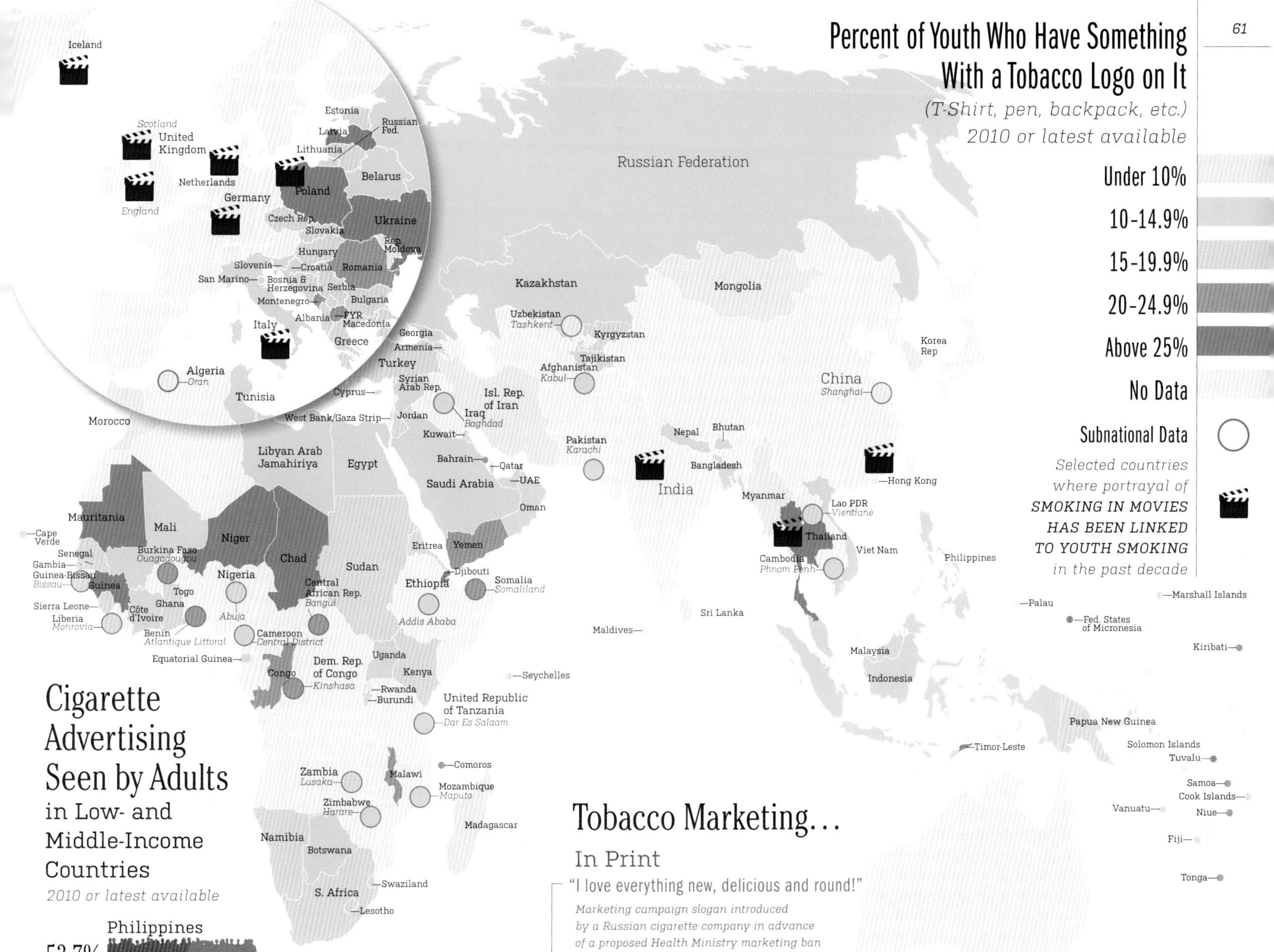

Iceland, Scotland, United Kingdom, England, Netherlands, Germany, Estonia, Latvia, Russian Fed., Lithuania, Belarus, Poland, Czech Rep., Slovakia, Ukraine, Rep. Moldova, Hungary, Slovenia, Croatia, Romania, San Marino, Bosnia & Herzegovina, Serbia, Montenegro, Bulgaria, Albania, FYR Macedonia, Italy, Greece, Georgia, Armenia, Turkey, Algeria, Oran, Tunisia, Morocco, Cyprus, Syrian Arab Rep., Isl. Rep. of Iran, Iraq, Baghdad, West Bank/Gaza Strip, Jordan, Kuwait, Bahrain, Qatar, UAE, Saudi Arabia, Oman, Libyan Arab Jamahiriya, Egypt, Russian Federation, Kazakhstan, Uzbekistan, Tashkent, Kyrgyzstan, Tajikistan, Afghanistan, Kabul, Mongolia, China, Shanghai, Korea Rep, Pakistan, Karachi, Nepal, Bhutan, India, Bangladesh, Hong Kong, Myanmar, Lao PDR, Vientiane, Thailand, Cambodia, Phnom Penh, Viet Nam, Philippines, Sri Lanka, Maldives, Malaysia, Indonesia, Palau, Marshall Islands, Fed. States of Micronesia, Kiribati, Papua New Guinea, Timor-Leste, Solomon Islands, Tuvalu, Samoa, Cook Islands, Vanuatu, Niue, Fiji, Tonga, New Zealand, Mauritania, Mali, Niger, Chad, Sudan, Cape Verde, Senegal, Gambia, Guinea-Bissau, Bissau, Guinea, Burkina Faso, Ouagadougou, Nigeria, Abuja, Togo, Ghana, Sierra Leone, Liberia, Monrovia, Côte d'Ivoire, Benin, Atlantique Littoral, Cameroon, Central District, Central African Rep., Bangui, Eritrea, Yemen, Djibouti, Ethiopia, Addis Ababa, Somalia, Somaliland, Equatorial Guinea, Congo, Dem. Rep. of Congo, Kinshasa, Uganda, Kenya, Rwanda, Burundi, Seychelles, United Republic of Tanzania, Dar Es Salaam, Comoros, Zambia, Lusaka, Malawi, Mozambique, Maputo, Zimbabwe, Harare, Madagascar, Namibia, Botswana, Swaziland, S. Africa, Lesotho

Cigarette Advertising Seen by Adults

in Low- and Middle-Income Countries

2010 or latest available

Percent of adults who noticed cigarette marketing in stores where cigarettes are sold

Country	Percent
Philippines	53.7%
Russian Federation	43.6%
Mexico	36.5%
Bangladesh	33.2%
Brazil	30.6%
Uruguay	20.9%
Ukraine	20.5%
Poland	13.9%
India	10.7%
Viet Nam	8.6%
Egypt	8.0%
Thailand	6.7%
Turkey	2.7%

Advertising was noticed in the 30 days prior to the survey.

Tobacco Marketing...

In Print

"I love everything new, delicious and round!"

Marketing campaign slogan introduced by a Russian cigarette company in advance of a proposed Health Ministry marketing ban on cigarettes, 2011

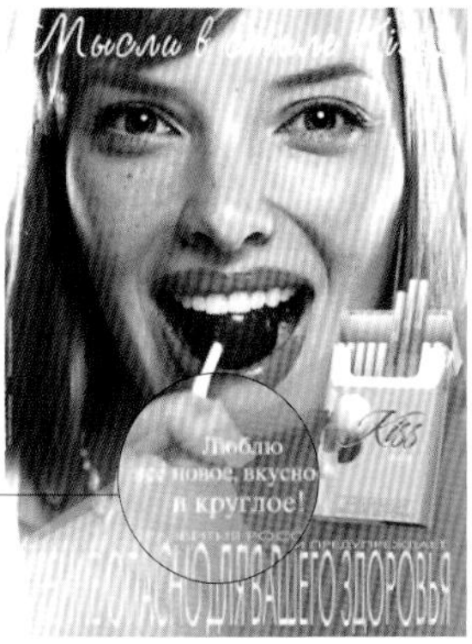

Мысли в...
Люблю всё новое, вкусное и круглое!

On Billboards

"Dying is better than leaving a friend; Sampoerna is a cool friend."

Indonesian billboard campaign by the tobacco company PT Sampoerna, 2011

In Films

"Smoking in films encourages children to take up smoking. And that's no surprise. That is why tobacco advertising was banned, because showing images of people, particularly glamorous young people, smoking encourages children to smoke."

Deborah Arnott, Action on Smoking and Health, UK, 2011

Online

"The Internet and social media websites are potentially the next frontier in tobacco company advertising strategy."

Campaign for Tobacco-Free Kids, US, 2011

Chapter 21

THE INDUSTRY SAYS:

"Portray the debate as one between the anti-smoking lobby and the smoker, instead of 'pro-health and public citizens' versus the tobacco industry."
Philip Morris USA, 1992

TOBACCO COMPANIES SPEND UNTOLD MILLIONS OF DOLLARS ANNUALLY TO INFLUENCE PUBLIC POLICY AND LEGISLATION. Reporting of tobacco industry political contributions is not required in most countries, so the complete picture of the tobacco industry's investment is not fully understood. In 2010, nineteen companies with tobacco interests spent $16.6 million and employed 168 lobbyists in an effort to directly influence political decisions in the US.

In addition to political influence, tobacco companies make charitable contributions under the guise of corporate social responsibility (CSR). Often these donations and efforts do more to benefit the image of tobacco companies than to benefit humanitarian efforts. In 2010 Philip Morris International contributed a fraction of a percent of the company's net profits in global charitable donations ($25 million in donations and $7.5 billion in profits).

Parties to the WHO FCTC are warned to "be alert to any efforts by the tobacco industry to undermine or subvert tobacco control efforts" and are obligated to protect their public health policies from commercial and other vested interests of the tobacco industry. The influence of the tobacco industry is monumental, and tobacco companies' contributions to socially responsible causes are of great concern. Not only are CSR contributions a form of tobacco advertising and promotion, but such contributions allow tobacco companies to legitimize themselves with policymakers and the public and counter the negative attention surrounding their deadly products.

The tobacco industry exerts undue influence through partnerships with other organizations, such as convenience stores, advertising, and farmers' associations, and the hospitality industry. Tobacco companies fund front groups and think tanks to promote tobacco or oppose tobacco legislation. While these organizations appear to be independent, governments must be wary of their involvement with Big Tobacco.

United States of America

In 2011, Lorillard, the largest producer of menthol cigarettes in the US, ***hired a former Food and Drug Administration employee*** who was a science and regulations expert. At the time of the hire, the FDA was considering restricting menthol cigarette sales.

! In 2010, Altria Group/Philip Morris USA spent over ***$10 million in lobbying expenditures*** in the US. This is more than all other tobacco companies spent combined.

"One thing the tobacco industry has done is stay out of the public view and disguise its efforts in politics...With the rise of this undisclosed money, it is hard to know what they're doing."
Stanton Glantz, University of California, San Francisco, US, 2011

Total Federal Election Contributions From Big Tobacco

1990–2010, US
to Republican Party
to Democratic Party

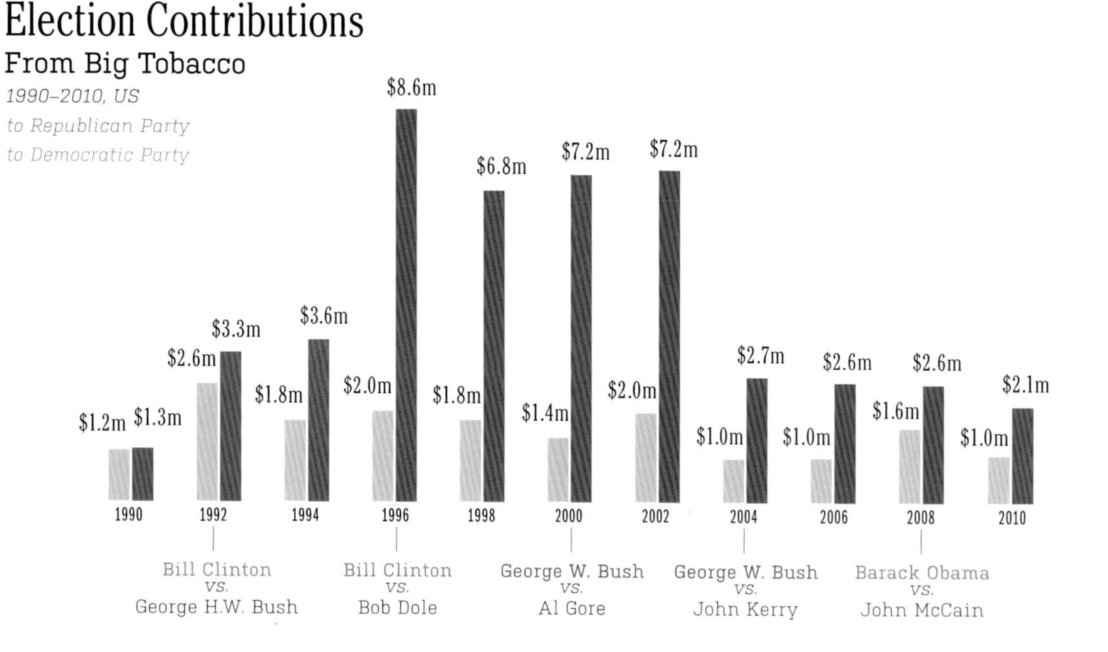

United Kingdom

BAT, Japan Tobacco International, and Imperial Tobacco ***contributed funds to the Tobacco Retailers Alliance,*** a front group that orchestrated the "Save Our Shop" campaign in 2008. ***Members of Parliament were inundated with postcards*** requesting they not support the Department of Health's proposed ban on cigarette display advertising.

China

China National Tobacco Corporation has sponsored at least 69 elementary schools, and thousands of students are exposed daily to pro-tobacco propaganda, names, and messages. School signage reads: ***"Genius comes from hard work / Tobacco helps you to be successful."***

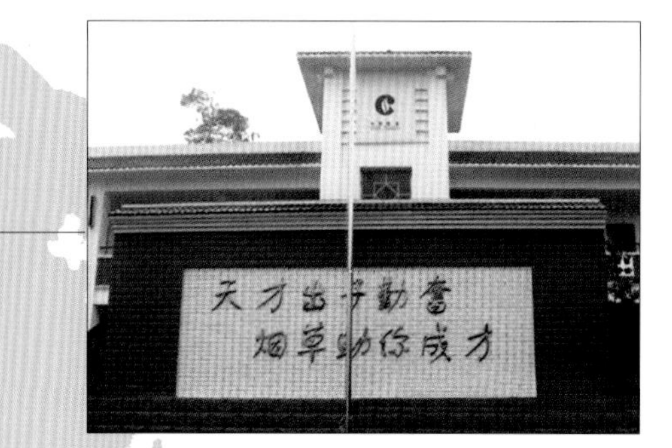

ADVOCATES SAY:

"We need to be alert and firm in protecting our tobacco control policies from the commercial and vested interests of the tobacco industry."

Evita Ricafort, lawyer with HealthJustice, Philippines, 2011

Philippines

Baguio City announced its intention to have smoke-free festivals in 2009. ***Philip Morris International responded by offering the mayor mechanized ashtrays,*** smoking tents, and recommendations on the number of designated smoking areas that should be allowed.

Indonesia

Sampoerna/Philip Morris International, Indonesia's largest tobacco company, sponsored a rescue camp on the slopes of Mount Merapi, a volcano that erupted in Central Java in 2010. Staff members at the camp wore uniforms with company logos and drove response vehicles and trucks with the same logos.

Malawi

In the early 1990s, a tobacco company consultant published a journal featuring articles criticizing the World Health Organization. One article from the Chief of Health Services in Malawi, who owned a tobacco farm, stated that "the list of economic benefits of tobacco is a long one. ***Tobacco-related deaths and illnesses are primarily problems of affluent societies.***" Philip Morris distributed thousands of copies of the journal.

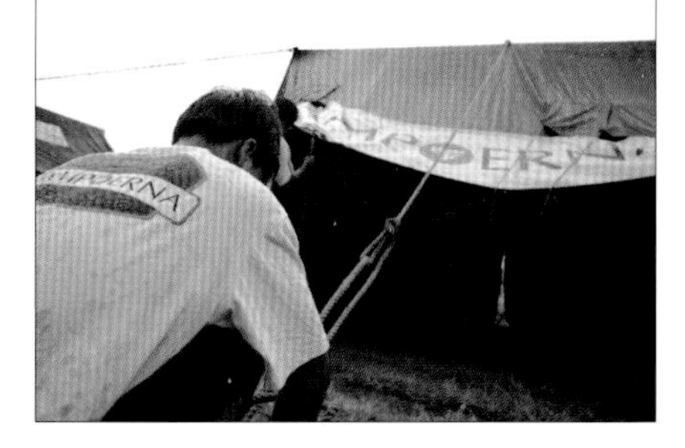

Australia

The Australian Government's world first legislation will require that all tobacco products sold in Australia are in plain, drab dark brown color packaging by 1 December 2012. ***Fourteen members of the World Trade Organization raised concerns that plain packages would restrict the trade of tobacco.***

"Ninety-seven percent of British American Tobacco's money is spent here on two parties: the Liberal Party and the National Party. And they are asking us to [believe] this has no influence on their decision on whether they are going to support plain packaging or not."

Nicola Roxon, Former Minister of Health and Ageing, Australia, 2011

RESEARCH SAYS:

"Recent attempts by large tobacco companies to represent themselves as socially responsible have been widely dismissed as image management."

Gary Fooks et al., University of Bath, UK, 2011

THE NUMBER OF PEOPLE COVERED BY AT LEAST ONE *MPOWER* MEASURE AT THE HIGHEST LEVEL OF ACHIEVEMENT

INCREASED BY 1.1 BILLION PEOPLE TO 3.8 BILLION BETWEEN 2008 AND 2010.

THIS MEANS THAT

More Than

OF THE WORLD'S POPULATION IS COVERED BY AT LEAST ONE *MPOWER* MEASURE.

See Glossary for details on MPOWER

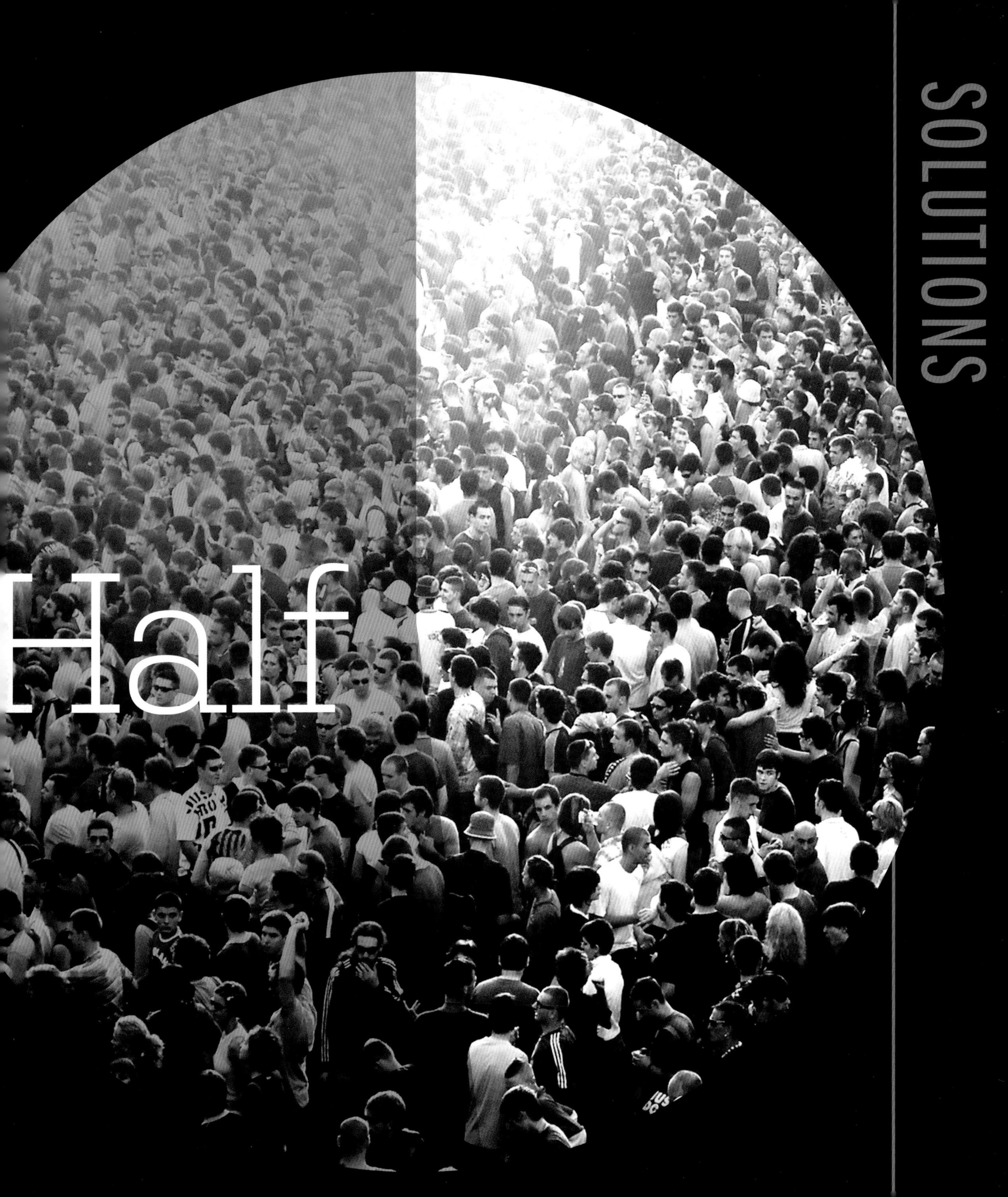
Half
SOLUTIONS

WISDOM SAYS:

"*Salus populi suprema est lex.*
The welfare of the people is the ultimate law."
Cicero, Italy, 106–43 BCE

Fifteen or more treaties touch upon issues related to tobacco control, such as health and human rights; poverty; economic development; gender; safe working environments; tobacco farming, land reform, and indebtedness; food insecurity; child labor; environmental degradation; and the behavior of industry. Evaluating these treaties is difficult because of the lack of precedence and rulings in relation to tobacco control. Even where public health provisions exist within treaties, it is uncertain whether their interpretation will always result in the implementation of effective tobacco control measures, although many do.

Additionally, some UN agencies have made recommendations that are short of being treaties. For example, in 1992 the International Civil Aviation Organization initiated measures to encourage its member states to restrict smoking on all air travel, then adopted resolutions urging states and airlines to act to prohibit smoking on all flights.

Some UN agencies have no treaty or codes of practice on tobacco. Among the International Labor Organization's nearly 200 treaties on worker and workplace safety, there is not one provision on smoke-free workplaces.

Most World Health Organization Member States have ratified the main treaty on tobacco, the WHO Framework Convention on Tobacco Control (WHO FCTC), **MAKING IT ONE OF THE MOST RAPIDLY EMBRACED INTERNATIONAL TREATIES OF ALL TIME.** The Conference of Parties' secretariat has been established and is currently developing protocols and guidelines.

Not surprisingly, the tobacco industry was and is against a strong, legally binding WHO FCTC. The industry prefers voluntary agreements and self-regulating market mechanisms, which are essentially ineffective in reducing tobacco use.

Contrary to tobacco industry arguments, implementing tobacco control measures will not harm national economies. The WHO FCTC has mobilized resources, rallied hundreds of nongovernmental organizations (NGOs), encouraged government action, led to the political maturation of health ministries, and raised tobacco control awareness in other government ministries and departments. A human-rights-based approach to tobacco control helps to expand the discussion of the harm caused by tobacco use.

UN High-Level Meeting on Noncommunicable Diseases *(NCDs)*
2011

- Only 28 such special sessions since 1945, and just one previously on health (AIDS).
- 34 world leaders attended the meeting.
- An agreement to tackle the world's major NCDs was approved by all member nations.
- The NCD Alliance formed of four federations uniting more than 2,000 organizations.

Next steps:

- WHO, as Secretariat, to prepare next steps (including recommendations for global targets, plans to liaise with other UN agencies, etc.) by the end of 2012.
- Countries to develop NCD policies by 2013.
- Civil society to support in myriad ways.

International Treaties, Conventions, and Agreements
That Directly or Indirectly Address Tobacco Issues

1948
UN UNIVERSAL DECLARATION ON HUMAN RIGHTS
Article 25: Everyone has the right to a standard of living adequate for the health and well-being of himself and of his family.

1957
TREATY OF ROME
European community is mandated to pursue a high degree of public health protection.

1959
UN CONVENTION ON THE RIGHTS OF THE CHILD
Defends children's right to health.

1976
INTERNATIONAL COVENANT ON ECONOMIC, SOCIAL, AND CULTURAL RIGHTS
References the right to safe and healthy working conditions.
INTERNATIONAL COVENANT ON CIVIL AND POLITICAL RIGHTS (ICCPR)
Article 19: Defends the curtailments of freedom of speech in the interests of public health.

1979
CONVENTION TO ELIMINATE DISCRIMINATION AGAINST WOMEN (CEDAW)
Article 11: Defends the right to health for women, including the right to protection of health and to safety in working conditions.

1995
WORLD TRADE ORGANIZATION (WTO)
Preamble: Replaced the 1947 General Agreement on Tariffs and Trade (GATT). In general, trade liberalization, without safeguards, has increased tobacco usage in low- and middle-income countries. The following five treaties entered into force with the establishment of the WTO.

WTO AGREEMENT ON THE TRADE-RELATED ASPECTS OF INTELLECTUAL PROPERTY RIGHTS (TRIPS)
Recognizes that WTO Members may adopt measures necessary to protect public health.

WTO AGREEMENT ON TECHNICAL BARRIERS TO TRADE (TBT AGREEMENT)
Requires WTO Members to ensure that all technical regulations are not more trade-restrictive than necessary to achieve a legitimate objective such as the protection of human health.

1945 1955 1965 1975 1985

WHO Framework Convention on Tobacco Control

Nonparticipating states as of 2012

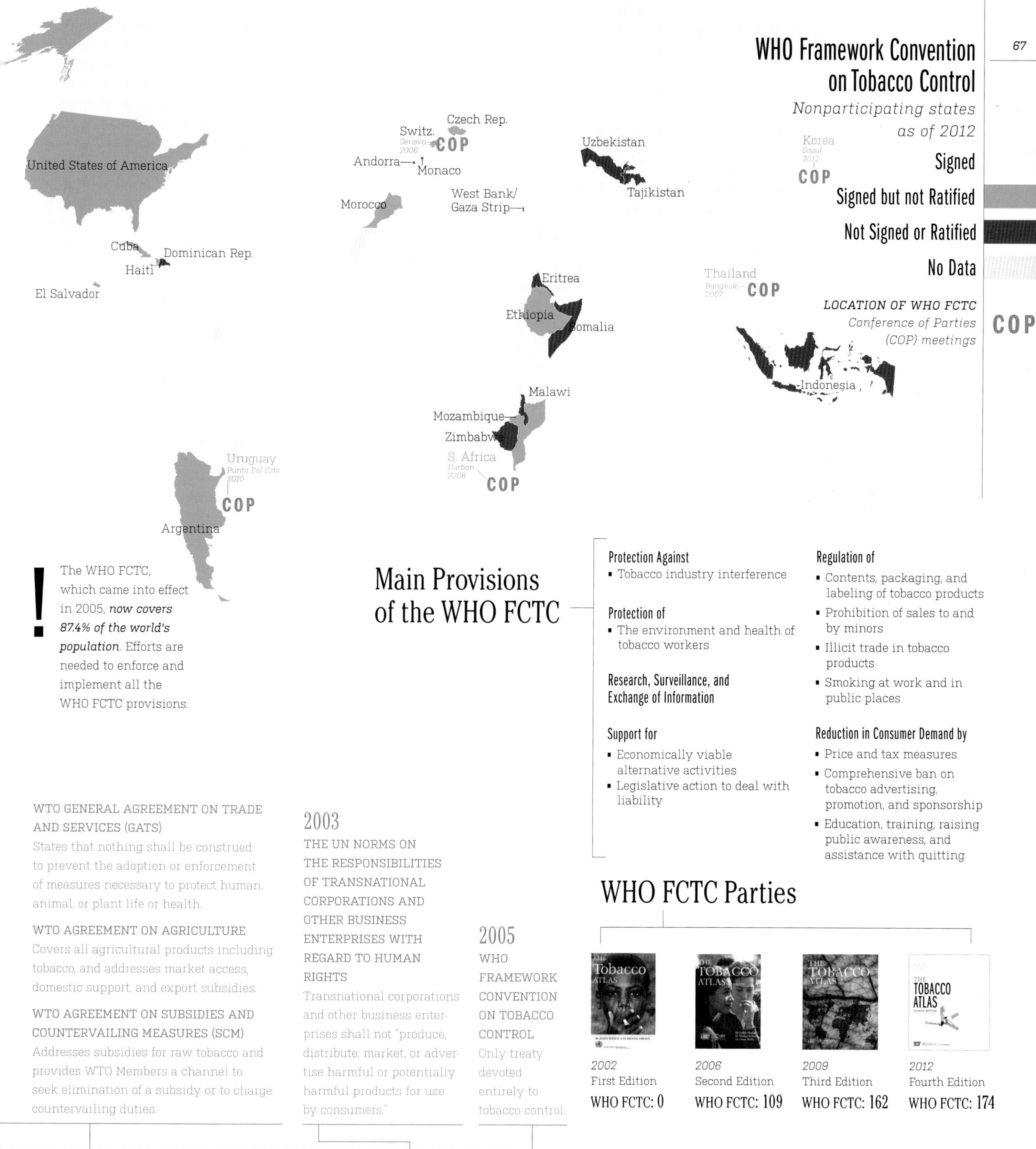

The WHO FCTC, which came into effect in 2005, *now covers 87.4% of the world's population*. Efforts are needed to enforce and implement all the WHO FCTC provisions.

Main Provisions of the WHO FCTC

Protection Against
- Tobacco industry interference

Protection of
- The environment and health of tobacco workers

Research, Surveillance, and Exchange of Information

Support for
- Economically viable alternative activities
- Legislative action to deal with liability

Regulation of
- Contents, packaging, and labeling of tobacco products
- Prohibition of sales to and by minors
- Illicit trade in tobacco products
- Smoking at work and in public places

Reduction in Consumer Demand by
- Price and tax measures
- Comprehensive ban on tobacco advertising, promotion, and sponsorship
- Education, training, raising public awareness, and assistance with quitting

WHO FCTC Parties

2002	2006	2009	2012
First Edition	Second Edition	Third Edition	Fourth Edition
WHO FCTC: 0	WHO FCTC: 109	WHO FCTC: 162	WHO FCTC: 174

WTO GENERAL AGREEMENT ON TRADE AND SERVICES (GATS)
States that nothing shall be construed to prevent the adoption or enforcement of measures necessary to protect human, animal, or plant life or health.

WTO AGREEMENT ON AGRICULTURE
Covers all agricultural products including tobacco, and addresses market access, domestic support, and export subsidies.

WTO AGREEMENT ON SUBSIDIES AND COUNTERVAILING MEASURES (SCM)
Addresses subsidies for raw tobacco and provides WTO Members a channel to seek elimination of a subsidy or to charge countervailing duties.

2003
THE UN NORMS ON THE RESPONSIBILITIES OF TRANSNATIONAL CORPORATIONS AND OTHER BUSINESS ENTERPRISES WITH REGARD TO HUMAN RIGHTS
Transnational corporations and other business enterprises shall not "produce, distribute, market, or advertise harmful or potentially harmful products for use by consumers."

2005
WHO FRAMEWORK CONVENTION ON TOBACCO CONTROL
Only treaty devoted entirely to tobacco control.

1995 2000 2005

HISTORY SAYS:

“Measure the distances. Estimate the expenses. Evaluate the forces. Assess the possibilities. Plan for victory.”

General Sun Tzu, Art of War, *China, Circa 500 BCE*

Tobacco control has evolved over the last 30 years from sporadic acts by activists and isolated action by some governments to a mainstream public health issue, with known, proven, cost-effective measures. Needed now is a coherent public health strategy designed to reduce tobacco consumption, involving international, regional, national, and local actors involved in strategic planning, policy-oriented research, capacity building, funding, enforcement, and evaluation.

Surveillance is essential to support sound policy. Almost half of all countries have monitoring systems enhanced by research initiatives such as GYTS, GATS, and STEPS. Yet research on tobacco continues to be underfunded throughout the world.

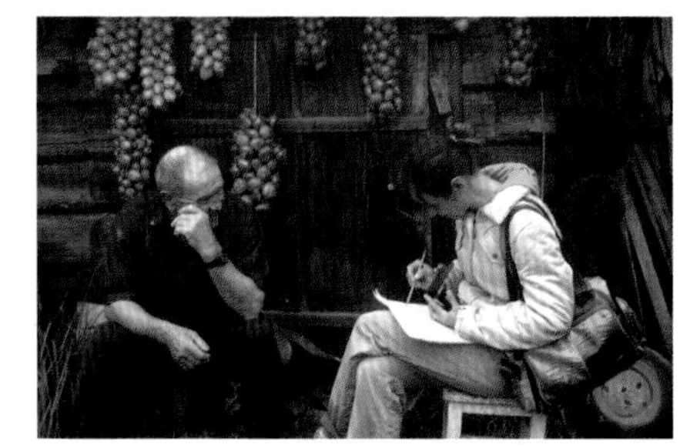

CORE FUNDING FOR THE DEVELOPMENT AND IMPLEMENTATION OF PUBLIC HEALTH POLICY MUST COME FROM GOVERNMENTS THEMSELVES. In addition to academic research, various philanthropic organizations have funded policy-oriented research and tobacco control projects. As of press time, Bloomberg Philanthropies has funded many projects in more than 40 countries. Philanthropist Michael Bloomberg and the Bill & Melinda Gates Foundation's commitment of $500 million over seven years (2006–2013) more than triples the available resources to control tobacco in low- and middle-income countries.

The UN High-Level Meeting on noncommunicable diseases in 2011 offered a unique opportunity to move tobacco forward strategically in the framework of other NCD issues, such as cancer, diabetes, heart disease, chronic lung disease, physical activity, alcohol, and unhealthy diets (see Chapter 22 – *Rights and Treaties*).

Field worker administers the Global Adult Tobacco Survey, Russia, 2009.

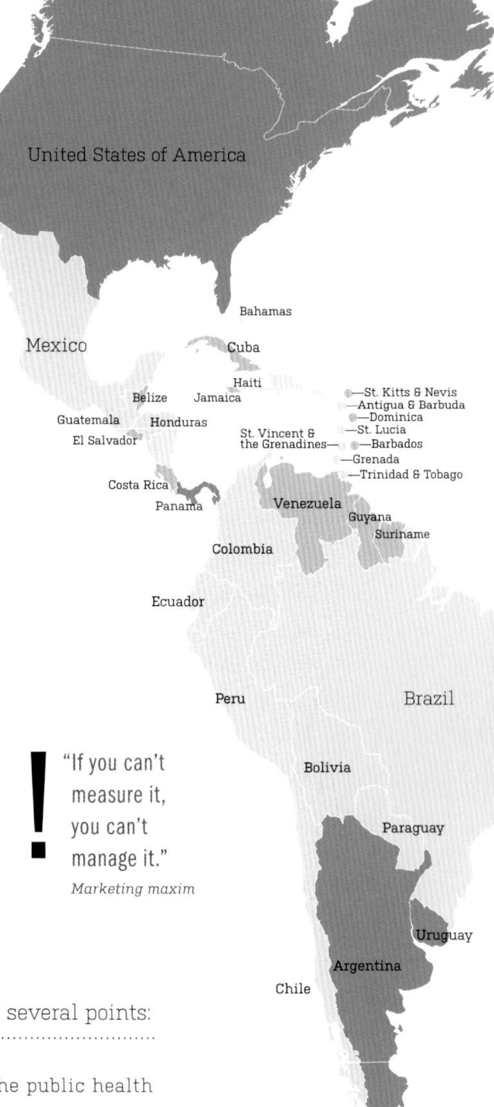

! “If you can't measure it, you can't manage it.”
Marketing maxim

Public Health Strategy

To mobilize public action on priority health issues, those involved with the process must identify several points:

The problem and the scale of the problem. Monitoring and surveillance, including prevalence, health, economic impact, actions taken, experience, and lessons learned from other countries.

The public health objectives, and how these should be framed.

The key decision makers, to whom they answer, if they can be influenced, and how.

Groups or individuals to be involved (inside and outside government) and how these may be most effectively used; whether there should be a coalition and how it could be managed; whether anyone should not be included; what roles are assigned to the leaders; what budget is required; and who should oversee it.

Obstacles to the public health objectives and how to overcome or circumvent them.

Strengths and weaknesses of **the opposition's position** and how to respond to it.

Media advocacy objectives.

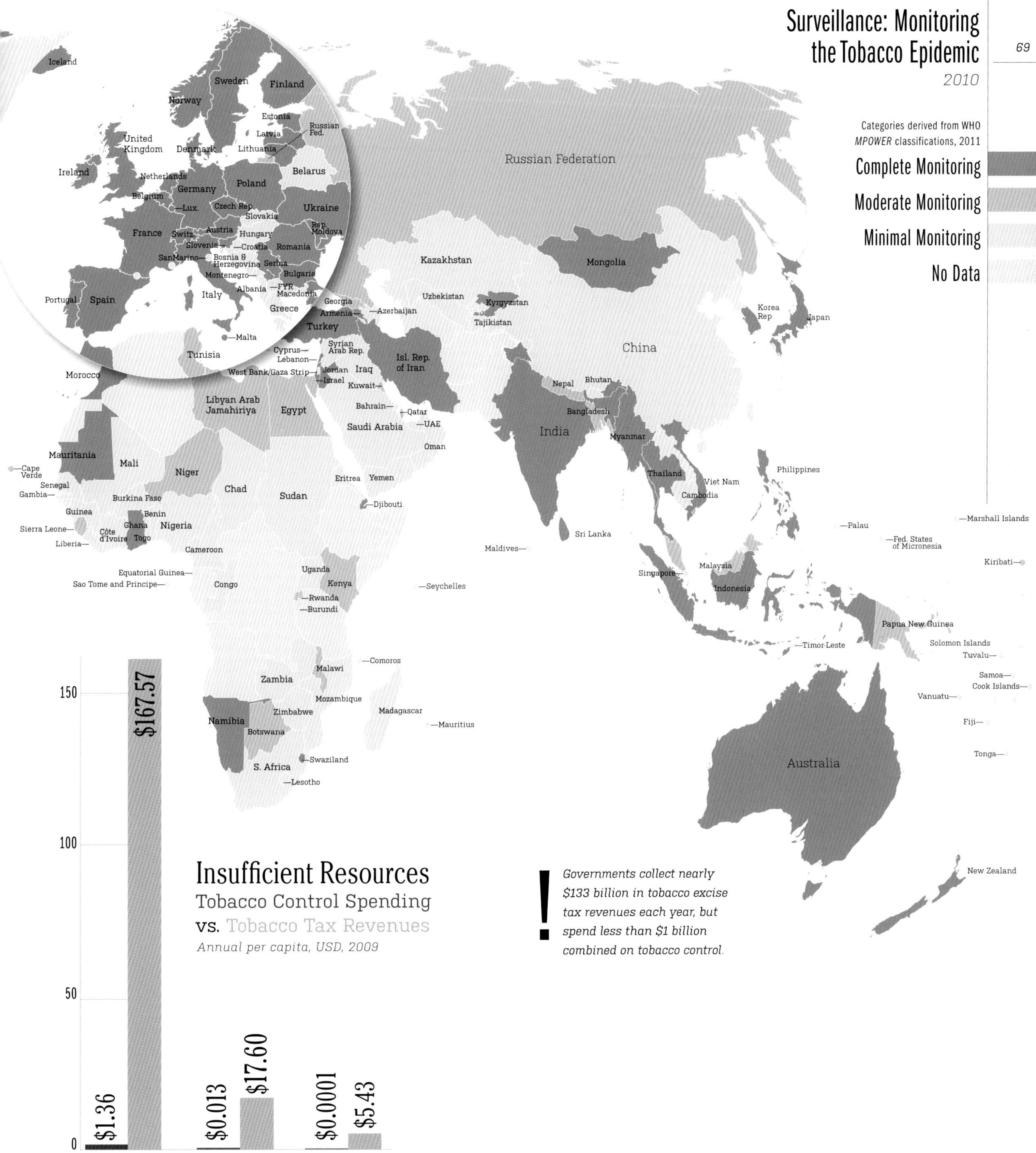
Surveillance: Monitoring the Tobacco Epidemic
2010
Categories derived from WHO MPOWER classifications, 2011
Complete Monitoring
Moderate Monitoring
Minimal Monitoring
No Data
Iceland
Sweden
Finland
Norway
Estonia
Latvia
Russian Fed.
United Kingdom
Denmark
Lithuania
Ireland
Belarus
Netherlands
Germany
Poland
Belgium
Lux.
Czech Rep.
Slovakia
Ukraine
France
Switz.
Austria
Hungary
Rep. Moldova
Slovenia
Croatia
Romania
San Marino
Bosnia & Herzegovina
Serbia
Montenegro
Bulgaria
Albania
FYR Macedonia
Portugal
Spain
Italy
Greece
Georgia
Armenia
Azerbaijan
Turkey
Malta
Tunisia
Cyprus
Lebanon
Syrian Arab Rep.
Morocco
West Bank/Gaza Strip
Jordan
Israel
Iraq
Isl. Rep. of Iran
Kuwait
Libyan Arab Jamahiriya
Egypt
Bahrain
Qatar
UAE
Saudi Arabia
Oman
Russian Federation
Kazakhstan
Mongolia
Uzbekistan
Kyrgyzstan
Tajikistan
Korea Rep
Japan
China
Nepal
Bhutan
Bangladesh
India
Myanmar
Thailand
Viet Nam
Cambodia
Philippines
Sri Lanka
Maldives
Palau
Marshall Islands
Fed. States of Micronesia
Kiribati
Singapore
Malaysia
Indonesia
Papua New Guinea
Timor-Leste
Solomon Islands
Tuvalu
Samoa
Cook Islands
Vanuatu
Fiji
Tonga
Australia
New Zealand
Mauritania
Mali
Niger
Cape Verde
Senegal
Gambia
Chad
Sudan
Eritrea
Yemen
Burkina Faso
Djibouti
Guinea
Benin
Sierra Leone
Ghana
Nigeria
Côte d'Ivoire
Togo
Liberia
Cameroon
Equatorial Guinea
Sao Tome and Principe
Congo
Uganda
Kenya
Rwanda
Burundi
Seychelles
Comoros
Malawi
Zambia
Mozambique
Madagascar
Namibia
Zimbabwe
Botswana
Mauritius
Swaziland
S. Africa
Lesotho
Insufficient Resources
Tobacco Control Spending vs. Tobacco Tax Revenues
Annual per capita, USD, 2009
150
100
50
0
$1.36
$167.57
$0.013
$17.60
$0.0001
$5.43
High-Income Countries
Middle-Income Countries
Low-Income Countries
!
Governments collect nearly $133 billion in tobacco excise tax revenues each year, but spend less than $1 billion combined on tobacco control.

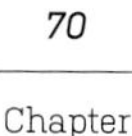

THE PUBLIC SAYS:

> “A few weeks before the [smoking] ban came into force in Ireland, Dublin banker Jimmy Fogarty asked the barman at his local pub: ‘What are you going to do when the ban comes in?’ ‘Breathe,’ the barman replied.”
>
> *Bulletin of the World Health Organization, Ireland, 2006*

BECAUSE THERE IS NO SAFE LEVEL OF EXPOSURE TO SECONDHAND SMOKE, SMOKE-FREE AREAS ARE THE ONLY WAY TO COMPLETELY PROTECT NONSMOKERS FROM THE HARM OF SECONDHAND SMOKE. When smoke-free areas are created, levels of smoke exposure are more than 90% lower than they are where smoking is permitted. When indoor smoking areas are allowed, ventilation is inadequate to eliminate secondhand smoke, and the reduction in smoking among smokers is less.

A 2010 Cochrane literature review assessed 31 studies measuring exposure to secondhand smoke after smoking bans, with 19 studies including biomarkers. The review concluded there is "CONSISTENT EVIDENCE THAT SMOKING BANS REDUCED EXPOSURE TO SECONDHAND SMOKE IN WORKPLACES, RESTAURANTS, PUBS, AND PUBLIC PLACES."

Some countries have now banned smoking in outdoor areas, such as those of restaurants and bars, and in beaches, parks, and campuses, on the rationale that smoking may expose workers, nonsmokers, patrons, and children to significant levels of secondhand smoke and readily preventable risks to health.

Public support is high for smoking bans in public places, including crowded outdoor areas. In regions where smoking bans have been mandated by law, employees, customers, and business owners report high compliance and satisfaction with the results, and compliance with smoke-free regulations increases over time. Independent studies consistently show no drop in employment or tax receipts.

Smoking bans, relatively inexpensive to implement, can produce immediate economic benefits to employers in the form of reduced accidental fire risk, lower insurance premiums, higher productivity, and less employee absenteeism.

Current challenges are how to decrease smoking in the home, and how to regulate smoking in multifamily homes and in vehicles with small children.

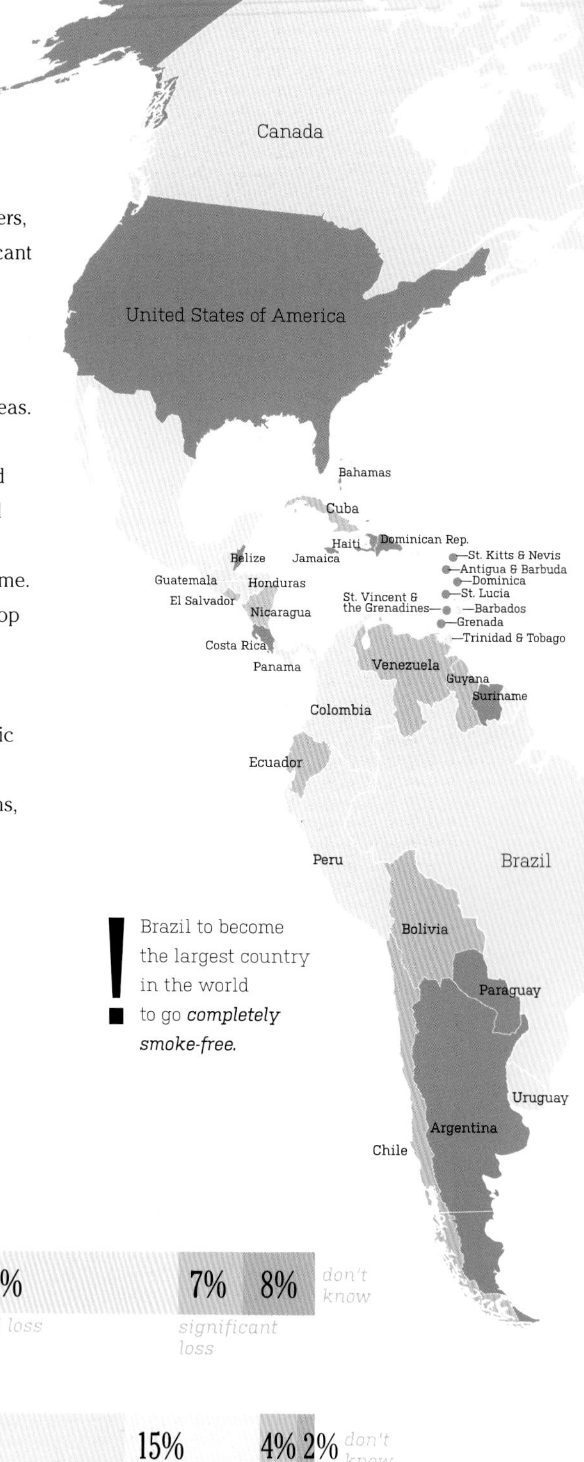

! Brazil to become the largest country in the world to go *completely smoke-free.*

Smoke-Free Policies Tend to Be Received Positively One Year Post-Ban

Impact, as reported by restaurant and bar owners, Italy, 2007

Changes in Revenue

61% gain/no effect · 24% mild loss · 7% significant loss · 8% don't know

Patron Opinion About the Law

79% positive · 15% neutral · 4% negative · 2% don't know

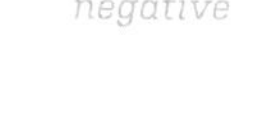

Owner Opinion About the Law

88% positive · 8% neutral · 4% negative

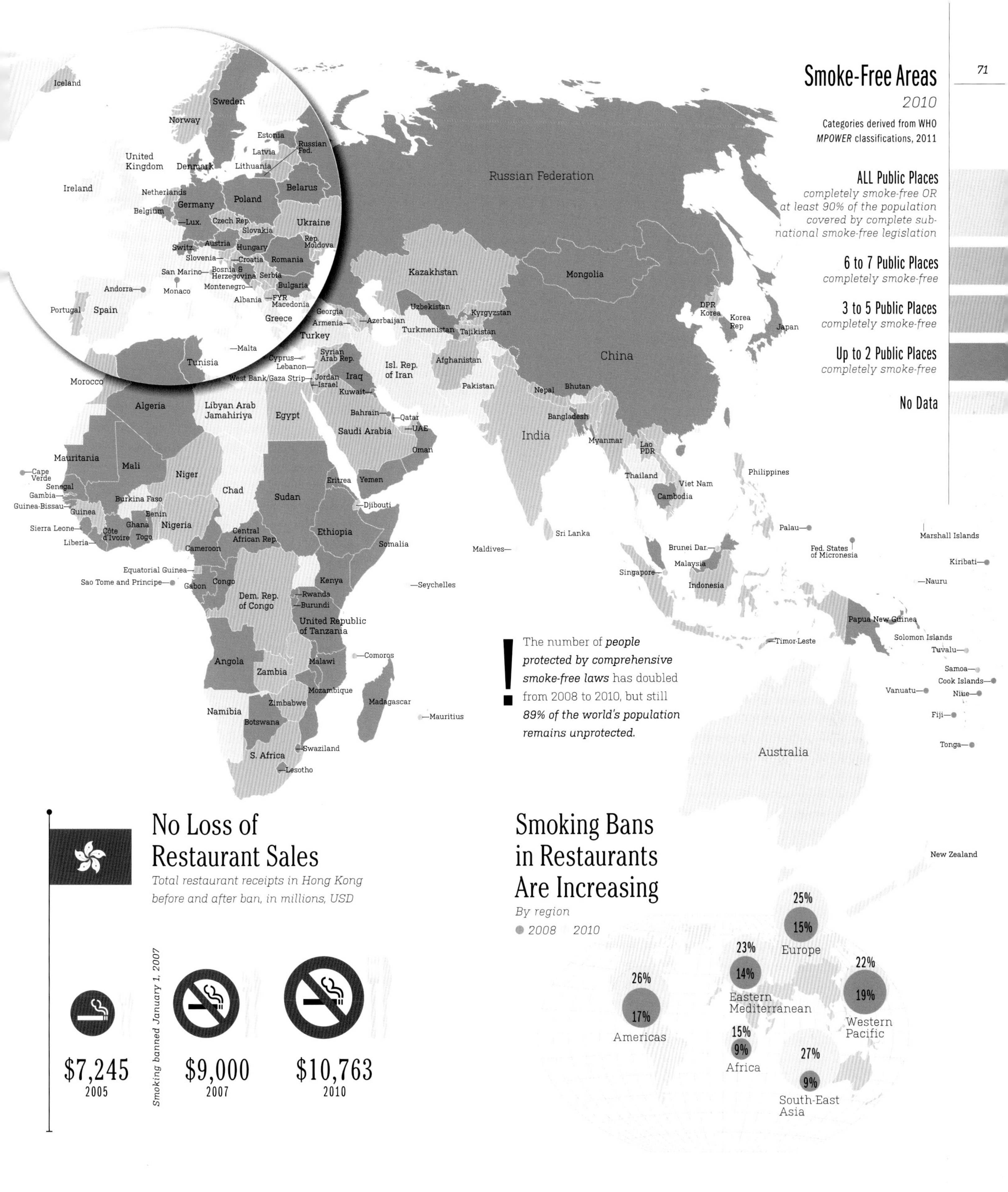
Smoke-Free Areas
2010
Categories derived from WHO MPOWER classifications, 2011
ALL Public Places
completely smoke-free OR at least 90% of the population covered by complete sub-national smoke-free legislation
6 to 7 Public Places
completely smoke-free
3 to 5 Public Places
completely smoke-free
Up to 2 Public Places
completely smoke-free
No Data
Iceland
Sweden
Norway
Estonia
Russian Fed.
Latvia
United Kingdom
Denmark
Lithuania
Ireland
Netherlands
Germany
Poland
Belarus
Belgium
Lux.
Czech Rep.
Slovakia
Ukraine
Rep. Moldova
Switz.
Austria
Hungary
Slovenia
Croatia
Romania
San Marino
Bosnia & Herzegovina
Serbia
Andorra
Monaco
Montenegro
Bulgaria
Albania
FYR Macedonia
Portugal
Spain
Greece
Georgia
Armenia
Azerbaijan
Turkey
Malta
Tunisia
Cyprus
Lebanon
Syrian Arab Rep.
West Bank/Gaza Strip
Jordan
Israel
Iraq
Kuwait
Isl. Rep. of Iran
Morocco
Algeria
Libyan Arab Jamahiriya
Egypt
Bahrain
Qatar
UAE
Saudi Arabia
Oman
Russian Federation
Kazakhstan
Mongolia
Uzbekistan
Kyrgyzstan
Turkmenistan
Tajikistan
Afghanistan
Pakistan
China
DPR Korea
Korea Rep
Japan
Nepal
Bhutan
Bangladesh
India
Myanmar
Lao PDR
Thailand
Viet Nam
Cambodia
Philippines
Mauritania
Mali
Niger
Cape Verde
Senegal
Gambia
Guinea-Bissau
Guinea
Burkina Faso
Chad
Sudan
Eritrea
Yemen
Djibouti
Benin
Sierra Leone
Ghana
Nigeria
Côte d'Ivoire
Togo
Liberia
Central African Rep.
Ethiopia
Somalia
Cameroon
Equatorial Guinea
Sao Tome and Principe
Gabon
Congo
Kenya
Dem. Rep. of Congo
Rwanda
Burundi
United Republic of Tanzania
Seychelles
Maldives
Sri Lanka
Palau
Marshall Islands
Fed. States of Micronesia
Kiribati
Nauru
Brunei Dar.
Malaysia
Singapore
Indonesia
Papua New Guinea
Solomon Islands
Tuvalu
Timor-Leste
Comoros
Angola
Malawi
Zambia
Mozambique
Madagascar
Zimbabwe
Namibia
Botswana
Mauritius
Swaziland
S. Africa
Lesotho
Australia
Samoa
Cook Islands
Vanuatu
Niue
Fiji
Tonga
New Zealand
The number of people protected by comprehensive smoke-free laws has doubled from 2008 to 2010, but still 89% of the world's population remains unprotected.
No Loss of Restaurant Sales
Total restaurant receipts in Hong Kong before and after ban, in millions, USD
Smoking banned January 1, 2007
$7,245
2005
$9,000
2007
$10,763
2010
Smoking Bans in Restaurants Are Increasing
By region
2008 2010
25%
15%
Europe
23%
14%
Eastern Mediterranean
22%
19%
Western Pacific
26%
17%
Americas
15%
9%
Africa
27%
9%
South-East Asia

RESEARCH SAYS:

“States can reduce death and disease by reducing smoking prevalence. It’s that simple.”

Gary Giovino, University of Buffalo, US, 2009

Quit Attempts

Percent of current smokers who have ever tried to quit, 2010

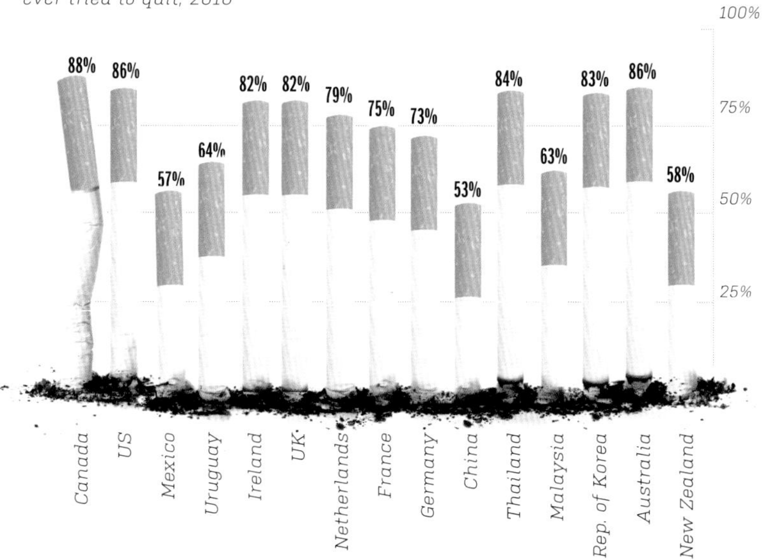

! A 2000 survey in Kuwait of 4,000 participants found 47% of all smokers stated that they wanted to stop smoking, and about 56% had attempted to quit. ***The biggest perceived barrier to quitting was uncertainty about "how to quit."***

There are only two ways to reduce tobacco use: prevent youth from starting to use tobacco and encourage and help users to quit. TO MAKE A SIGNIFICANT REDUCTION IN GLOBAL TOBACCO-RELATED DEATHS, CURRENT SMOKERS MUST QUIT. UNLESS THEY DO, TOBACCO DEATHS WILL RISE DRAMATICALLY OVER THE NEXT 40 YEARS, IRRESPECTIVE OF WHETHER YOUTH UPTAKE IS REDUCED.

Some improvement of health is seen soon after quitting, and much of the harm can be eliminated over time, even for lifelong smokers.

General tobacco control policies, such as disseminating health information, mandating smoke-free areas, and implementing tax increases, can encourage smokers to quit. Most ex-smokers quit successfully on their own ("cold turkey"), but an increasing number of programs and aids are available to help smokers stop, some more effective than others. Nicotine replacement therapies (gum, patch, and inhaler) and pharmacologic agents such as bupropion, varenicline, and newer agents such as cystisine are now available in many countries. Some jurisdictions, such as Hong Kong, have even introduced quitting services for teens. Many people change their health behaviors easily, while others struggle through a difficult cycle of addiction.

Communication technologies—such as telephone quit lines, text messaging, online counseling, and social media—offer support. Psychological and behavioral therapies, particularly behavior modification, but also less-tested modalities such as hypnosis, meditation, and acupuncture, also have been employed.

Canada
United States of America
Mexico
Bahamas
Cuba
Dominican Rep.
Haiti
Jamaica
Belize
Guatemala
Honduras
El Salvador
Nicaragua
Costa Rica
Panama
St. Kitts & Nevis
Antigua & Barbuda
Dominica
St. Lucia
St. Vincent & the Grenadines
Barbados
Grenada
Trinidad & Tobago
Venezuela
Guyana
Suriname
Colombia
Ecuador
Peru
Brazil
Bolivia
Paraguay
Chile
Uruguay
Argentina

Quitting Calendar
The Benefits of Stopping Smoking

1 week later
Heart, blood pressure, circulation, breathing show improvement
1 year later
Excess risk of coronary heart disease is half th
of a continuing smoker

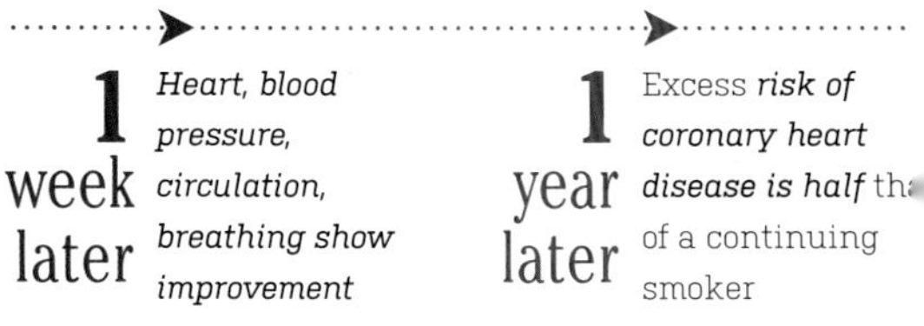

Quitting Resources Available by Country

2010

Categories derived from WHO *MPOWER* classifications, 2011

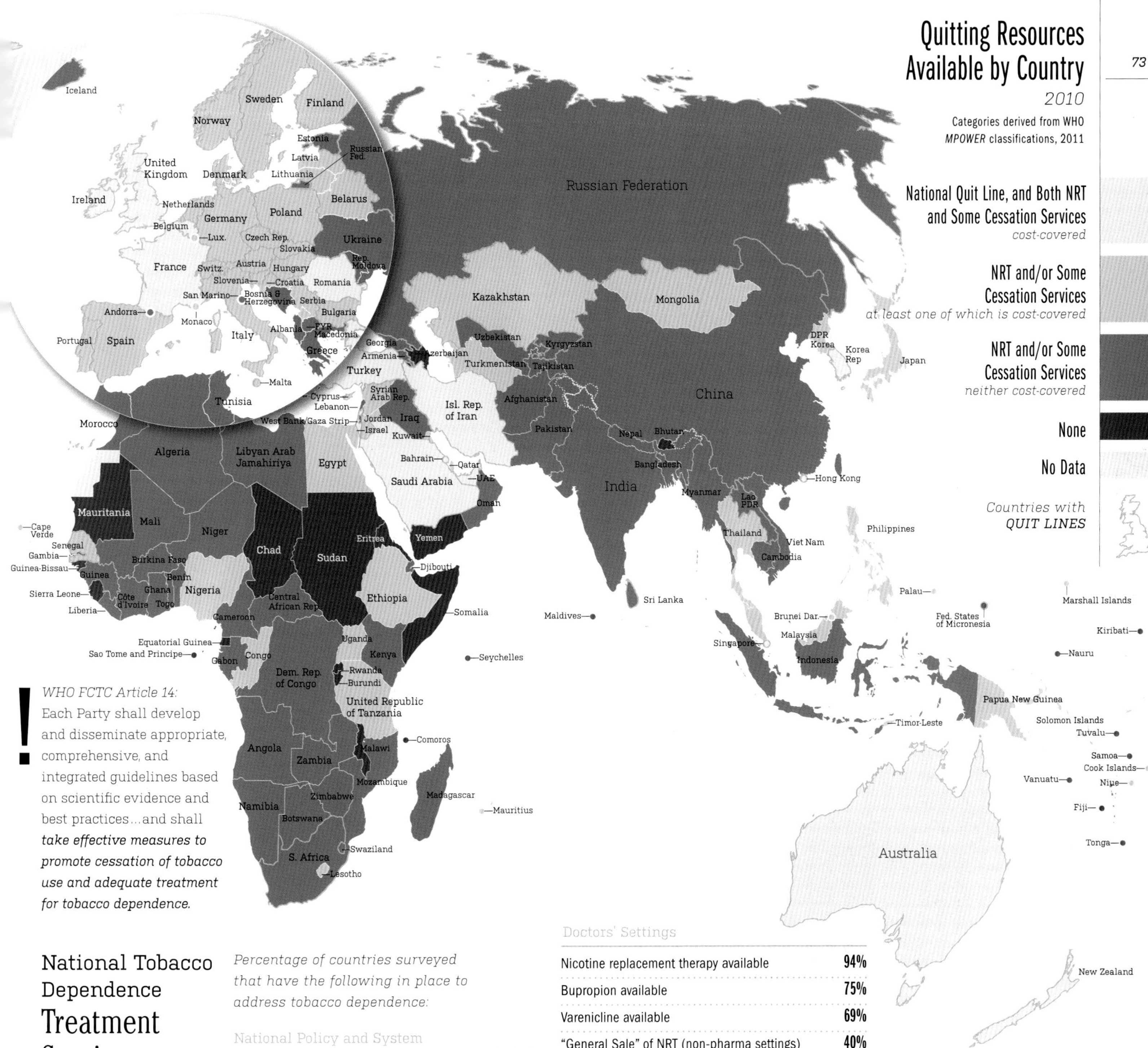

! *WHO FCTC Article 14:* Each Party shall develop and disseminate appropriate, comprehensive, and integrated guidelines based on scientific evidence and best practices…and shall ***take effective measures to promote cessation of tobacco use and adequate treatment for tobacco dependence.***

National Tobacco Dependence Treatment Services

36 sampled countries, 2007

Percentage of countries surveyed that have the following in place to address tobacco dependence:

National Policy and System	
Official written policy on treatment	44%
Specialized national treatment system	19%
Help easily available in general-practice settings	24%

Doctors' Settings	
Nicotine replacement therapy available	94%
Bupropion available	75%
Varenicline available	69%
"General Sale" of NRT (non-pharma settings)	40%
Fully reimbursed brief quitting advice	45%
Fully reimbursed intensive specialist support	29%
Mandatory recording of patients' smoking status in medical notes	31%

5-15 years later — *Risk of a stroke is **reduced*** to that of never-smokers

10 years later — *Risk of lung cancer is **reduced*** to less than half that of continuing smokers; risk of many other cancers decrease

15 years later — *Risk of coronary heart disease is **similar to that of never-smokers**,* and the overall risk of death is almost the same, especially if the smoker quits before illness develops

RESEARCH SAYS:

“Mass-media campaigns about the harms of tobacco can induce quitting and prevent young people from taking up the habit, especially if implemented as part of a comprehensive tobacco-control program.”

Sandra Mullin, World Lung Foundation, US, 2011

Legislative and tax interventions for tobacco control are unlikely to reduce smoking rates without public awareness and support. Mass communication, health education, and reliable information are essential elements for tobacco control success. SUSTAINED USE OF MASS MEDIA CAMPAIGNS CONTRIBUTES TO POPULATION-LEVEL DECREASES IN SMOKING PREVALENCE BY INCREASING KNOWLEDGE ABOUT THE HARM OF TOBACCO USE, ENCOURAGING QUIT ATTEMPTS, AND IMPROVING QUIT RATES.

Funding for mass media campaigns is often cited as a barrier, yet mass media is a cost-efficient way to reduce smoking, because it reaches large segments of the population. Countries can save time and resources by adapting campaigns that have performed well in other jurisdictions for use in their own, subject to appropriate local pretesting. Of the 23 countries reporting at least one best-practice campaign, 16 were low- or middle-income, suggesting that mass media need not be a tool of only high-income countries.

Public education is a core provision of the WHO Framework Convention on Tobacco Control. Yet, as shown by the WHO Report on the Global Tobacco Epidemic 2011, most countries should be doing more to inform their citizens adequately about the illnesses and deaths caused by tobacco. In nearly 150 countries surveyed, including 110 low- and middle-income countries, there is a paucity of anti-tobacco public education via mass media.

The scale of the tobacco epidemic warrants that governments give priority to implementing strong and effective campaigns.

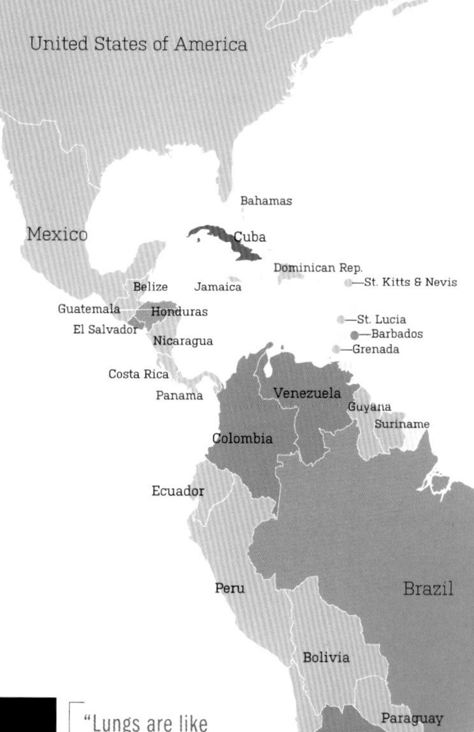

Ads With Visceral Images Are the Most Effective

! *TV is the preferred medium for anti-tobacco advertising,* but in low-income countries, where TV has minimal coverage, radio is an alternative, albeit less effective option.

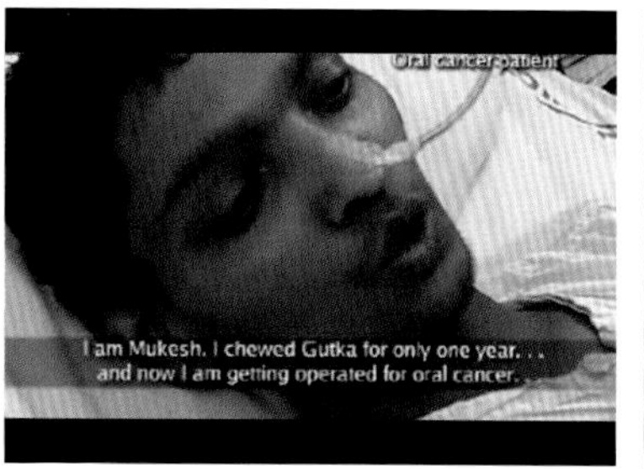

Mukesh, India, 2009

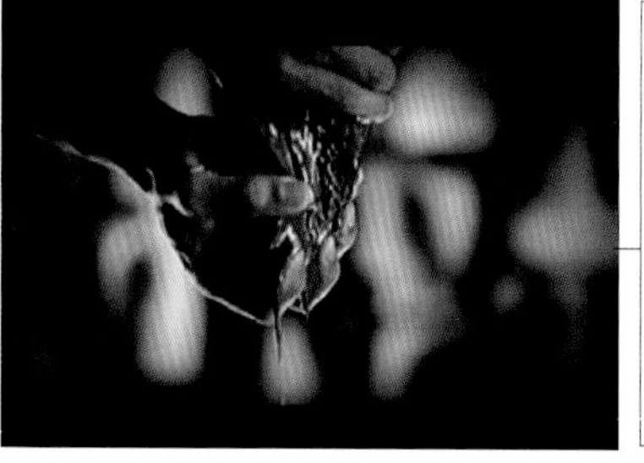

Sponge, Produced by Cancer Institute, New South Wales, Australia

“Lungs are like sponges. If you could wring out the cancer-producing tar that goes into the lungs of a pack-a-day smoker every year, this is how much you would get.”

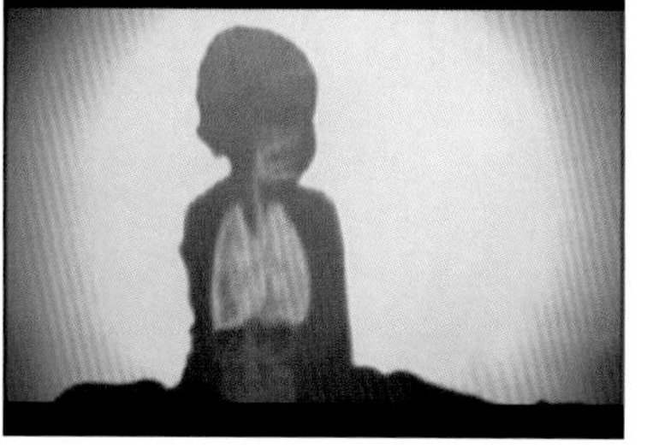

Cigarettes Are Eating Your Baby Alive, US and Various Countries

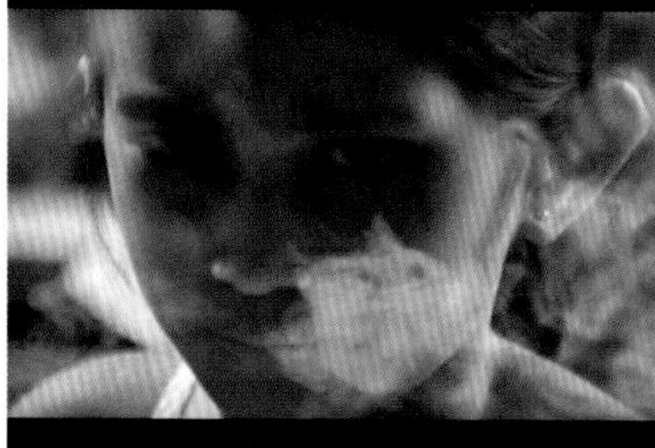

Say No to Secondhand Smoke, Philippines, 2009

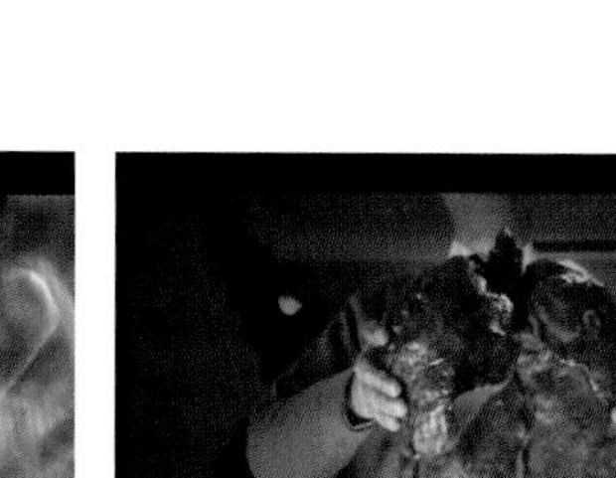

Gift-Giving, China, 2009

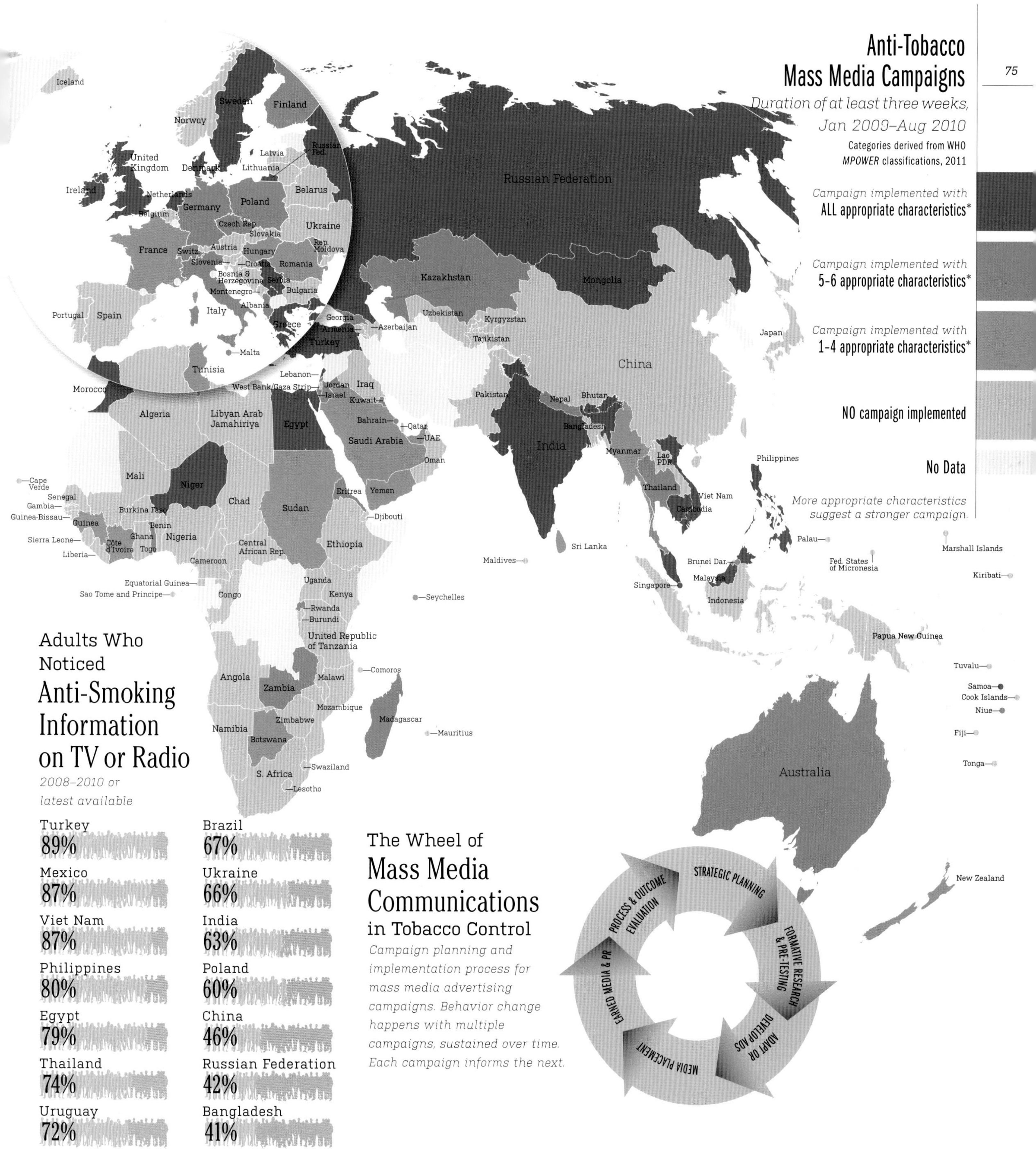

Information was noticed in the 30 days prior to the survey.

*APPROPRIATE CHARACTERISTICS are based on whether the campaign was part of a comprehensive tobacco control program; whether research informed an understanding of the target audience; and whether materials were pretested; as well as how the campaign was promoted, placed, and publicized; and the extent to which campaigns were evaluated.

GOVERNMENT SAYS:

"Plain packaging means that the glamour is gone from smoking."

Nicola Roxon, Former Minister of Health and Ageing, Australia, 2011

Health warnings on the packaging of all tobacco products have progressed from simple, small, weak text warnings 30 years ago to strong, graphic warnings introduced by Canada in 2001. **CURRENTLY, PICTORIAL WARNINGS HAVE BEEN ADOPTED BY ABOUT ONE-QUARTER OF COUNTRIES, WITH SEVERAL IN THEIR SECOND ROUND OF SUCH WARNINGS.**

Health messages on cigarette packaging deliver important information directly to smokers. The message is repeated and reinforced every time a smoker reaches for a cigarette.

In one of its strongest provisions, Article 11 of the World Health Organization Framework Convention on Tobacco Control compels Parties, within three years of becoming a Party, to require tobacco product health warnings that cover at least 30%, and preferably 50%, of the visible area on a cigarette pack. Warnings should be extended to all forms of smoking and smokeless tobacco.

In 2012, plain packaging—specifically, the standardization of cigarette packaging that removes all product advertising including colors, logos, and brand imagery, and enforces restrictions on font size and type—is a major battleground between the industry and governments.

Australia was the first country to adopt legislation to require plain packaging, and did so in the face of bitter opposition from the tobacco industry, including legal threats.

Action on Smoking and Health UK, a tobacco control advocacy group, explained, "Of all the laws on tobacco control, there are few the tobacco industry fears more than plain or standardized packaging. Even where tobacco advertising is banned, the pack is the tobacco's silent salesman, calling out from retailers' shelves and displayed by smokers 20 times a day. The ad men don't simply use the pack to tell us which brand is for women and which for men, or which brands are youthful and which are sophisticated. They can also use them to send out misleading, illegal signals giving the impression that one is less harmful or less addictive than another."

THE INDUSTRY SAYS:

"BAT Australia is opposed to the introduction of plain packaging. It is unfair and unworkable and will inevitably bring with it significant unintended consequences."

David Crow, CEO, BAT Australia, 2011

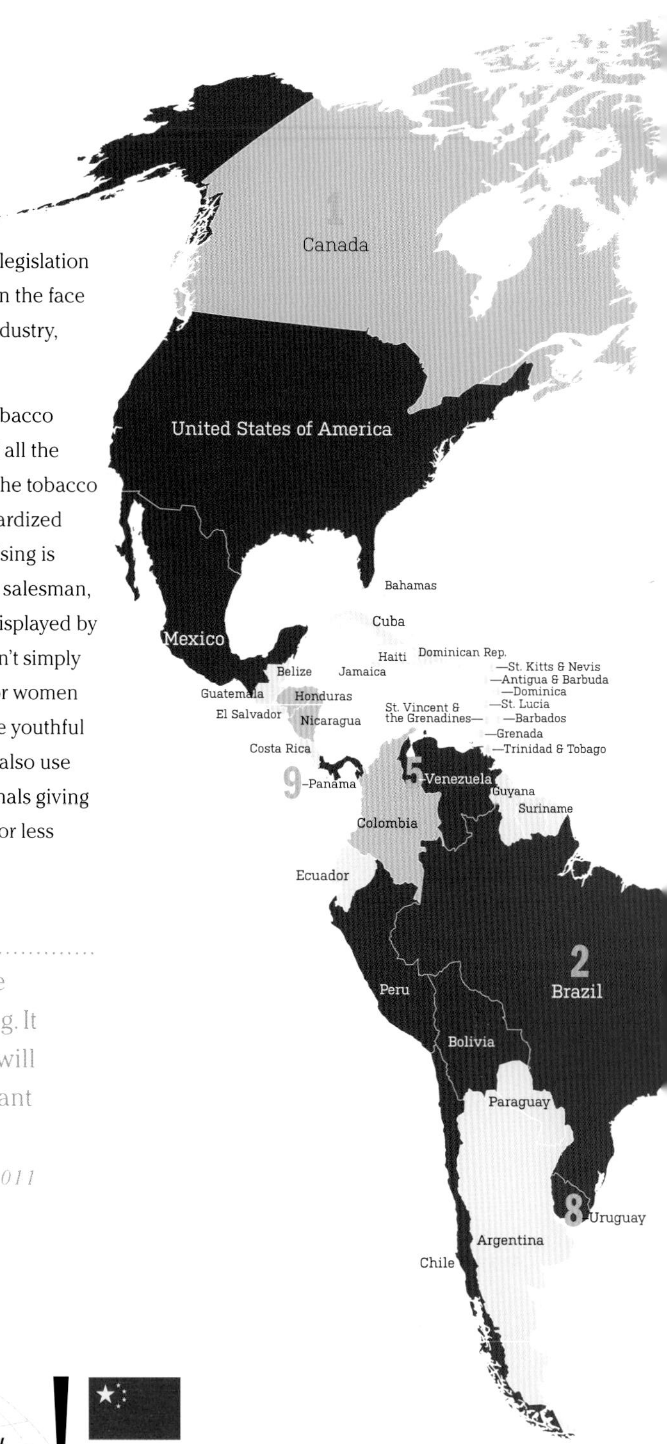

Canada
1
United States of America
Mexico
Bahamas
Cuba
Haiti
Dominican Rep.
Belize
Jamaica
Guatemala
Honduras
El Salvador
Nicaragua
St. Vincent & the Grenadines
—St. Kitts & Nevis
—Antigua & Barbuda
—Dominica
—St. Lucia
—Barbados
—Grenada
—Trinidad & Tobago
Costa Rica
9
Panama
5
Venezuela
Guyana
Suriname
Colombia
Ecuador
Peru
2
Brazil
Bolivia
Paraguay
8
Uruguay
Argentina
Chile

Product Labeling Laws

Prohibition of the Use of "Light," "Mild," and Similar Misleading Descriptors

Percentage of countries by region, 2010

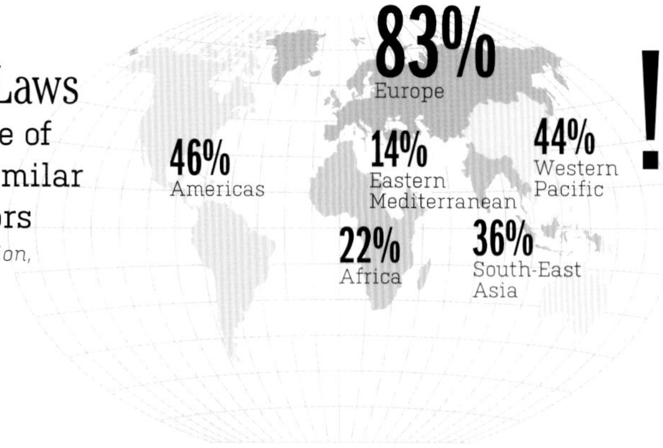

83% Europe
46% Americas
14% Eastern Mediterranean
44% Western Pacific
22% Africa
36% South-East Asia

!

In 2006 about 70% of Chinese smokers, irrespective of age, income, and education, ***believed "light"/"low tar" cigarettes are less harmful*** compared with "full flavor" cigarettes.

Package Warning Labels, Proposed and/or Implemented

2010

Categories derived from WHO *MPOWER* classifications, 2011

Large Warnings[1] *with all appropriate characteristics**

Medium Warnings[2] *with all appropriate characteristics* OR* **Large Warnings**[1] *missing some appropriate characteristics**

Medium Warnings[2] *missing some appropriate characteristics* OR* **Large Warnings**[1] *missing many appropriate characteristics**

No Warnings *OR* **Small Warnings**[3]

No Data

FIRST TEN COUNTRIES to require graphic health warnings

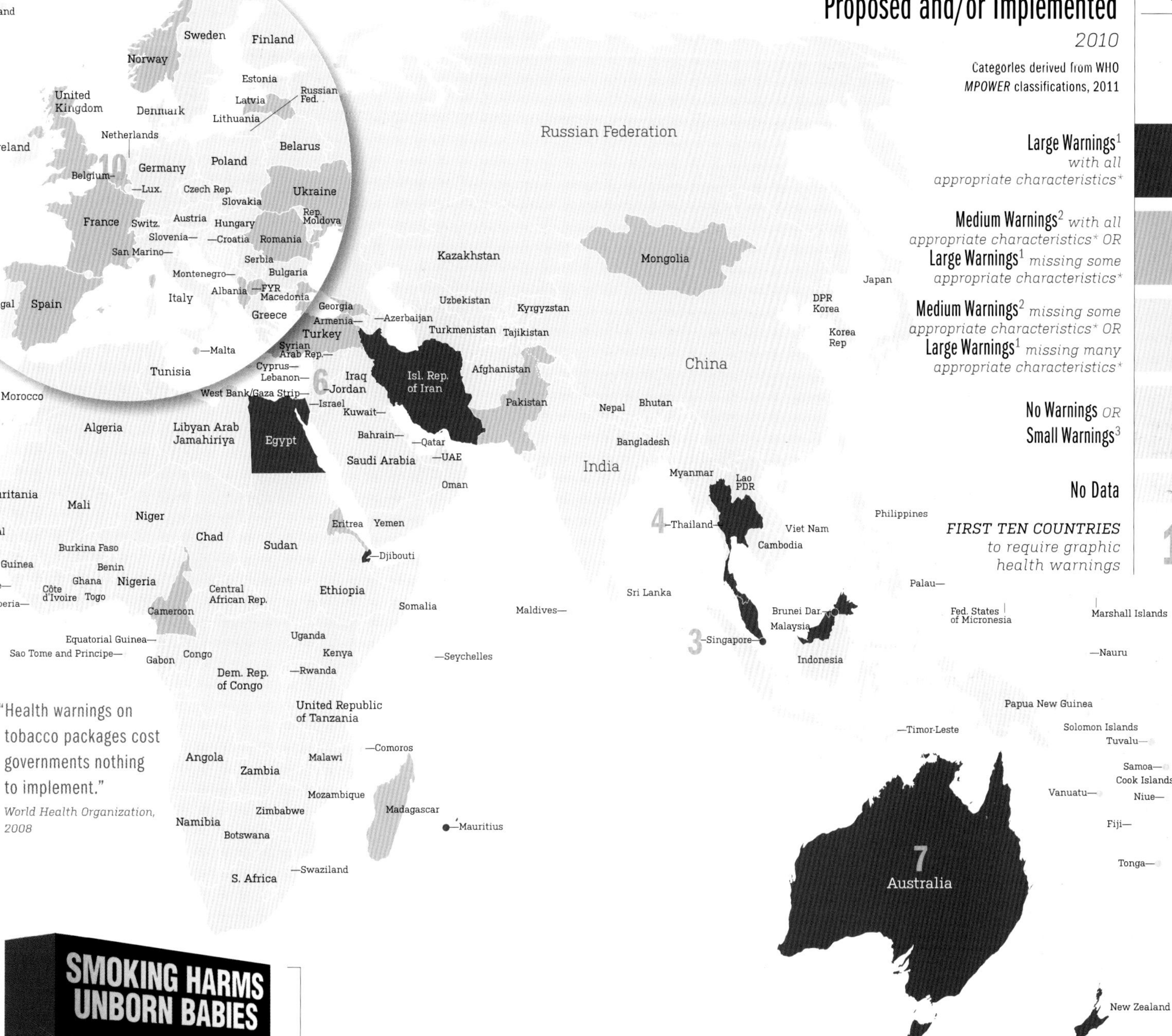

> **!** "Health warnings on tobacco packages cost governments nothing to implement."
>
> *World Health Organization, 2008*

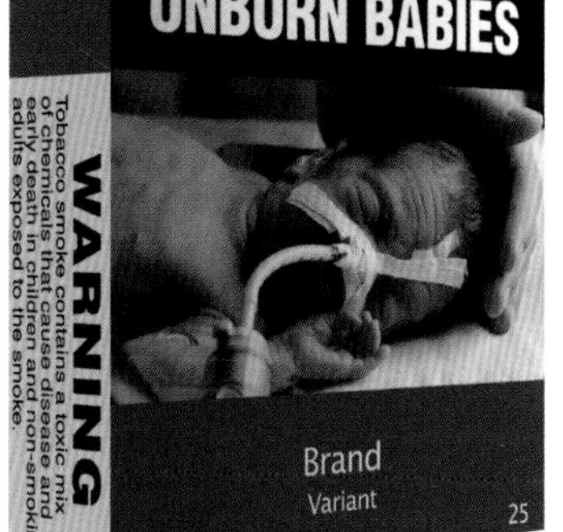

Example of Australian tobacco plain packaging as required by 2011 Australian law.
© Commonwealth of Australia

> **!** "Plain packaging of all tobacco products would remove a key remaining means for the industry to promote its products to billions of the world's smokers and future smokers."
>
> *Becky Freeman, Simon Chapman, and Matthew Rimmer, University of Sydney, Australia, 2008*

[1] LARGE WARNING = Average of front and back of the package is at least 50%. [2] MEDIUM WARNING = Average of front and back of package is between 30 and 49%. [3] SMALL WARNING = Average of front and back of package is less than 30%.
* APPROPRIATE CHARACTERISTICS are based on percentage of package covered; whether warnings are mandated; whether they appear on packets and external packaging; whether they describe specific harm; are large, clear, visible, and legible; rotate; are written in principal language of country; and include pictures.

LEGAL JUDGMENT SAYS:

“Defendants have marketed and sold their lethal products with zeal, with deception, with a single-minded focus on their financial success, and without regard for the human tragedy or social costs that success exacted.”

US District Judge Gladys Kessler, 2006

Over 60% of countries have imposed some restriction on tobacco marketing. ONLY COMPREHENSIVE BANS ON ALL FORMS OF TOBACCO ADVERTISING, MARKETING, SPONSORSHIP, AND PROMOTION ARE EFFECTIVE AT REDUCING POPULATION SMOKING RATES. Partial restrictions are ineffective in reducing smoking because tobacco companies redirect their marketing efforts to other available venues. Voluntary agreements are also inadequate because they are unenforceable.

In the face of broadening advertising bans, tobacco companies have become ever more creative in their attempts to lure new consumers into addiction. Use of new media, brand-stretching, event promotion, retailer incentives, sponsorship and advertising through international media, cross-border advertising, and promotional packaging are some of the ways that the tobacco industry circumvents the intent of advertising bans. An example of this is the SHANGHAI TOBACCO COMPANY, WHICH CREATED A BRAND CALLED "I LOVE CHINA." The slogan was then used on generic billboards and advertisements and may not be directly considered to be tobacco advertising.

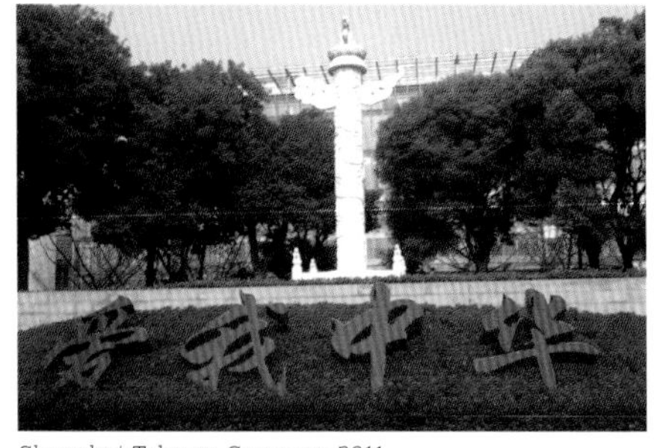

Shanghai Tobacco Company, 2011

Bans deny the tobacco industry one of its tools to recruit new tobacco users to replace those who have quit or died, to maintain or increase use among current users, to reduce tobacco users' willingness to quit, and to encourage former users to start using tobacco again.

Comprehensive bans protect youth from the onslaught of tobacco marketing in sports, music venues, the Internet, and elsewhere. Advertising bans also help reduce the social acceptability of smoking and tobacco use.

Parents can also do their part at the individual level by protecting children from exposure to depictions of smoking in various contexts, including in movies and television and online.

THE INDUSTRY SAYS:

“[Following advertising bans, marketing] evolved to a more focused, direct one-to-one approach. Philip Morris uses the database to target smokers for discount coupons and even chances to win a vacation in 'experiential programs.' The Marlboro brand is often associated with Marlboro Country, and the great outdoors and the West. We own a ranch, and Marlboro smokers can win an opportunity to visit that ranch and experience Marlboro Country.”

Bill Phelps, Altria, US, 2008

***PUBLIC STATEMENTS BY BIG TOBACCO** deny that their marketing targets youth or affects youth smoking incidence and initiation, despite overwhelming evidence to the contrary.*

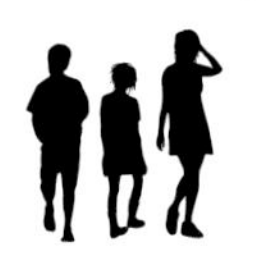

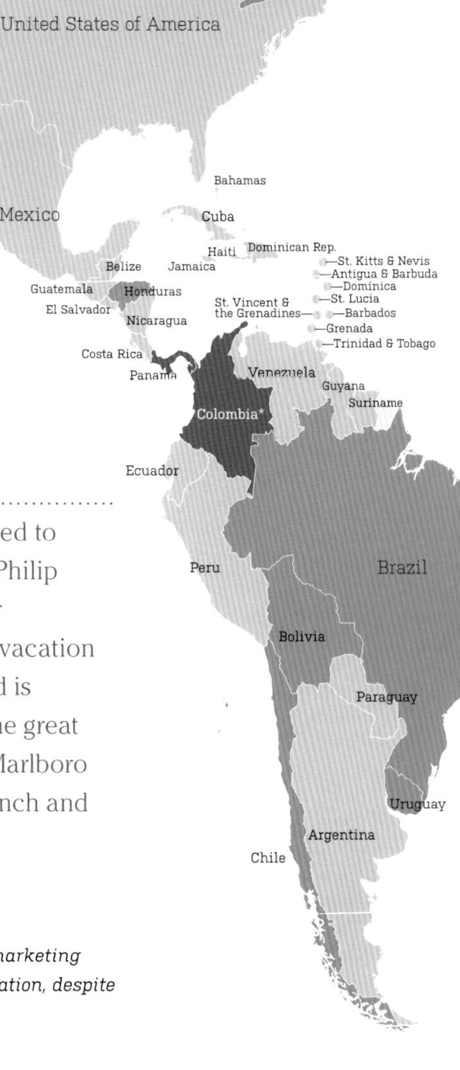

Excerpts From Marketing Findings Against the Tobacco Industry

Kessler trial summary, 2006

EXCERPTS

- Tobacco marketing is a substantial contributing factor to youth smoking initiation.
- Tobacco marketing employs themes that resonate with youth and successfully reach youth.
- The industry has continually increased its investment in marketing.
- The industry markets to youth through direct mail and an array of retail promotions and other means that attract youth.
- Industry-sponsored Youth Smoking Prevention Programs are not designed to effectively prevent youth smoking.

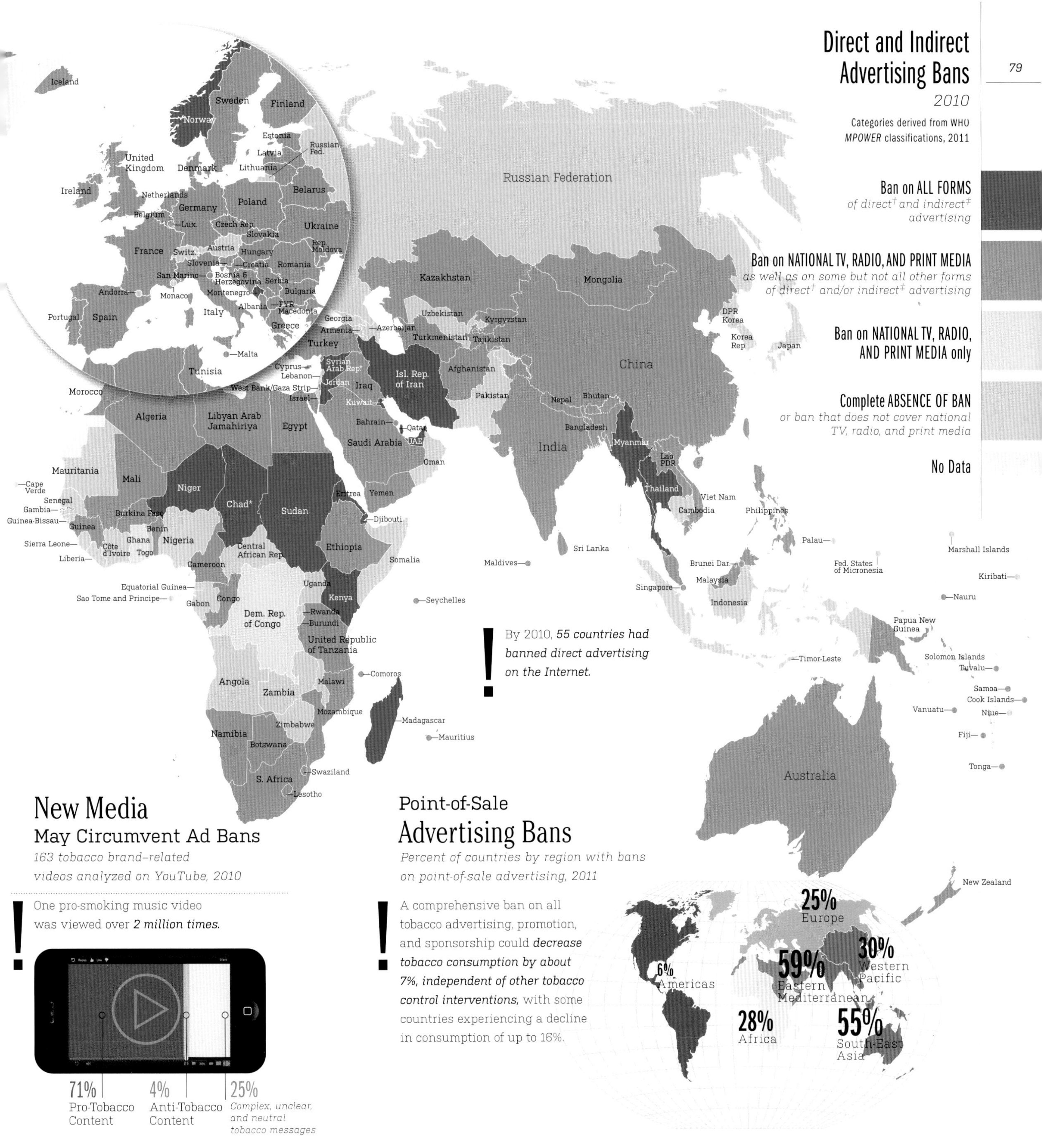

† DIRECT ADVERTISING includes television, radio, magazine, direct mail, email, telemarketing, coupons, sweepstakes, brand loyalty programs, and other methods to promote tobacco products directly to consumers. ‡ INDIRECT ADVERTISING uses brand names, trade names, trademarks, emblems, etc., to indirectly promote tobacco products through "brand stretching" (where tobacco brand names are used as part of other product names), event sponsorships, product placement in television and films, and other methods.

*Between 2008 and 2010, three additional countries—Chad, Colombia, and Syria—banned tobacco advertising, promotion, and sponsorship.

FUNDERS SAY:

“Among the revenue proposals I have examined, tobacco taxes are especially attractive because they encourage smokers to quit and discourage people from starting to smoke, as well as generate significant revenues. It's a win-win for global health.”

Bill Gates, G20 Summit, France, 2011

Cigarette Consumption Goes Down
as Tobacco Taxes Go Up

Real (inflation-adjusted) price of a pack of cigarettes in 1990 Shekels (NIS) in Israel. Increases in cigarette prices were driven by tax increases.

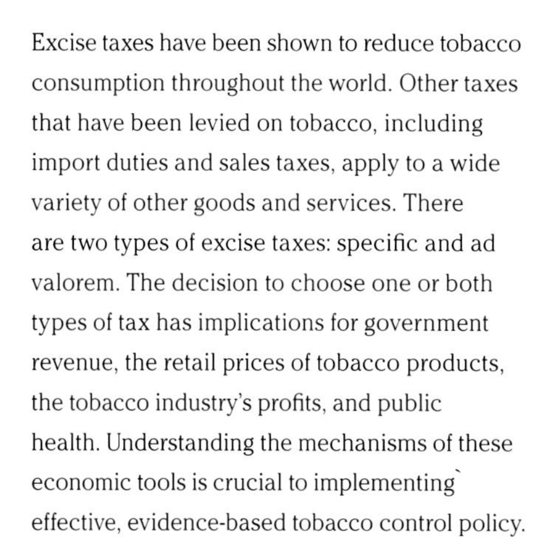

When administered correctly, tobacco tax increases are among the most effective and important tobacco control policies. INCREASES IN TOBACCO TAXES THAT LEAD TO HIGHER CIGARETTE PRICES ENCOURAGE SMOKERS TO QUIT, INCREASE SUCCESSFUL QUIT ATTEMPTS, REDUCE THE NUMBER OF CIGARETTES SMOKED PER PERSON, AND PREVENT INITIATION AMONG YOUTH. A 10% increase in cigarette prices reduces cigarette demand by 2–6% in high-income countries and by 2–8% in low- and middle-income countries. Youth, minorities, and low-income smokers are more likely than others to quit or smoke less in response to cigarette price increases. Because cigarette prices influence youth smoking initiation, increases in price significantly reduce long-term trends in cigarette consumption.

In addition to reducing cigarette consumption, higher tobacco taxes increase tax revenues, which can be used to implement and enforce tobacco control measures or to pay for tobacco-related health-care services or other social programs. On the other hand, tax cuts allow the industry to raise their profit margins.

Excise taxes have been shown to reduce tobacco consumption throughout the world. Other taxes that have been levied on tobacco, including import duties and sales taxes, apply to a wide variety of other goods and services. There are two types of excise taxes: specific and ad valorem. The decision to choose one or both types of tax has implications for government revenue, the retail prices of tobacco products, the tobacco industry's profits, and public health. Understanding the mechanisms of these economic tools is crucial to implementing effective, evidence-based tobacco control policy.

The WHO Framework Convention on Tobacco Control obligates signatories to adopt tax and price policies that reduce tobacco consumption. Furthermore, the World Health Organization recommends that AT LEAST 70% OF THE RETAIL PRICE OF TOBACCO PRODUCTS COMES FROM EXCISE TAXES. ONLY FIVE NATIONS HAVE ACHIEVED THIS BEST-PRACTICE STANDARD.

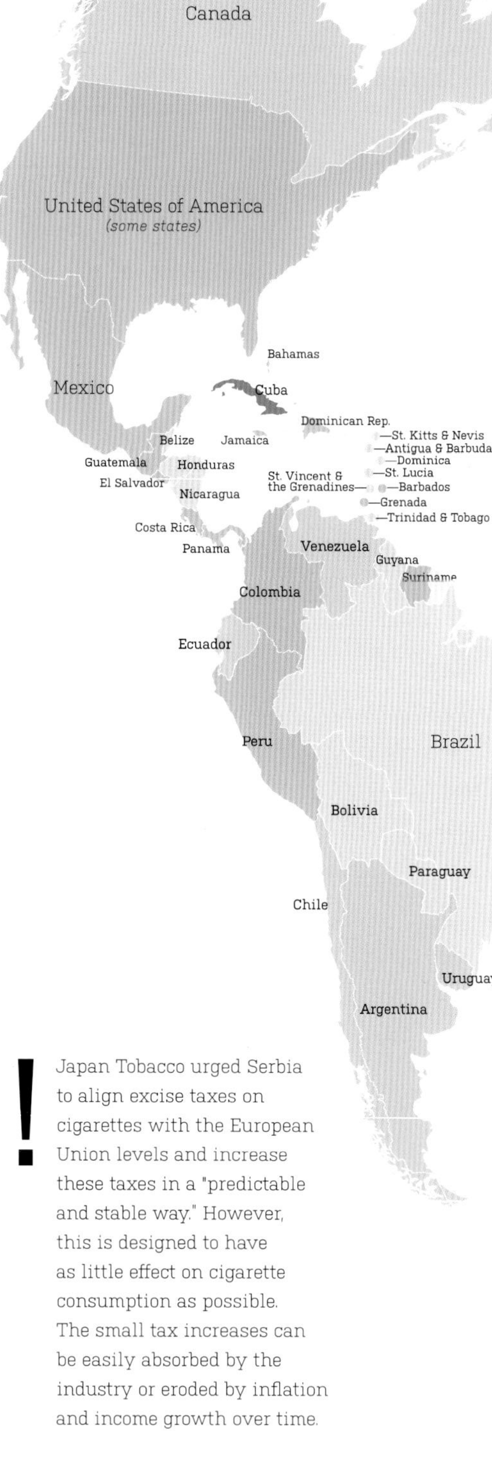

! Japan Tobacco urged Serbia to align excise taxes on cigarettes with the European Union levels and increase these taxes in a "predictable and stable way." However, this is designed to have as little effect on cigarette consumption as possible. The small tax increases can be easily absorbed by the industry or eroded by inflation and income growth over time.

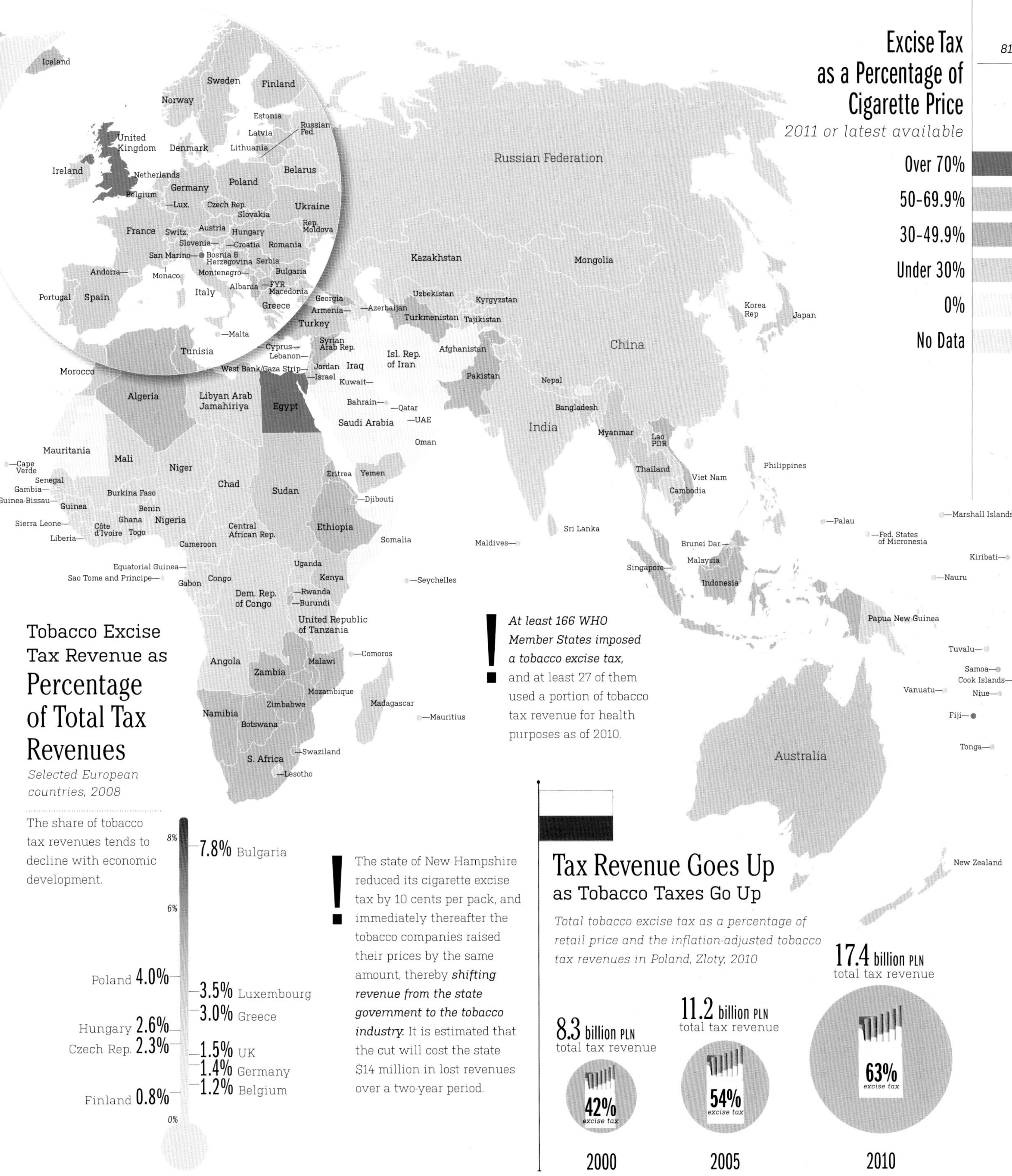
Excise Tax
as a Percentage of
Cigarette Price
2011 or latest available
Over 70%
50-69.9%
30-49.9%
Under 30%
0%
No Data
Iceland
Sweden
Finland
Norway
Estonia
Russian Fed.
Latvia
United Kingdom
Denmark
Lithuania
Ireland
Belarus
Netherlands
Poland
Germany
Belgium
Lux.
Czech Rep.
Ukraine
Slovakia
Rep. Moldova
France
Switz.
Austria
Hungary
Slovenia
Croatia
Romania
San Marino
Bosnia & Herzegovina
Serbia
Andorra
Monaco
Montenegro
Bulgaria
Albania
FYR Macedonia
Portugal
Spain
Italy
Greece
Georgia
Armenia
Azerbaijan
Turkey
Malta
Tunisia
Cyprus
Lebanon
Syrian Arab Rep.
Morocco
West Bank/Gaza Strip
Jordan
Iraq
Israel
Kuwait
Isl. Rep. of Iran
Russian Federation
Kazakhstan
Mongolia
Uzbekistan
Kyrgyzstan
Turkmenistan
Tajikistan
Afghanistan
Pakistan
China
Korea Rep
Japan
Nepal
Bangladesh
India
Myanmar
Lao PDR
Thailand
Viet Nam
Cambodia
Philippines
Algeria
Libyan Arab Jamahiriya
Egypt
Bahrain
Qatar
UAE
Saudi Arabia
Oman
Mauritania
Mali
Niger
Cape Verde
Senegal
Gambia
Guinea-Bissau
Guinea
Chad
Sudan
Eritrea
Yemen
Djibouti
Burkina Faso
Benin
Sierra Leone
Côte d'Ivoire
Ghana
Togo
Nigeria
Liberia
Central African Rep.
Cameroon
Ethiopia
Somalia
Maldives
Sri Lanka
Equatorial Guinea
Sao Tome and Principe
Gabon
Congo
Uganda
Kenya
Seychelles
Dem. Rep. of Congo
Rwanda
Burundi
United Republic of Tanzania
Singapore
Brunei Dar.
Malaysia
Indonesia
Palau
Fed. States of Micronesia
Marshall Islands
Kiribati
Nauru
Papua New Guinea
Angola
Zambia
Malawi
Comoros
Mozambique
Zimbabwe
Madagascar
Namibia
Botswana
Mauritius
Swaziland
S. Africa
Lesotho
Australia
Tuvalu
Samoa
Cook Islands
Vanuatu
Niue
Fiji
Tonga
New Zealand
Tobacco Excise Tax Revenue as
Percentage of Total Tax Revenues
Selected European countries, 2008
The share of tobacco tax revenues tends to decline with economic development.
8%
6%
0%
7.8% Bulgaria
Poland 4.0%
3.5% Luxembourg
3.0% Greece
Hungary 2.6%
Czech Rep. 2.3%
1.5% UK
1.4% Germany
1.2% Belgium
Finland 0.8%
!
At least 166 WHO Member States imposed a tobacco excise tax, and at least 27 of them used a portion of tobacco tax revenue for health purposes as of 2010.
!
The state of New Hampshire reduced its cigarette excise tax by 10 cents per pack, and immediately thereafter the tobacco companies raised their prices by the same amount, thereby shifting revenue from the state government to the tobacco industry. It is estimated that the cut will cost the state $14 million in lost revenues over a two-year period.
Tax Revenue Goes Up
as Tobacco Taxes Go Up
Total tobacco excise tax as a percentage of retail price and the inflation-adjusted tobacco tax revenues in Poland, Zloty, 2010
8.3 billion PLN
total tax revenue
42%
excise tax
2000
11.2 billion PLN
total tax revenue
54%
excise tax
2005
17.4 billion PLN
total tax revenue
63%
excise tax
2010

THE INDUSTRY SAYS:

"We will continue to use all necessary resources ... and where necessary litigation, to actively challenge unreasonable regulatory proposals."

Louis Camilleri, Chairperson and CEO, Philip Morris International, 2010

Litigation against the tobacco industry has been based on grounds such as "health harms, wrongful death, health-care costs, involvement in smuggling, racketeering, conspiracy, defective product, concealment of scientific evidence, fraud, deception, misconduct, failure to warn consumers adequately of the dangers of tobacco smoke, negligence, and exposing the public to unreasonable danger." **THE WORLD HEALTH ORGANIZATION ENCOURAGES INDIVIDUALS AND GOVERNMENTS TO TAKE LEGAL ACTION FOR THE PURPOSE OF TOBACCO CONTROL.**

Litigation puts the industry on the political defensive, forces tobacco companies to the bargaining table, and may result in large settlements. Beyond dollar amounts, other effects of awards or settlements may include the release of internal industry documents; agreements from the industry to restrict marketing; the channeling of settlement money to public health; increased media attention to the problem of tobacco use; decreased youth access to tobacco products; and improvements in protection from secondhand smoke. However, policy changes as a direct result of litigation have been limited.

Increasingly, tobacco companies and their allies are challenging effective legislative measures adopted by countries seeking to protect the health of their citizens. These legal challenges are expensive to defend and invariably delay implementation of laws passed in the interest of public health.

In November 2010 the WHO Framework Convention on Tobacco Control (WHO FCTC) Conference of Parties adopted the Punta del Este Declaration in support of FCTC Parties that are facing legal attacks for implementing the treaty and its guidelines.

! Cases pending against *British American Tobacco* and its subsidiaries, as of December 31, 2010:

3,161

! Smokers' rights and neo-libertarian groups, funded by the tobacco industry, are being used globally to challenge tobacco control legislation.

History of Tobacco Tort Litigation

Strategies in the US

Individual plaintiffs vs. tobacco companies

	1950 — WAVE I — 1970	1980 — WAVE II — 1990	1998 — WAVE III — Present
Legal Strategies Employed	The industry used three arguments: (a) smoking could not be proven to have caused plaintiffs' individual injuries; (b) if smoking is dangerous, the industry didn't know it when they made the cigarettes the plaintiffs smoked; (c) if the victims changed brands over time, there could be no proof their product had caused the claimed harm.	As an outgrowth of the concerns about smoking initiated by the 1964 Surgeon General's Report and the subsequent law requiring warning labels, the tobacco industry used the presence of such labels as a defense in the claims brought by smokers. While continuing to deny a causal link between smoking and plaintiffs' illnesses, tobacco companies also began to claim that, because of the warning labels and publicity about the claimed dangers of smoking, smokers knew as much as they did, a strategy known as the "assumption of risk" defense.	In 1998, 6 million confidential tobacco industry documents became available to the public as a result of legal action, providing damning evidence that the industry had long known about the harms of smoking. Plaintiffs now argued that the industry had covered up the reality of the dangers of smoking at a time when the general public was unaware of this danger, suggesting negligence, product liability, fraud, and intentional misrepresentation on the industry's part. Claimants began arguing that the industry also hid the fact that smoking was highly addictive, and that the industry deliberately marketed to minors.
Results	*Plaintiffs lost all cases.*	*Plaintiffs lost all cases.*	In 1998, in the historic Master Settlement Agreement, cigarette companies agreed to pay *46 US States $206 billion over 25 years, to settle litigation on the cost of smoking-related health care.*

Legal Challenges Against Tobacco Control Legislation

Selected countries, recent, pending, or under appeal

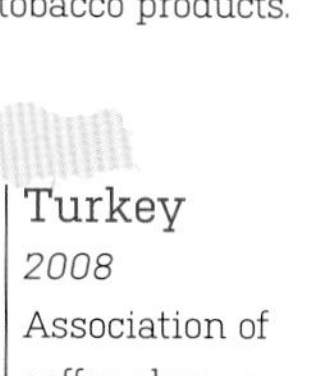

US
2010
Tobacco company and a retailer challenging law related to event sponsorships, merchandising, health warnings, and advertising.

Guatemala
2010
Chamber of Commerce challenged smoke-free law. *Law upheld.*

Colombia
2010
Tobacco company challenged tobacco advertising, promotion, and sponsorship law. *Law upheld.*

Argentina
2008
Tobacco company affiliate challenging smoke-free law in Santa Fe province.

Ireland
2009
Tobacco company challenging the ban on display of tobacco products at retail stores.

Panama
2010
Tobacco company challenging an executive decree banning point-of-sale display.

Peru
2010
Individual, on behalf of more than 5,000 citizens, challenging smoke-free law.

Brazil
2010
Tobacco company challenging smoke-free laws in four states as well as the national law restricting tobacco advertising, promotion, and sponsorship.

Uruguay
2010
Tobacco companies challenging packaging regulations at the International Centre for Settlement of International Disputes (ICSID) using a bilateral investment agreement between Switzerland and Uruguay.

Norway
2010
Tobacco company challenging point-of-sale display restrictions.

Scotland
2010
Tobacco company challenged bans on point-of-sale displays and vending machine sales. *Law upheld.*

Finland
2009
Tobacco company challenging the ban on the display of tobacco products.

Turkey
2008
Association of coffee shop owners challenging smoke-free law.

2009
Tobacco companies challenging packaging and labeling regulations.

South Africa
2009
Tobacco company challenging amendments to advertising, promotion, and sponsorship law.

India
2007
Tobacco company challenging law on packaging and labeling through 31 suits.

2008
Hotel and restaurant associations challenging smoke-free law through four suits.

Indonesia
2010
Tobacco farmers challenging law on tobacco advertising, promotion, and sponsorship.

2010
Tobacco farmers challenging law on packaging and labeling.

Philippines
2010
Tobacco company challenging a Department of Health Administrative Order on graphic health warnings and a ban on misleading descriptors.

Australia
2011
Tobacco company challenging government on trademark and other intellectual property issues.

THE GOVERNMENT SAYS:

> "It is fair to say that we are being targeted by what can only be described as subversive and disgraceful tactics by the tobacco industry, including using every available vehicle and opportunity to try and intimidate and/or threaten us to withdraw the legislation."

Jane Halton, Secretary of the Department of Health and Ageing, Australia, 2011

THE OPTIMIST SAYS:

"In years to come, people will shake their heads in disbelief that there was ever smoking in homes where children live, eat, sleep and breathe."

Jonathan Winickoff, Harvard Medical School, US, 2010

In July 2011, the World Health Organization suggested a target of a 40% relative reduction in prevalence of current daily tobacco smoking among adults over 15 years of age by 2025 (from a 2010 baseline). This does not include smokeless tobacco or some of the new forms of tobacco. The reduction has yet to be adopted by Member States, but it is a start in encouraging countries to set targets within the overall parameter.

The future is mixed. On the one hand, many nations are beginning to take even stronger measures, and smoking prevalence is forecast to reach single figures, below 5 percent in 2040—the "2040 end game." On the other hand, even if smoking prevalence rates decline and youth uptake is reduced, the number of smokers in the world will most likely rise for the foreseeable future, due principally to world population growth in low- and middle-income countries.

One major future issue is that of smokeless products and alternative nicotine delivery systems. Tobacco companies are shifting from marketing traditional cigarettes to marketing alternative products, and this will have an effect on current tobacco control strategies, such as clean indoor-air policies. Will e-cigarettes be allowed in previously smoke-free areas, and will tax rates be modified to encourage non-combustible products?

Many countries, including low-income ones, have shown that tobacco can be controlled and smoking rates can be reduced. These successes can be reproduced by any responsible nation, but only through concerted, comprehensive, and sustained governmental and community action. It is clear that preventing youth initiation and encouraging cessation require steadfast political will to tackle the tobacco industry and allocate appropriate resources proportional to the health and economic magnitude of the tobacco problem.

THE MEANS TO CURB THIS PANDEMIC ARE CLEAR AND WITHIN REACH.

Future Policy Directions

Since the first edition of *The Tobacco Atlas*, huge strides have been made in the global effort to reduce smoking prevalence and harm, with many countries experiencing a reduction in smoking prevalence in the past 10 years. Nevertheless, it is projected that smoking will still cause 1 billion deaths in the 21st century (see Chapter 1 – *Deaths*). As overwhelming evidence about the great costs of tobacco use to human health and life, as well as to the global economy, continue to emerge and be disseminated, countries will need to become increasingly engaged in strategies to reduce the burden of tobacco use—and it is also likely the tobacco industry will continue to resist and obstruct such measures.

Recommended Future Policies and Actions

1 WHO FCTC
All countries that have not signed or ratified the World Health Organization Framework Convention on Tobacco Control should do so immediately. Those that have ratified it should implement all the Articles forthwith. This includes the whole range of legislative, tax, and other measures.

2 MILLENNIUM DEVELOPMENT GOALS
Given the evidence and global consensus on the negative impact of tobacco on a broad range of health and economic outcomes, tobacco control goals and targets should be included in the second round of the Millennium Development Goals in 2015.

3 UN HIGH-LEVEL MEETING
Following the UN High-Level Meeting on noncommunicable diseases, tobacco issues should be strategically placed in national policies and action plans on NCDs.

4 FUNDING
Government funding for health research, surveillance, and action still lags behind the enormity of the problem of tobacco as a health issue (see Chapter 23 – *Public Health Strategies*). Substantially increased funding—ideally from a percentage of tobacco tax—at country level is needed to reflect the burden that tobacco poses to health and economies, and particularly to combat the issue in geographic areas where the number of tobacco users is increasing.

5 TOBACCO INDUSTRY REGULATIONS
Given the wealth of evidence showing that nicotine is a highly addictive drug, governments should move to regulate the tobacco industry, as well as any other industry producing nicotine products, as rigorously as possible, including licensing nicotine as an addictive drug.

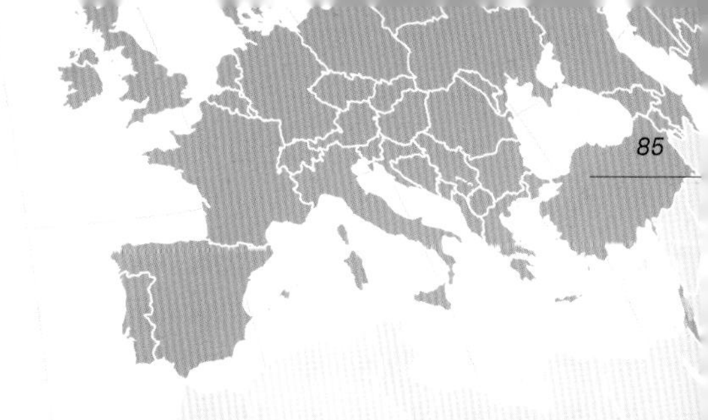

THE REALIST SAYS:

“My prediction for the 2020s is that most of the types of cancer that were killing many people in 2010 will still be killing many people, and that **the trends in premature death from cancer will be driven mainly by the extent to which people choose to stop smoking, rather than by improvements in treatment.**”

Sir Richard Peto, University of Oxford, UK, 2010

6 TOBACCO TAXES

National tobacco taxes serve as a major deterrent to initiating and maintaining a smoking habit (see Chapter 29 – *Tobacco Taxes*). Countries that have yet to implement rigorous tobacco tax policies should seek to increase excise taxes to at least 70% of the retail price. 'Duty-free' tobacco, currently sold worldwide in the international terminals of airports and elsewhere, should be prohibited.

7 HEALTH PROFESSIONALS

Based on the high level of smoking among health-care professionals (see Chapter 12 – *Health Professionals*) and the need for health professionals to set an example, they should not smoke; medical and other health professions schools should be smoke-free; and teaching on tobacco control should be systematically introduced into the health-care curriculum.

8 QUITTING

Research supports that most people who smoke want to quit (see Chapter 25 – *Quitting Smoking*), but many find it difficult to do so, and quitting rates remain low. Support for individual efforts to quit must be improved. Future quitting incentives may include monetary savings through rebates and lower health-insurance premiums.

9 MESSAGING

Health education messages and mass media campaigns have been shown to be replicable and effective in a range of cultural contexts. These messages should continue to be developed and disseminated more effectively.

10 NEW TOBACCO PRODUCTS

Research reflects a general confusion among the public about a range of tobacco products and their true harm (see Chapter 5 – *Nicotine Delivery Systems*). As the tobacco industry introduces novel products, often purporting that these products reduce harm, awareness campaigns and media attention are sorely needed to inform the public about the true dangers of these products and reiterate that there is no safe way to use tobacco.

11 TOBACCO FARMING

Economies with large tobacco-farming sectors need assistance and support in diversifying crops. New, commercially profitable uses for tobacco that contribute to, rather than harm, human health should be pursued.

12 HOT SPOTS

Media and advocates should partner to bring increased attention and assistance to rapidly expanding geographic "tobacco hot spots," particularly when litigation is being pursued and statements, legislation, taxation, and other tobacco control action is being challenged.

13 TOBACCO INDUSTRY BEHAVIOR

The tobacco industry has recently and increasingly taken to using legal and trade challenges to national legislation. A global strategy and support for countries that find themselves under legal threat need to be developed (see Chapter 30 – *Legal Challenges and Litigation*). In addition, the industry has introduced corporate social responsibility programs promoting voluntary measures as an effective way to address tobacco control, create an illusion of being a "changed" company, and establish partnerships with health interests. It has also employed the use of seemingly independent front groups to challenge science and action funded business analysts to make its legislative case, and engaged in political lobbying. The behavior of the industry must be exposed and regulated, and the industry should have no place in discussions of tobacco control at any level.

14 POLITICAL WILL

What works in reducing smoking rates has been known for decades. Political will is needed to implement such policies, to protect the public from Big Tobacco, to permit victims of the industry to protect themselves from products that are highly addictive and enormously harmful, and to seek legal remedies against the manufacturers of these products.

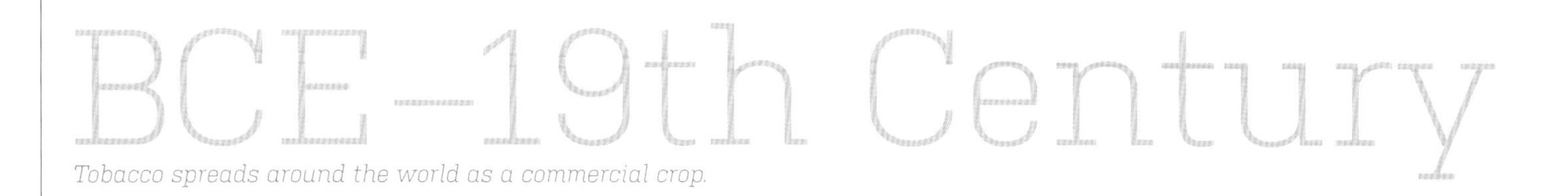

BCE–19th Century

Tobacco spreads around the world as a commercial crop.

6000 BCE
Americas First cultivation of the tobacco plant.

Circa 1 BCE
Americas Indigenous Americans begin smoking tobacco and using tobacco enemas.

Americas Huron Indian myth: "In ancient times, when the land was barren and the people were starving, the Great Spirit sent forth a woman to save humanity. As she traveled over the world everywhere her right hand touched the soil, there grew potatoes. And everywhere her left hand touched the soil, there grew corn. And in the place where she had sat, there grew tobacco."

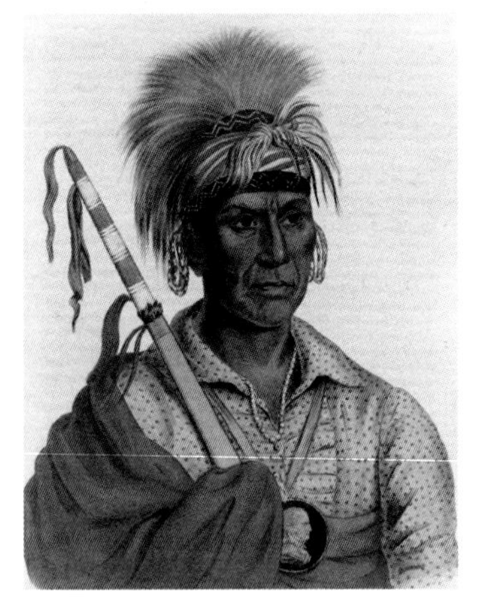

1493
Christopher Columbus and his crew return to Europe from the Americas with the first tobacco leaves and seeds ever seen on the continent. A crew member, Rodrigo de Jerez, is seen smoking and is imprisoned by the Inquisition, which believes he is possessed by the devil.

Early 1500s
Middle East Tobacco is introduced to Egypt by Turkish traders.

1530-1600
China Tobacco is introduced via Japan or the Philippines.

1558
Europe Tobacco plant is brought to Europe. Attempts at cultivation fail.

1560
Africa Portuguese and Spanish traders introduce tobacco to Sub-Saharan Africa.

France Diplomat Jean Nicot, Lord of Villemain, introduces tobacco from Portugal. Queen Catherine de Medici uses it to treat her migraines.

1577
Europe European doctors recommend tobacco as a cure for toothaches, falling fingernails, worms, halitosis, lockjaw, and cancer.

1592-1598
Korea The Japanese Army introduces tobacco to Korea.

Circa 1600
India Tobacco is first introduced.

1600s
China Philosopher Fang Yizhi points out that long years of smoking "scorches one's lung."

1603
Japan Use of tobacco is well-established.

1604
England King James I writes *A Counterblaste to Tobacco:* "Smoking is a custom loathsome to the eye, hateful to the nose, harmful to the brain, dangerous to the lungs, and in the black, stinking fume thereof nearest resembling the horrible Stygian smoke of the pit that is bottomless."

1608-1609
Japan Ban on smoking is introduced to prevent fires.

1612
Americas Tobacco is first grown commercially.

1614
England Seven thousand tobacco shops open following the first sale of Virginia tobacco.

1633
Turkey Death penalty is imposed for smoking.

1634
China Qing dynasty decrees a smoking ban, during which a violator is executed. The ban is not to protect health, but to address the inequality of trade with Korea.

1650s
South Africa European settlers grow tobacco and use it as a form of currency.

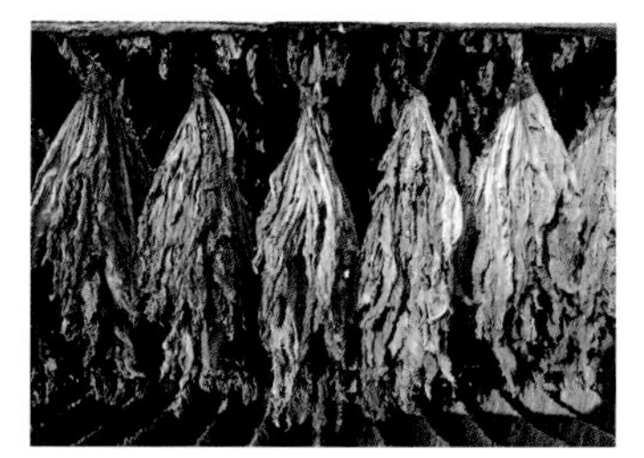

1692 & 1717
Korea Bans on smoking in Choson are introduced to reduce fire risk.

1700s

Africa/Americas African slaves are forced to work in tobacco fields.

Europe Snuff becomes the most popular mode of tobacco use.

Circa 1710

Russia Peter the Great encourages his courtiers to smoke tobacco and drink coffee, which is seen as fashionable and pro-European.

1719

France Smoking is prohibited in many places.

1753

Sweden Botanist Carolus Linnaeus names the plant genus *Nicotiana* and describes two species, *Nicotiana rustica* and *Nicotiana tabacum*.

1761

England John Hill conducts the first study of the malignant effects of tobacco, showing that snuff users could contract nasal polyps.

1769

New Zealand Captain James Cook arrives smoking a pipe, and is promptly doused in case he is a demon.

1771

France A French official is condemned to be hanged for admitting foreign tobacco into the country.

1788

Australia Tobacco arrives with the First Fleet, 11 ships that sailed from England carrying mostly convicts and crew.

1795

Germany Samuel Thomas von Soemmerring reports cancers of the lip afflicting pipe smokers.

1800

Canada Tobacco is first grown commercially.

1833

UK Phosphorus friction matches are introduced on a commercial scale, making smoking more convenient.

1840

France Frederic Chopin's mistress, the Baroness de Dudevant, becomes one of the first women to smoke in public (in Paris).

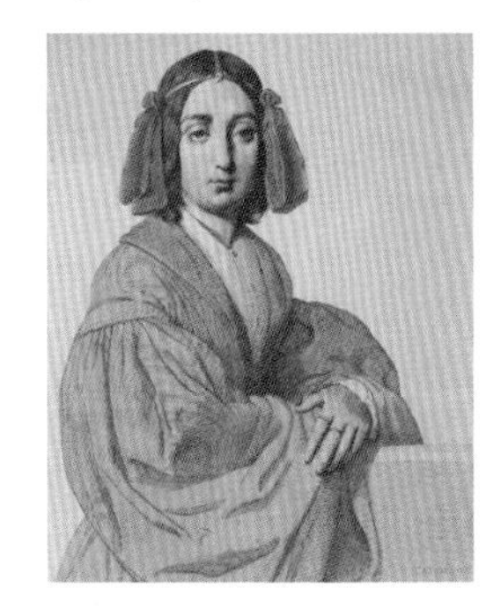

1847

England Philip Morris, Esq., a tobacconist and importer of fine cigars, opens a shop in London selling hand-rolled Turkish cigarettes.

1854

England Philip Morris begins making his own cigarettes. Old Bond Street soon becomes the center of Britain's retail tobacco trade.

1858

China Treaty of Tianjin allows cigarettes to be imported into China duty-free.

1862

US First federal tobacco tax is introduced to help finance the Civil War.

1876

Korea Foreign cigarettes and matches are introduced.

1880s

England Richard Benson and William Hedges open a tobacco shop near Philip Morris's in London.

1881

US First practical cigarette-making machine is patented by James Bonsack, producing 100,000 cigarettes a day, replacing the labor of 50 people. Production costs plummet, and cigarette smoking begins its explosive growth.

Circa 1890s

Indonesia Clove cigarette, the kretek, is invented.

Pre-1900

Lung cancer is still extremely rare.

20th Century

As tobacco becomes big business, science finds evidence of tobacco-related illness.

1900-1910

China, Japan, and Korea
BAT introduces cigarettes, using films as a promotional vehicle.

1901-1902

England Imperial Tobacco Company Limited (ITL) and British American Tobacco (BAT) are founded.

1903

Brazil Tobacco company Souza Cruz is founded.

1911

US American Tobacco empire is broken up by exercise of the Sherman Antitrust Act.

1913

US Birth of the "modern" blended cigarette: R.J. Reynolds launches Camel brand.

1915

Japan At Tokyo University, cancer is induced in laboratory animals by applying coal tar to the skin of rabbits.

1921

Korea Korea Ginseng Corporation becomes Korea Tobacco and Ginseng, and a monopoly is formed.

1924

US Philip Morris introduces Marlboro as a women's cigarette—"mild as May."

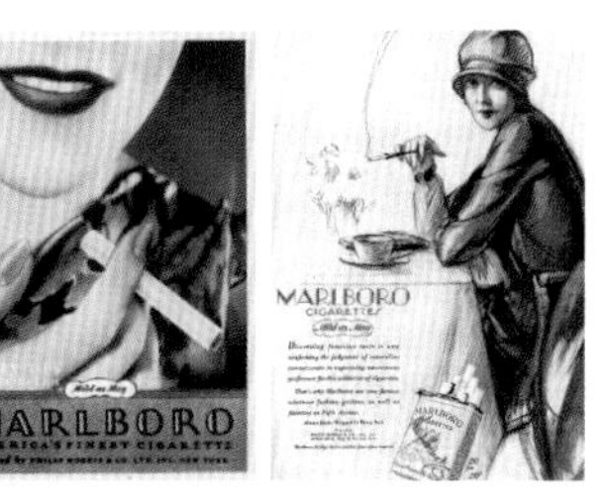

US *Reader's Digest* publishes "Does Tobacco Injure the Human Body," launching a campaign by the magazine to make people think before starting to smoke.

1929

US Edward Bernays mounts a "freedom march" of smoking debutantes/fashion models who walk down New York City's Fifth Avenue during the Easter parade holding aloft their Lucky Strike cigarettes as "torches of freedom."

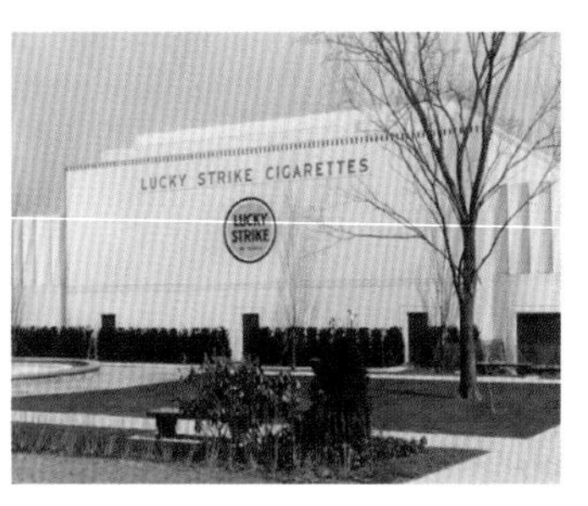

Germany Fritz Lickint of Dresden publishes the first formal statistical evidence of a lung cancer–tobacco link, based on a case series showing that lung cancer sufferers are likely to be smokers.

1931

Argentina Angel Roffo of Buenos Aires contributes to a growing body of evidence on the harms of smoking, showing that tobacco tars rubbed onto the ears of rabbits produce tumors.

1936

Germany Fritz Lickint first uses the term *Passivrauchen* (passive smoking) in his *Tabakgenuss und Gesundheit.*

1938

US Dr. Raymond Pearl, from the Medical School and the School of Hygiene and Public Health of Johns Hopkins University, publishes a paper in *Science* describing the premature deaths of heavy smokers as compared to nonusers and moderate smokers.

1939

US Tobacco companies are found in violation of price-fixing laws.

Germany Franz Herman Müller of Cologne City Hospital launches the field of case-control epidemiology, showing that smokers are far more likely to suffer from lung tumors than nonsmokers. Abstract of his work is published in *JAMA.*

US Alton Ochsner and Michael DeBakey report an association between smoking and lung cancer.

1947

Canada Norman Delarue compares 50 patients with lung cancer with 50 patients hospitalized with other diseases, finding that over 90% of the first group—but only half of the second—were smokers. Delarue predicts that by 1950, no one will be smoking.

1950s

China State monopoly takes control of the tobacco business, and foreign tobacco companies leave China. BAT, almost half of whose revenues came from China, is especially hurt.

1950

US The link between smoking and lung cancer is reconfirmed. "Tobacco Smoking as a Possible Etiologic Factor in Bronchogenic Carcinoma" by E. L. Wynder and Evarts Graham is published in *JAMA*; the same issue features a full-page ad for Chesterfields with the actress Gene Tierney and golfer Ben Hogan. *JAMA* accepts tobacco ads until 1953; some state medical journals accept ads into the late 1960s.

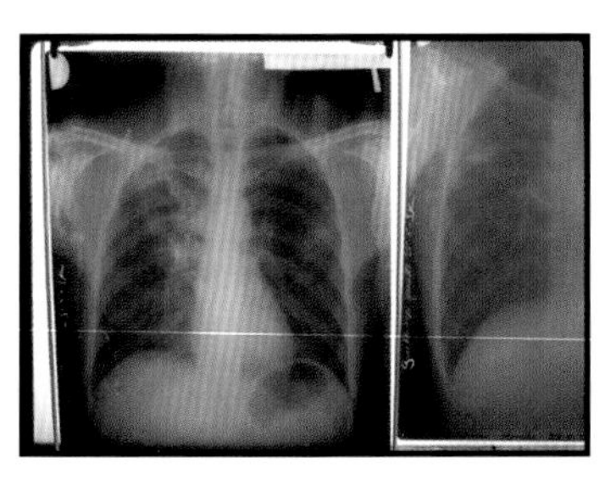

UK Richard Doll and A. Bradford Hill publish a case-control study linking smoking and lung cancer. Doll and Hill also launch a large-scale prospective study.

1953

US Ernst Wynder, Evarts Graham, and Adele Croninger show that tumors can be produced by painting tobacco tars on the shaved skins of mice; tobacco stocks plummet in response, and the tobacco industry faces its biggest crisis in decades.

US Tobacco executives meet at the Plaza Hotel in New York City to organize a campaign to respond to recent scientific data indicating health harms from cigarettes. Public relations firm Hill & Knowlton is hired to orchestrate denialist campaign.

1954

US Tobacco Industry Research Committee places nationwide full-page ad, "A Frank Statement to Cigarette Smokers," reassuring them that it is safe to smoke.

US St. Louis factory worker Ira C. Lowe files first product liability action against a tobacco company on behalf of her smoker husband, who died from cancer. The tobacco company wins this, and the next couple of hundred cases filed against it.

US The Marlboro cowboy is created for Philip Morris by Chicago ad agency Leo Burnett.

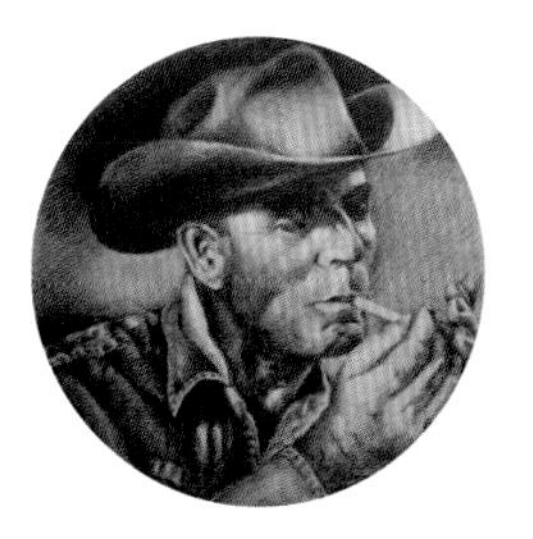

1957

Vatican Pope Pius XII suggests that the Jesuit order give up smoking.

1958

US Tobacco Institute is formed in Washington as a trade organization by US cigarette manufacturers, with a broad mission to put out good news about tobacco, especially economic news to attack scientific studies by casting doubt on them rather than by rebutting them directly, and to lobby Congress.

1960

US Framingham Heart Study is published finding cigarette smoking to increase the risk of heart disease.

1962

UK First report of the Royal College of Physicians of London on Smoking and Health is published.

1963

World Tobacco and *Tobacco Journal International,* tobacco industry trade journals, first published.

1964

US First US Surgeon General's report on smoking and health announces that smoking causes lung cancer in men.

1965

WHO establishes International Agency for Research on Cancer (IARC) in Lyon, France.

UK Cigarette advertising on TV is banned.

1967

US First World Conference on Smoking and Health held in New York.

1969

US Surgeon General's report confirms link between maternal smoking and low birth weight. Philip Morris President and CEO Joseph Cullman claims shortly thereafter that "some women would prefer having smaller babies."

1971

UK Action on Smoking and Health (ASH) UK establishes national tobacco control organization.

US Cigarette manufacturers agree to put health warnings on advertisements. This agreement is later made law.

1972

Marlboro becomes the best-selling cigarette in the world.

International Association for the Study of Lung Cancer is inaugurated.

1974

France Joe Camel is born—and used in French poster campaign for Camel cigarettes.

1976

US *Shimp v. New Jersey Bell Telephone Co.* is the world's first lawsuit claiming damages from secondhand smoke. The office worker is granted an injunction to ensure a smoke-free area in her workplace.

1977

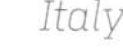

Italy The Martignacco Project community-prevention trial results in a reduction of coronary heart disease.

US First Great American Smokeout is held nationally, during which smokers quit smoking on the third Thursday of November.

1978

Australia The three-year community study North Coast Healthy Lifestyle Programme shows a significant reduction in smoking.

US A Roper Report prepared for the Tobacco Institute concludes that the nonsmokers' rights movement is "the most dangerous development to the viability of the tobacco industry that has yet occurred."

Switzerland Nicorette chewing gum is approved for use as nicotine replacement therapy.

1979

The Freedom Organization for the Right to Enjoy Smoking Tobacco (FOREST) is formed.

US Tobacco Control Resource Center and its Tobacco Products Liability Project are formed.

Australia Activist group BUGA UP (Billboard Utilising Graffitists Against Unhealthy Promotions) is formed, re-facing tobacco and alcohol billboards.

20th Century

Government agencies and international organizations act to protect public health.

1981

Japan Professor Takeshi Hirayama publishes first report linking passive smoking and lung cancer in the nonsmoking wives of men who smoked.

1983

Europe ERC Group Plc, an independent market research group, publishes first European Tobacco Market Report.

1984

US FDA approves nicotine gum as prescription medicine, following efforts to suppress its use by Philip Morris.

1985

US Lung cancer surpasses breast cancer as number-one cancer killer of women.

By 1985, 73% of the world's tobacco is grown in low- and middle-income countries.

US Washington, D.C.: First International Summit of Smoking Control Leaders is organized by the American Cancer Society.

1987

US Smoke-free Educational Services is founded, advocating the right of all employees to work in a safe, healthy, smoke-free environment.

1988

First WHO report on the effects of smokeless tobacco is published.

US Framingham Heart Study finds cigarette smoking increases risk of stroke.

First WHO World No Tobacco Day, subsequently an annual event on May 31, with different annual themes and awards of commemorative medals.

Make every day World No Tobacco Day.
www.who.int/tobacco
31 MAY
World Health Organization

1989

Asia The Asia Pacific Association for the Control of Tobacco (APACT) is established by David Yen of the John Tung Foundation in Taiwan, China.

Thailand U.S. Trade Representative (USTR) launch a petition under section 301 of the 1975 Trade Act. The General Agreement on Tariffs and Trade (GATT) panel rules that an import ban on foreign cigarettes was not justified, but Thailand could raise its tobacco tax, impose laws (e.g. advertising bans, labelling, ingredient disclosure) if imported products were given equal treatment.

1990s

Cigars become fashionable again in high-income countries.

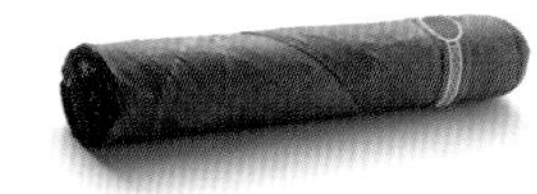

1990

Western Pacific Region First five-year WHO Action Plan on Tobacco or Health is published.

GLOBALink, the international interactive website and marketplace founded by the International Union Against Cancer, is inaugurated for the international tobacco control community.

International Network of Women Against Tobacco (INWAT) is formed.

China Chinese Association on Smoking and Health is inaugurated, changing its name to the Chinese Association on Tobacco Control in 2004.

Tobacco control in the Third World: A resource atlas, edited by Simon Chapman and Wong Wai Leng, is published by the International Organisation of Consumers Unions, Penang, Malaysia.

1991

UK International Agency on Tobacco and Health (IATH) is formed to act as an information and advisory service for low-income countries. IATH ceases its operations in 2007 in view of the fact that so many new, similar resources have become available, mostly as a result of the WHO FCTC.

Geneticists determine that chemicals in cigarette smoke switch on a gene that makes lung cells vulnerable to the chemicals' cancer-causing properties.

International Network Towards Smoke-free Hospitals is inaugurated.

1992

Tobacco Control is founded by the British Medical Journals group. This is the first international peer-reviewed journal on tobacco control.

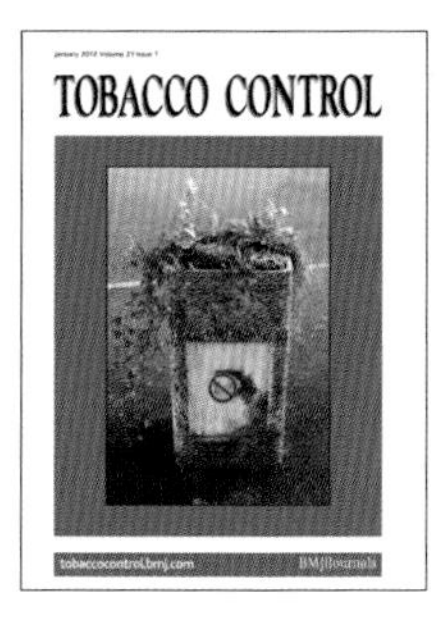

Northern Ireland First conference on women and tobacco is initiated by the UICC (International Union Against Cancer), the Ulster Cancer Foundation, and the Health Promotion Agency of Northern Ireland.

Thailand Major comprehensive tobacco control laws come into effect, including first ingredient disclosure provisions.

1993

US Environmental Protection Agency (EPA) declares cigarette smoke a Class-A carcinogen.

South Africa Tobacco Products Control Amendment Act is passed.

Europe European Network on Young People and Tobacco (ENYPAT) is founded.

1994

US Society for Research on Nicotine and Tobacco is founded.

US Cigarette executives testify before Congress that in their opinion nicotine is not addictive.

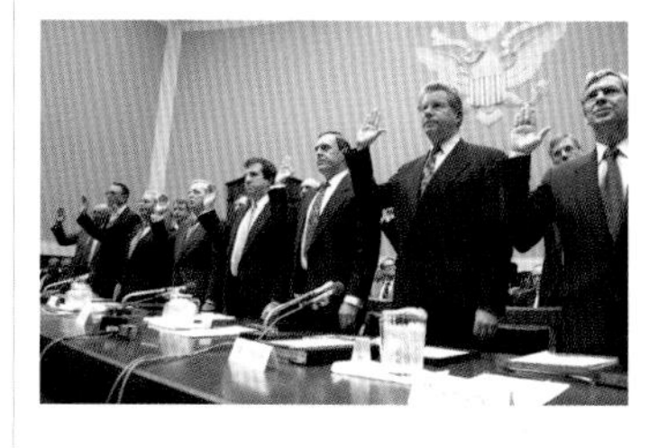

US Confidential internal tobacco industry documents are leaked to Professor Stan Glantz.

Austria First TABEXPO held in Vienna. TABEXPO stages exhibitions and congresses for the international tobacco industry.

International Non Governmental Coalition Against Tobacco (INGCAT) is founded.

First international "Quit & Win" campaign is run, with successful quitters competing for a monetary award.

Canada Research for International Tobacco Control (RITC) is inaugurated, with a major focus on low- and middle-income countries.

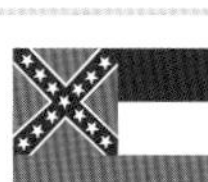

US State of Mississippi files first lawsuit by a health authority for reimbursement of money expended to treat smokers with smoking-caused illnesses. It ends with an out-of-court settlement.

1995

US Smokescreen.org (later Smokefree.net) is inaugurated. Focusing on the right to breathe clean air, this is the first web-based advocacy site that enables visitors to send faxes directly to their elected officials. Mainly used by US citizens, but also by 10,000 international participants.

Italy The Bellagio Statement that tobacco is a major threat to sustainable and equitable development is issued by members of a retreat at the Rockefeller Foundation's Bellagio Study and Conference Centre.

International Council of Nurses publishes a position statement on tobacco.

US Federal Drug Administration declares cigarettes to be "drug delivery devices." Restrictions are proposed on marketing and sales to reduce smoking by young people.

FORCES International (Fight Ordinances and Restrictions to Control and Eliminate Smoking), an ostensibly grassroots pro-tobacco organization, is established.

US "Marlboro Man" David McLean dies of lung cancer.

1996

US First smoking cessation guidelines are issued by the federal Public Health Service.

1997

Europe European Network for Smoking Prevention is created.

Scotland Doctors and Tobacco: Tobacco Control Resource Centre is formed by the European Forum Medical Associations, based at the British Medical Association in Edinburgh.

US Congress passes a bill prohibiting the Departments of State, Justice, and Commerce from promoting the sale or export of tobacco.

1998

Studies confirm the harmfulness of smoking fewer than 10 cigarettes a day.

WHO's Tobacco Free Initiative is established.

United Nations Foundation funds its first tobacco control project.

Australia Tobacco Control Supersite website is inaugurated, enabling exploration of internal, previously private tobacco industry documents, and providing access to a wide range of information relevant to smoking prevention and control in Australia.

US Master Settlement Agreement between attorneys general of 46 states and five territories with tobacco companies to settle lawsuits.

1999

US Network for Accountability of Tobacco Transnationals (NATT) is founded by Corporate Accountability International (formerly Infact), comprising environmental, consumer, human rights, and corporate accountability organizations working together to prevent life-threatening abuses by transnational corporations.

Global Youth Tobacco Surveys (GYTS) commence by the US Centers for Disease Control and Prevention. These are followed by the Global School Personnel Surveys (GSPS) started in 2000, the Global Health Professions Student Survey (GHPSS) started in 2005, and the Global Adult Tobacco Survey (GATS) started in 2007.

World Bank report "Curbing the Epidemic: Governments and the Economics of Tobacco Control" is published.

Sweden Swedish International Development Cooperation Agency first supports tobacco control projects.

UK Britain's royal family orders the removal of its seal of approval and royal crest from Gallaher's Benson and Hedges cigarettes by 2000.

US US Justice Department sues the tobacco industry to recover billions of government dollars spent on smoking-related health care, accusing cigarette makers of "fraud and deceit."

21st Century

Serious efforts are undertaken to reduce the global harm caused by tobacco use.

2000

Framework Convention Alliance (FCA) of NGOs is formed to support the WHO Framework Convention on Tobacco Control (WHO FCTC) and related protocols.

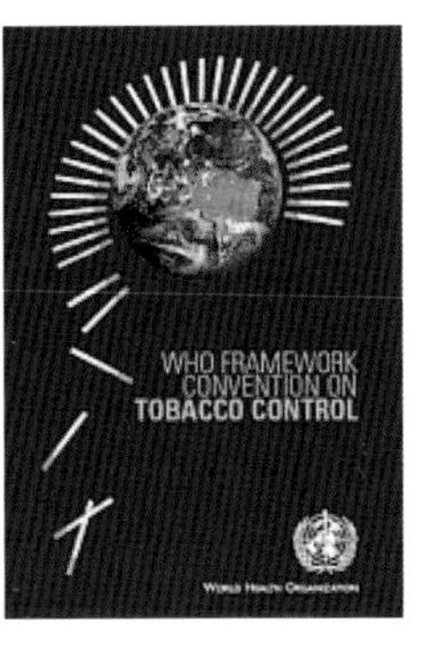

US First Luther L. Terry Awards are given for contributions to tobacco control.

Global Partnerships for Tobacco Control is founded by Essential Action to help support and strengthen international tobacco control activities at the grassroots level.

International Tobacco Evidence Network (ITEN) is established, with the goal of expanding global research.

Rockefeller Foundation International Health Research Awards are established for "Trading Tobacco for Health" in selected Association of South-East Asian Nations countries.

South Africa Tobacco Products Control Amendment Act comes into effect, strictly regulating smoking and advertising.

2001

US A new report, *Clearing the Smoke: Assessing the Science Base for Tobacco Harm Reduction*, from the Institute of Medicine (IOM) is released.

WHO publishes *Tobacco & the Rights of the Child.*

Czech Republic Philip Morris releases a report to the government concluding that smokers save the state money by dying early.

Thailand ThaiHealth Promotion Foundation is established, funded by a percentage of tobacco taxation. The Southeast Asia Tobacco Control Alliance (SEATCA) is also established for regional and sustainable funding of tobacco control activity in SE Asia.

2002

TobaccoPedia, the online tobacco encyclopedia, is inaugurated.

US Global Tobacco Research Network is founded by the Institute for Global Tobacco Control at Johns Hopkins University.

Switzerland WHO publishes the first edition of *The Tobacco Atlas*, made available by Myriad Editions.

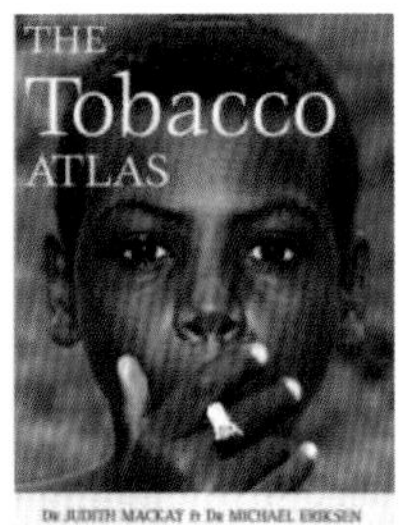

US Fogarty International Center, National Institutes of Health, allocates funding for tobacco research projects.

2003

World Medical Association launches the Doctors' Manifesto for Global Tobacco Control.

Treatobacco web-based database and educational resource for treatment of tobacco dependence established by the Society for Research on Nicotine and Tobacco.

The Global Network of Pharmacists Against Tobacco is launched.

2004

Ireland Workplace smoking ban, including pubs and restaurants, is implemented, showing significantly reduced salivary cotinine concentrations among nonsmoking staff.

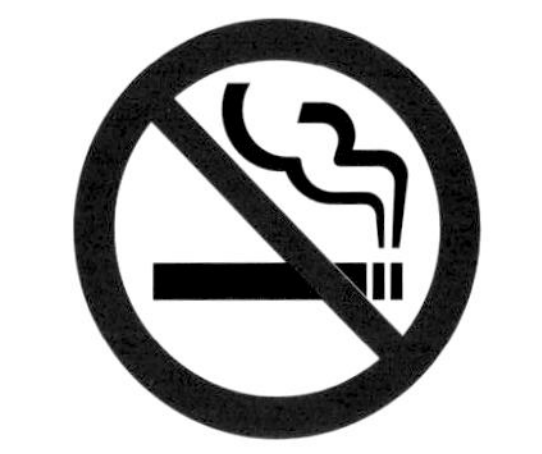

First textbook for health professionals on tobacco is published by Oxford University Press: *Tobacco: Science, Policy and Public Health.*

Europe The EU Commission publishes the ASPECT report, "Tobacco or Health in the European Union: Past, Present and Future," the first comprehensive overview of tobacco control in the 25 EU member countries plus Norway, Iceland, and Switzerland.

Uganda Environment Minister Kahinda Otafiire announces a ban on smoking in restaurants, educational institutions, and bars.

Canada Non-Smokers' Rights Association, the first such association, celebrates its 30th anniversary.

WHO's Code of Practice on Tobacco Control for Health Professional Organizations is launched.

IARC Monograph on Tobacco Smoke and Involuntary Smoking is released, conclusively refuting extensive tobacco industry disinformation by classifying secondhand smoke as a carcinogen.

India Complete ban on tobacco advertising and promotion comes into effect.

2005

World Dental Federation (FDI) launches *Tobacco or Oral Health* publication.

WHO Framework Convention on Tobacco Control (WHO FCTC), initiated by Ruth Roemer in 1993, comes into force, using international law to reduce tobacco use.

2006

US *United States v. Philip Morris.* Racketeer Influenced and Corrupt Organizations (RICO) case is the largest litigation ever undertaken by the US government, and Judge Gladys Kessler finds tobacco companies guilty of racketeering and defrauding the American public.

US Second edition of *The Tobacco Atlas* is published by the American Cancer Society and launched at the 13th World Conference on Tobacco or Health in Washington, D.C.

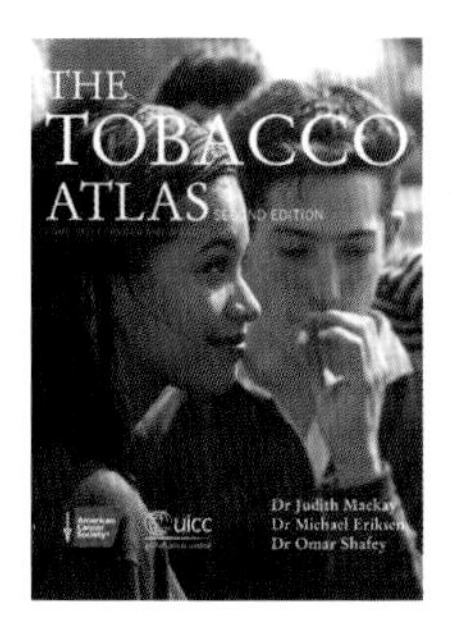

US Bloomberg Initiative to Reduce Tobacco Use in low- and middle-income countries is launched with $125 million donation from Bloomberg Philanthropies.

2007

The Global Adult Tobacco Survey, launched in February, is designed to produce standardized data on adult tobacco use, including exposure to secondhand smoke and quit attempts among adults.

2008

The Global Smokefree Partnership is formed to promote effective smoke-free air policies worldwide.

The first WHO *MPOWER* report on the global status of the tobacco epidemic is published, and published every two years thereafter.

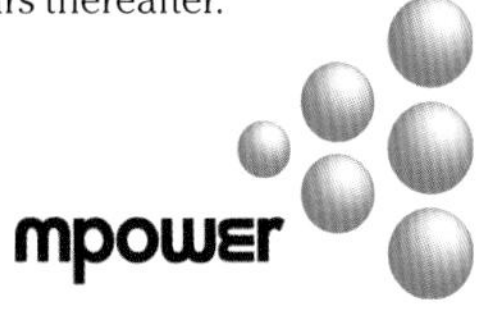

The Bill & Melinda Gates Foundation and Bloomberg Philanthropies jointly pledge additional financial resources to reduce tobacco use in low- and middle-income countries, bringing the total outlay to $500 million over seven years, 2006–2013.

2009

India Third edition of *The Tobacco Atlas* is published by the American Cancer Society and World Lung Foundation and launched at the 14th World Conference on Tobacco or Health in Mumbai.

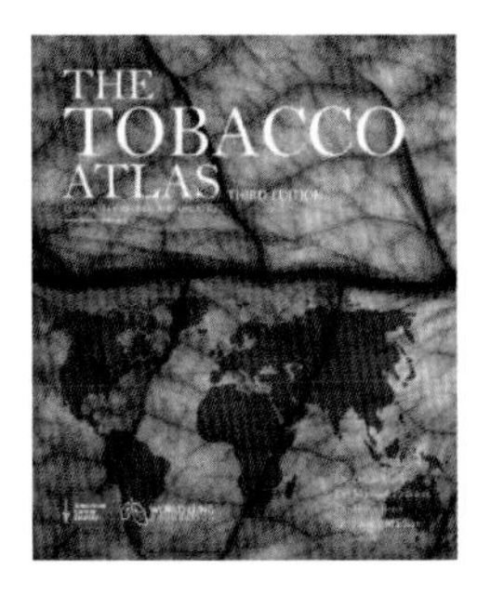

2011

US First UN High-Level Meeting on noncommunicable diseases includes tobacco as a major risk factor for the four main NCDs (cancer, cardiovascular disease, chronic lung disease, and diabetes).

2012

Singapore Fourth edition of *The Tobacco Atlas* is published by the American Cancer Society and World Lung Foundation and launched at the 15th World Conference on Tobacco or Health in Singapore.

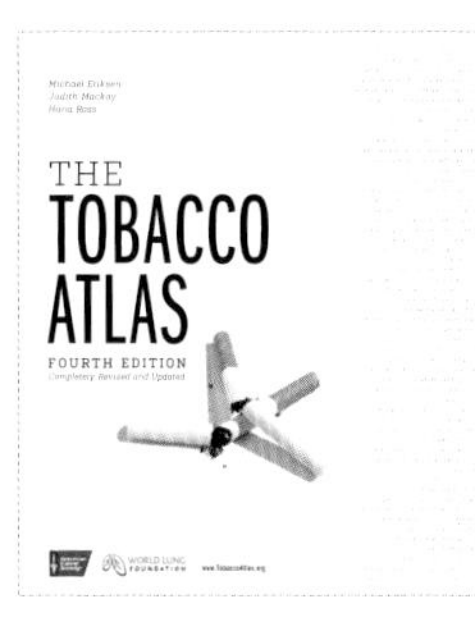

“Never let the future disturb you. You will meet it, if you have to, with the same weapons of reason which today arm you against the present.”

Marcus Aurelius Antoninus, Roman emperor (AD 121–180)

ADDICTION
Physiological or psychological dependence on a substance characterized by neurochemical changes, compulsive drug-seeking behaviors, dose tolerance, withdrawal symptoms, uncontrolled cravings, and self-destructive behaviors. Common addictive drugs include alcohol, stimulants, cocaine, heroin, and nicotine.

ADVERTISING
Any commercial effort to promote tobacco consumption, including the display of trademarks, brand names, and manufacturer logos; marketing of tobacco products; sponsorship of sports and other social and cultural activities; and other methods.

BCE
Before the Common Era.

BILLION
1,000 million, or 1,000,000,000.

BRAND STRETCHING
A marketing approach by tobacco companies in which cigarette brand names are attached to advertisements for nontobacco products (such as clothing).

BUPROPION
An antidepressant pharmaceutical used as a smoking-cessation aid. Brand names include Wellbutrin and Zyban.

CANCER
A type of disease in which abnormal cells divide uncontrollably. Cancer cells can invade nearby tissue and spread through the bloodstream and lymphatic system to other parts of the body. Tobacco consumption significantly increases the risk of developing many types of cancers, especially lung and oral cancers. Tobacco is also associated with cancers of the pharynx, larynx, esophagus, pancreas, kidney, bladder, and other organs.

CARCINOGEN
A substance that causes cancer. Tobacco contains many potent chemical carcinogens, including tobacco-specific nitrosamines (TSNs), polyaromatic hydrocarbons (PAHs), and volatile organic compounds (VOCs).

CHRONIC BRONCHITIS
Inflammation of the bronchial mucus membrane over a long period of time, characterized by cough, hypersecretion of mucus, and expectoration of sputum; associated with increased vulnerability to bronchial infection.

CHRONIC OBSTRUCTIVE PULMONARY DISEASE (COPD)
A chronic lung disease, such as asthma or emphysema, in which breathing becomes slowed or forced. See also *Chronic bronchitis*.

CONSUMPTION
Total cigarette consumption is the number of cigarettes sold annually in a country, usually in millions of sticks. Total cigarette consumption is calculated by adding a country's cigarette production and imports and subtracting exports.

Per adult cigarette consumption is calculated by dividing total cigarette consumption by the total population of those ages 15 years and older. Smuggling may account for inaccuracies in these estimates.

CORONARY ARTERY DISEASE
The narrowing or blockage of the coronary arteries (blood vessels that carry blood and oxygen to the heart) usually caused by atherosclerosis (a buildup of fatty material [cholesterol] and plaque inside the coronary arteries). Also known as *coronary heart disease*.

COSTS
Macroeconomic costs associated with tobacco use.

Direct costs: Health costs related to diseases caused by tobacco, including health-service costs, such as hospital services, physician and outpatient services; prescription drugs; nursing home services; home health care and allied health care; and changed expenditures due to increased utilization of services.

Indirect costs: Productivity costs caused by tobacco-related illness or premature death; loss of productivity and earnings.

Total costs: The sum of direct and indirect tobacco-attributable costs to society.

COTININE
Nicotine's major metabolite, which has a significantly longer half-life than nicotine. Cotinine measurement is often used to estimate a smoker's tobacco/nicotine usage prior to quitting, and to confirm abstinence self-reports during follow-up. Also, cotinine is commonly used as an indicator of exposure to secondhand smoke among nonsmokers. Cotinine is commonly measured in blood serum, urine, and saliva.

E-CIGARETTE (ELECTRONIC CIGARETTE)
An electrical device that attempts to simulate the act of cigarette smoking by producing an inhaled mist bearing the physical sensation, appearance, and often the flavor and nicotine content of inhaled cigarette smoke.

ELECTRONIC NICOTINE DELIVERY SYSTEMS (ENDS)
Scientific term describing electronic cigarettes and other products that deliver nicotine without combustion.

EMPHYSEMA
A pathological condition of the lungs marked by an abnormal increase in the size of the air spaces, resulting in labored breathing and an increased susceptibility to infection. It can be caused by irreversible expansion of the alveoli or by the destruction of alveolar walls. See *Chronic obstructive pulmonary disease (COPD)*.

ENVIRONMENTAL TOBACCO SMOKE (ETS)
See *Secondhand smoke (SHS)*.

EXCESS MORTALITY
Absolute difference between two rates of mortality. The amount by which death rates for a given population group (e.g., smokers) exceeds that of another population group chosen as a reference or standard (e.g., nonsmokers).

FRAMEWORK CONVENTION ON TOBACCO CONTROL

The World Health Organization Framework Convention on Tobacco Control (WHO FCTC) is the first treaty negotiated under the auspices of the WHO. WHO FCTC establishes the international public health and legal template for national tobacco control activities.

GLOBAL TOBACCO SURVEILLANCE SYSTEM (GTSS)

The World Health Organization (WHO) and the US Centers for Disease Control and Prevention (CDC) developed these surveys to track tobacco use using a common methodology and core questionnaire. The GTSS includes the Global Youth Tobacco Survey (GYTS), Global School Personnel Survey (GSPS), Global Health Professional Student Survey (GHPSS), and Global Adult Tobacco Survey (GATS).

HARM REDUCTION

A public health philosophy that seeks to mitigate health hazards by replacing high-risk products with lower-risk products or activities. In tobacco control, harm reduction is proposed for smokers who do not want to stop smoking or are unable to do so despite many attempts. Harm reduction seeks to reduce the adverse health effects of smoking by removing harmful constituents or encouraging smokers to switch to alternative modes of tobacco consumption that are considered less harmful than smoking—e.g., smokeless tobacco. Some consider the approach controversial and believe the main focus should be on smoking cessation.

HEALTH PROFESSIONALS

Dentists, health science practitioners, hospital staff, medical doctors, nurses, pharmacists, ancillary medical staff, and students in these disciplines.

HEALTH WARNINGS

Government-mandated medical statements or graphic images placed on tobacco products, packaging, or advertisements.

INGREDIENT

Every component of the tobacco product that is smoked, chewed, or inhaled, including all genetically modified, blended, and introduced components, additives, flavorings, and other constituents, including paper, ink, adhesives, hardening agents, filters, and other materials used in the manufacturing process and present in the finished product in burned or unburned form.

MARKETING

A range of activities aimed at identifying, anticipating, and satisfying customer requirements profitably.

MPOWER

To make the WHO Framework Convention on Tobacco Control (WHO FCTC) a reality, WHO introduced the *MPOWER* measures, intended to assist in country-level implementation of effective interventions to reduce the demand for tobacco. Measures are:

Monitor tobacco use and prevention policies;
Protect people from tobacco smoke;
Offer help to quit tobacco use;
Warn about the dangers of tobacco;
Enforce bans on tobacco advertising, promotion, and sponsorship; and
Raise taxes on tobacco.

NICOTIANA TABACUM

The tobacco plant. Its leaves contain high levels of the addictive chemical nicotine and many cancer-causing chemicals, especially polyaromatic hydrocarbons (PAHs). The leaves may be smoked (in cigarettes, cigars, and pipes), used orally (as dipping and chewing tobacco), or inhaled (as snuff).

NICOTINE

An addictive, poisonous alkaloid chemical found in tobacco that acts as a stimulant, increasing heart rate and use of oxygen by the heart. Also used as an insecticide. The lethal dose for an adult is about 50mg.

NICOTINE REPLACEMENT THERAPY (NRT)

A type of smoking cessation treatment that provides a low dose of nicotine to ease cravings experienced by addicted smokers. NRTs include devices such as transdermal patches, nicotine gum, nicotine nasal sprays, and inhalers.

NOVEL NICOTINE PRODUCTS

Newly marketed products including items such as nicotine water, wafers, candy, and e-cigarettes. These products deliver nicotine to consumers in an innovative yet unregulated manner, and the side effects and potential benefits and dangers are largely unknown.

OPPORTUNITY COST

The cost associated with the lost opportunity of using resources in an alternative way. For example, the resources used for treating smoking-related illnesses could be used to build schools.

PASSIVE SMOKING

Inhaling cigarette, cigar, or pipe smoke produced by another individual. See also *Secondhand smoke (SHS)*.

POLYAROMATIC HYDROCARBON (PAH)

A type of organic compound composed of several benzene rings. PAHs, many of which are carcinogenic, are produced during charbroiling of meat, incomplete combustion of fossil fuels, and the burning of tobacco. Tobacco smoke is the most common source of human exposure.

PREVALENCE

Smoking prevalence is the percentage of smokers in the total population. Prevalence of current smokers and prevalence of current daily smokers are two common point estimates of prevalence. Meanwhile, the prevalence of ever-smokers is a measure of lifetime prevalence. Commonly, estimates of prevalence are presented separately by groups of age, gender, and location (urban/rural), although overall estimates also are informative. Adult smoking prevalence is usually defined as the percentage of smokers among those ages 15 years and older.

PROMOTION

Includes special offers, gifts, price discounts, coupons, company websites, specialty item distribution, and telephone advertising used to facilitate the sale or placement of any tobacco product. Also includes allowances paid to retailers, wholesalers, full-time company employees, or any other persons involved in tobacco distribution.

RELATIVE INCOME PRICE (RIP) OF CIGARETTES

A percentage of annual per capita income (measured by per capita GDP) required for purchase of 100 packs of cigarettes. The lower the RIP, the more affordable cigarettes are.

RETAILER

A person engaged in a business that includes the sale of tobacco products to consumers.

RISK

The probability of incurring a particular event or circumstance (e.g., risk of disease measures the chances of an individual contracting a disease).

SECONDHAND SMOKE (SHS)

Smoke resulting from the combustion of tobacco products. SHS is composed of mainstream smoke (exhaled by smokers) and side-stream smoke (from the tip of the cigarette, cigar, or pipe). Secondhand smoke contains the same harmful chemicals that smokers inhale. Also known as environmental tobacco smoke (ETS).

SMOKE-FREE AREA

Area where smoking or holding a lighted cigarette, cigar, or pipe is banned, and where it is expected that no evidence of SHS will be found, if measured.

SMOKELESS TOBACCO

Includes snuff and chewing tobacco; not a safe alternative to smoking. Smokeless tobacco is as addictive as smoking and can cause cancers of the gum, cheek, lip, mouth, tongue, and throat.

SMOKER

Someone who smokes any tobacco product either daily or occasionally.

STROKE

A condition in which a blood vessel in the brain bursts or is clogged by a blood clot. This leads to an inadequate blood supply to the brain and to the death of brain cells, and usually results in temporary or permanent neurological deficits. Smoking significantly increases the risk of stroke.

SUFFICIENT EVIDENCE

Term used by the US Surgeon General to indicate that current available evidence strongly supports the inference of a causal relationship between smoking and specific health outcomes.

SUGGESTIVE EVIDENCE

Term used by the US Surgeon General to indicate that current available evidence, although indicative, is not sufficient to infer a causal relationship between smoking and specific health outcomes.

TAR

The raw anhydrous nicotine-free condensate of smoke.

TAR AND NICOTINE YIELD

The amount of tar and nicotine in one cigarette, as determined by a machine designed to measure the chemical content of cigarette smoke. Machine yields of cigarette tar and nicotine levels do not reflect the actual level of exposure experienced by smokers. See also *Tobacco smoke condensate (TSC)*.

TOBACCO-ATTRIBUTABLE MORTALITY

The number of deaths attributable to tobacco use within a specific population.

TOBACCO CONTROL ORGANIZATION

An organization with a goal of reducing tobacco consumption and/or protecting nonsmokers from the effects of secondhand smoke, as well as monitoring compliance with legislation and reporting tobacco industry maneuvers.

TOBACCO INDUSTRY DOCUMENTS

Previously secret internal industry records that are now available in the public domain as a result of court rulings.

TOBACCO PRODUCT

Any product manufactured wholly or partly from tobacco that is ingested by smoking, inhalation, chewing, sniffing, or sucking.

TOBACCO PRODUCTION

The volume of actual tobacco leaves harvested from the field, excluding harvesting and threshing losses and any part of the unharvested tobacco crop.

TOBACCO SMOKE CONDENSATE (TSC)

Sticky particles comprising thousands of chemicals created by burning tobacco.

TOBACCO-SPECIFIC NITROSAMINE (TSN OR TSNA)

A group of toxic chemicals found only in tobacco products. The most carcinogenic include

- N'-nitrosonornicotine (NNN)
- (4-methylnitrosamino)-1-(3-pyridyl)-1-butanone (NNK)
- N-oxide, 4-(methylnitrosamino)-1-(3-pyridylN-oxide)-1-butanol (NNAL; a metabolic product of NNK).

TOBACCO EXCISE TAX

A tax levied specifically on tobacco products. There are two basic types of tobacco excise tax:

Specific tax: set as a specific amount of money per unit (e.g., cigarette, pack, etc.) or per weight (e.g., gram) of tobacco.

Ad valorem tax: set as a percentage markup on some determined value (tax base), usually the retail selling price or the wholesale (ex-factory) price of tobacco products.

Excise taxes are often differentiated according to the type of tobacco product (e.g., filtered vs. nonfiltered cigarettes, pipe tobacco vs. cigars).

In addition to the excise tax, other taxes may apply (e.g., VAT, sales tax), but these are not tobacco-product-specific taxes.

TOBACCO TAX AVOIDANCE

Legal methods of circumventing tobacco taxes.

Cross-border shopping involves individual tobacco users residing in higher-tax jurisdictions purchasing tobacco products in nearby lower-tax jurisdictions for their own consumption within the customs constraints.

Tourist shopping is similar to cross-border shopping, but involves the purchase of tobacco products in more distant jurisdictions.

Duty-free shopping involves the purchase of tax-free tobacco products purchased in airports, on airplanes, and in other travel-related venues. Most governments impose limits on how much an individual can purchase and bring home from duty-free sources.

Industry reformulation and/or repositioning refers to strategies of tobacco companies to reduce the tax imposed on their products—for example, by increasing the length of cigarettes when the taxes are based on quantity.

TOBACCO TAX EVASION

Illegal methods of circumventing tobacco taxes.

Small-scale smuggling involves the purchase, by individuals or small groups, of tobacco products in low-tax jurisdictions in amounts that exceed the limits set by customs regulations, for smuggling or resale in high-tax jurisdictions.

Large-scale smuggling involves the illegal transportation, distribution, and sale of large quantities of tobacco products that generally avoid all taxes.

Illicit manufacturing refers to the production of tobacco products contrary to law.

Counterfeiting involves the production and distribution of products bearing a trademark without the approval of the trademark owner.

TOBACCO USE

The consumption of tobacco products by burning, chewing, inhaling, or other forms of ingestion.

VARENICLINE

A smoking cessation aid that works by blocking nicotine receptors so nicotine is not needed for dopamine release. Brand name: Chantix in the US, Champix in Europe and Canada.

VOLATILE ORGANIC COMPOUND (VOC)

An organic (carbon-containing) compound that evaporates at room temperature. VOCs contribute significantly to indoor air pollution and respiratory disease.

WORLD HEALTH ORGANIZATION REGIONS

WHO Member States are grouped into six regions:

- African Region (AFRO)
- Region of the Americas (AMRO)
- Eastern Mediterranean Region (EMRO)
- European Region (EURO)
- South-East Asia Region (SEARO)
- Western Pacific Region (WPRO)

Data from these regions are included throughout *The Tobacco Atlas*.

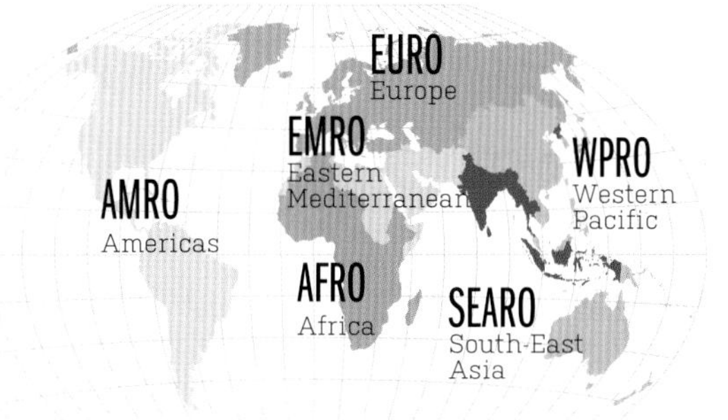

COUNTRY			HARM: DEATHS		HARM: SECONDHAND SMOKE	PRODUCTS & THEIR USE: CIGARETTE CONSUMPTION	PRODUCTS & THEIR USE: MALE TOBACCO USE				
	WHO REGION	World Bank Income Group^	Male Deaths	Female Deaths	Youth Exposed to Secondhand Smoke in Home	Per Capita Consumption	Current Cigarette Use	Currently Smoking ANY Tobacco Product	Type of Tobacco Use	Age Group	Crude Male Prevalence
			% 2004, Due to Tobacco (Estimates)		*% Ages 13–15*	*Cigarettes Per Person*	*% 2009, Male Age Standardized (or country-specific data)*		*Male Crude, Latest Available*	*years*	*%*
Afghanistan	EMRO	Low	24	6	38.8**	61	-	-	-	-	-
Albania	EURO	Middle	25	8	84.8	1,116	60.1	60.1	Current tobacco smoking	15+	60.1
Algeria	AFRO	Middle	17	0	33.2**	775	28.8	-	Current tobacco smoking	15+	33.9
Andorra	EURO	High	-	-	-	784	38.4	38.4	Current tobacco smoking	15+	42.2
Angola	AFRO	Middle	9	5	-	414	-	-	-	-	-
Antigua and Barbuda	AMRO	Middle	2	3	18.0	375	-	-	-	-	-
Argentina	AMRO	Middle	19	6	54.7	1,042	31.2	31.7	Current cigarette smoking	18+	32.4
Armenia	EURO	Middle	33	8	89.8	1,620	50.9	50.9	Current tobacco smoking	20-60	55.7
Australia	WPRO	High	17	14	17.2	1,034	19.9	19.9	Daily tobacco smoking	14+	16.4
Austria	EURO	High	19	10	-	1,650	47.4	47.4	Current tobacco smoking	14-99	48.0
Azerbaijan	EURO	Middle	22	7	-	1,877	41.2	41.2	Current cigarette smoking	-	49.6
Bahamas	AMRO	High	6	5	21.6	288	-	-	-	-	-
Bahrain	EMRO	High	14	14	38.7	661	28.8	34.3	Current tobacco smoking	20-64	33.4
Bangladesh	SEARO	Low	24	12	34.7	154	28.3	46.4	Current tobacco smoking	15+	44.7
Barbados	AMRO	High	4	0	25.9	344	13.1	13.4	Current tobacco smoking	25+	14.2
Belarus	EURO	Middle	28	0	75.3	2,266	48.9	48.9	Current tobacco smoking	16+	52.3
Belgium	EURO	High	31	8	-	1,455	30.0	30.0	Current tobacco smoking	15+	28.6
Belize	AMRO	Middle	10	1	25.7	367	23.2	23.2	Current cigarette smoking	20+	17.7
Benin	AFRO	Low	3	-	21.5	71	11.4	15.2	Current tobacco smoking	25-64	15.8
Bhutan	SEARO	Middle	13	1	31.9	120	8.7	-	Current tobacco smoking	25-74	8.4
Bolivia (Plurinational State of)	AMRO	Middle	8	2	34.3**	179	41.7	41.7	Current cigarette smoking	15+	40.7
Bosnia and Herzegovina	EURO	Middle	30	10	77.3	2,278	46.5	46.5	Current tobacco smoking	18+	54.2
Botswana	AFRO	Middle	3	0	38.5	336	20.1	-	Current tobacco smoking	25-64	32.8
Brazil	AMRO	Middle	15	6	35.5**	504	21.6	21.6	Current tobacco smoking	15+	21.6
Brunei Darussalam	WPRO	High	-	-	-	751	27.3	31.9	Current tobacco smoking	9+	31.8
Bulgaria	EURO	Middle	22	5	63.9	2,822	47.5	47.5	Current tobacco smoking	15+	50.3
Burkina Faso	AFRO	Low	6	2	32.9**	109	12.6	18.2	Current tobacco smoking	18+	23.6
Burundi	AFRO	Low	3	0	33.9	137	-	-	-	-	-
Cambodia	WPRO	Low	17	8	47.0	452	41.0	41.6	Current tobacco smoking	15+	39.1
Cameroon	AFRO	Middle	5	-	23.4**	93	11.2	13.8	Current tobacco smoking	15+	12.7
Canada	AMRO	High	23	20	-	809	19.1	23.8	Current tobacco smoking	15+	23.0
Cape Verde	AFRO	Middle	3	-	13.9	339	10.1	13.5	Current tobacco smoking	25-64	15.9
Central African Republic	AFRO	Low	4	-	35.2**	102	-	-	-	-	-
Chad	AFRO	Low	6	-	33.9	86	17.8	22.3	Current tobacco smoking	25-64	20.2
Chile	AMRO	Middle	11	8	51.7**	860	36.9	37.5	Current cigarette smoking	15+	44.2
China	WPRO	Middle	12	-	47.0**	1,711	50.4	51.2	Current tobacco smoking	15+	52.9
Colombia	AMRO	Middle	9	8	27.6**	412	-	-	Current cigarette smoking	12-65	23.8
Comoros	AFRO	Low	3	-	35.2	583	19.2	24.0	Current tobacco smoking	18+	27.8
Congo	AFRO	Middle	7	-	22.8	-	8.1	9.5	Current tobacco smoking	18+	13.0
Congo (Democratic Republic of)	AFRO	Low	4	-	30.2**	105	8.8	10.5	Current tobacco smoking	15+	14.2
Cook Islands	WPRO	Middle	6	5	61.9	-	43.0	43.0	Current tobacco smoking	25-64	46.6
Costa Rica	AMRO	Middle	6	6	21.6	529	24.0	24.0	Current tobacco smoking	15-70	23.0
Côte d'Ivoire	AFRO	Middle	9	0	33.1	148	12.9	17.3	Current tobacco smoking	15-64	22.4
Croatia	EURO	High	28	8	73.4	1,621	36.5	36.5	Daily tobacco smoking	18+	33.8
Cuba	AMRO	Middle	21	18	51.5	1,261	42.9	-	Current tobacco smoking	15+	31.1
Cyprus	EURO	High	14	2	96.1	1,620	-	-	Daily tobacco smoking	15+	38.1
Czech Republic	EURO	High	26	10	38.0	2,125	35.6	42.9	Current tobacco smoking	15-64	42.5
Denmark	EURO	High	23	21	-	1,413	30.0	30.0	Current tobacco smoking	15+	28.0
Djibouti	EMRO	Middle	2	0	39.5	309	-	-	Daily tobacco smoking	15+	41.1

PRODUCTS & THEIR USE

FEMALE TOBACCO USE					TOTAL (MALE AND FEMALE) CRUDE TOBACCO USE			BOYS' & GIRLS' TOBACCO USE			COUNTRY
Current Cigarette Use	Currently Smoking ANY Tobacco Product	Type of Tobacco Use	Age Group	Crude Female Prevalence	Type of Tobacco Use	Age Group	Crude Male and Female Prevalence	Boys' Current Cigarette Use	Girls' Current Cigarette Use	Total Current Cigarette Use	
% 2009, Female Age Standardized (or country-specific data)		*Female Crude, Latest Available*	*years*	*%*	*Total Crude, Latest Available*	*years*	*% Total*	*% Ages 13–15*			
-	-	-	-	-	-	-	-	7.6**	-	4.8**	Afghanistan
19.4	19.4	Current tobacco smoking	15+	18.3	Current tobacco smoking	15+	40.2	11.9	5.8	8.5	Albania
0.2	-	Current tobacco smoking	15+	2.4	Current tobacco smoking	15+	19.3	18.0	1.4	9.2	Algeria
32.3	32.3	Current tobacco smoking	15+	30.2	Current tobacco smoking	15+	-	-	-	-	Andorra
-	-	-	-	-	-	-	-	-	-	-	Angola
-	-	-	-	-	-	-	-	8.2	6.1	7.4	Antigua and Barbuda
20.1	21.7	Current cigarette smoking	18+	22.4	Current cigarette smoking	18+	27.1	21.1	27.3	24.5	Argentina
2.1	2.1	Current tobacco smoking	20-60	2.9	Current tobacco smoking	20-60	28.3	10.3	0.9	5.0	Armenia
16.3	16.3	Daily tobacco smoking	14+	13.9	Daily tobacco smoking	14+	15.1	3.0	4.6	3.8	Australia
45.1	45.1	Current tobacco smoking	14-99	47.0	Current tobacco smoking	14-99	47.0	-	-	-	Austria
0.6	-	Current cigarette smoking	-	-	Current cigarette smoking	-	-	-	-	-	Azerbaijan
-	-	-	-	-	-	-	-	6.2	3.7	5.2	Bahamas
6.8	8.1	Current tobacco smoking	20-64	7.0	Current tobacco smoking	20-64	19.9	17.5	3.9	10.6	Bahrain
<1	2.0	Current tobacco smoking	15+	1.5	Current tobacco smoking	15+	23.0	2.9	1.1	2.0	Bangladesh
1.2	1.4	Current tobacco smoking	25+	1.6	Current tobacco smoking	25+	7.5	14.3	9.3	11.6	Barbados
8.8	8.8	Current tobacco smoking	16+	9.3	Current tobacco smoking	16+	27.5	31.2	21.7	26.5	Belarus
22.0	22.0	Current tobacco smoking	15+	20.7	Current tobacco smoking	15+	24.5	-	-	-	Belgium
2.8	2.8	Current cigarette smoking	20+	1.4	Current cigarette smoking	20+	10.2	11.7	4.4	7.7	Belize
<1	1.4	Current tobacco smoking	25-64	1.4	Current tobacco smoking	25-64	8.7	3.3	1.6	2.8	Benin
4.9	-	Current tobacco smoking	25-74	4.7	Current tobacco smoking	25-74	6.8	18.3	6.3	12.1	Bhutan
17.8	17.8	Current cigarette smoking	15+	18.3	Current cigarette smoking	15+	-	20.3**	12.0**	16.3**	Bolivia (Plurinational State of)
35.6	35.6	Current tobacco smoking	18+	34.2	Current tobacco smoking	18+	44.0	14.3	9.4	11.7	Bosnia and Herzegovina
1.5	-	Current tobacco smoking	25-64	7.8	Current tobacco smoking	25-64	19.7	18.1	10.9	14.3	Botswana
13.1	13.0	Current tobacco smoking	15+	13.1	Current tobacco smoking	15+	17.2	9.2**	13.2**	11.6**	Brazil
3.2	4.4	Current tobacco smoking	9+	2.9	Current tobacco smoking	9+	-	-	-	-	Brunei Darussalam
26.9	26.9	Current tobacco smoking	15+	28.2	Current tobacco smoking	15+	38.8	24.4	31.6	28.2	Bulgaria
<1	8.0	Current tobacco smoking	18+	11.1	Current tobacco smoking	18+	16.9	14.1**	2.4**	8.4**	Burkina Faso
-	-	-	-	-	-	-	-	5.8	3.2	4.6	Burundi
3.3	3.4	Current tobacco smoking	15+	3.4	Current tobacco smoking	15+	19.5	0.5**	-	0.2**	Cambodia
<1	1.6	Current tobacco smoking	15+	2.0	Current tobacco smoking	15+	6.3	8.8**	3.0**	5.7**	Cameroon
15.8	16.8	Current tobacco smoking	15+	16.0	Current tobacco smoking	15+	19.5	13.0	14.0	14.0	Canada
<1	3.4	Current tobacco smoking	25-64	4.0	Current tobacco smoking	25-64	9.9	3.7	3.1	3.5	Cape Verde
-	-	-	-	-	-	-	-	10.4**	4.3**	8.1**	Central African Republic
1.5	2.8	Current tobacco smoking	25-64	1.2	Current tobacco smoking	25-64	11.2	8.4	4.3	7.5	Chad
30.2	33.2	Current cigarette smoking	15+	37.1	Current cigarette smoking	15+	40.6	28.0**	39.9**	34.2**	Chile
2.1	2.2	Current tobacco smoking	15+	2.4	Current tobacco smoking	15+	28.1	2.7**	0.8**	1.7**	China
-	-	Current cigarette smoking	12-65	11.1	Current cigarette smoking	12-65	17.0	28.6**	30.7**	29.9**	Colombia
3.5	9.4	Current tobacco smoking	18+	17.0	Current tobacco smoking	18+	22.3	13.5	6.9	9.6	Comoros
<1	<1	Current tobacco smoking	18+	1.3	Current tobacco smoking	18+	6.6	15.0	8.1	11.4	Congo
<1	1.8	Current tobacco smoking	15+	1.2	Current tobacco smoking	15+	6.4	11.7**	3.6**	8.2**	Congo (Democratic Republic of)
31.2	31.2	Current tobacco smoking	25-64	41.1	Current tobacco smoking	25-64	43.9	19.9	19.4	19.7	Cook Islands
7.8	7.8	Current tobacco smoking	15-70	8.6	Current tobacco smoking	15-70	15.8	10.4	8.4	9.5	Costa Rica
<1	3.6	Current tobacco smoking	15-64	7.3	Current tobacco smoking	15-64	13.6	19.3	7.1	13.6	Côte d'Ivoire
29.6	29.6	Daily tobacco smoking	18+	21.7	Daily tobacco smoking	18+	27.4	21.7	25.6	24.1	Croatia
29.4	-	Current tobacco smoking	15+	16.4	Current tobacco smoking	15+	23.7	8.7	13.1	10.6	Cuba
-	-	Daily tobacco smoking	15+	10.5	Daily tobacco smoking	15+	23.9	3.7	4.2	3.9	Cyprus
22.7	30.9	Current tobacco smoking	15-64	30.1	Current tobacco smoking	15-64	36.3	29.8	32.7	31.1	Czech Republic
27.6	27.6	Current tobacco smoking	15+	26.0	Current tobacco smoking	15+	26.0	13.0	14.0	13.5	Denmark
-	-	Daily tobacco smoking	15+	9.2	Daily tobacco smoking	15+	25.4	3.7	2.8	3.3	Djibouti

*** Subnational data used   ^ Countries classified as "middle low income" or "middle high income" by World Bank are classified here as "middle"   † See male/female crude data for age range*

COUNTRY			HARM			PRODUCTS & THEIR USE					
			DEATHS		SECONDHAND SMOKE	CIGARETTE CONSUMPTION	MALE TOBACCO USE				
	WHO REGION	World Bank Income Group^	Male Deaths	Female Deaths	Youth Exposed to Secondhand Smoke in Home	Per Capita Consumption	Current Cigarette Use	Currently Smoking ANY Tobacco Product	Type of Tobacco Use	Age Group	Crude Male Prevalence
			% 2004, Due to Tobacco (Estimates)		*% Ages 13–15*	*Cigarettes Per Person*	*% 2009, Male Age Standardized (or country-specific data)*		*Male Crude, Latest Available*	*years*	*%*
Dominica	AMRO	Middle	9	13	26.3	339	10.2	10.6	*Current tobacco smoking*	15-64	12.2
Dominican Republic	AMRO	Middle	9	8	33.1	234	15.6	17.1	*Current tobacco smoking*	18+	17.2
Ecuador	AMRO	Middle	-	-	28.9**	227	23.4	-	*Current cigarette smoking*	18+	36.3
Egypt	EMRO	Middle	10	1	38.7	1,104	33.1	39.7	*Current tobacco smoking*	15+	37.6
El Salvador	AMRO	Middle	1	0	14.8	209	-	-	*Current tobacco use*	12-64	21.5
Equatorial Guinea	AFRO	High	6	-	47.5	391	-	-	-	-	-
Eritrea	AFRO	Low	3	-	18.4	74	8.8	10.5	*Current tobacco smoking*	15-64	-
Estonia	EURO	High	26	7	41.1	1,523	45.7	45.7	*Current tobacco smoking*	15+	46.0
Ethiopia	AFRO	Low	2	1	14.9**	42	7.5	8.1	*Current tobacco smoking*	18+	6.3
Fiji	WPRO	Middle	-	-	47.1	530	17.7	17.7	*Daily tobacco smoking*	15-85	26.0
Finland	EURO	High	16	6	-	671	28.1	28.1	*Current tobacco smoking*	15-64	29.8
France	EURO	High	22	5	-	854	35.6	35.6	*Current tobacco smoking*	12-75	33.3
Gabon	AFRO	Middle	10	0	-	501	15.5	18.9	*Current tobacco smoking*	15-64	21.0
Gambia	AFRO	Low	7	-	45.8	85	25.4	31.3	*Current tobacco smoking*	25-64	31.3
Georgia	EURO	Middle	16	1	62.7	1,039	56.6	56.6	*Current tobacco smoking*	18-64	55.5
Germany	EURO	High	22	9	-	1,045	34.8	-	*Current tobacco smoking*	15+	30.5
Ghana	AFRO	Middle	3	-	19.1	44	7.6	10.6	*Daily cigarette smoking*	15-59	7.3
Greece	EURO	High	25	7	89.8	2,795	63.0	63.0	*Current cigarette smoking*	18-89	51.0
Grenada	AMRO	Middle	10	5	27.3	229	-	-	-	-	-
Guatemala	AMRO	Middle	7	4	23.1	235	21.7	21.7	*Current tobacco smoking*	18+	23.9
Guinea	AFRO	Low	9	1	27.7	9	19.7	25.1	*Current tobacco smoking*	15-64	23.2
Guinea-Bissau	AFRO	Low	4	-	31.0**	97	-	-	-	-	-
Guyana	AMRO	Middle	3	1	33.4	49	26.4	26.7	*Current cigarette smoking*	15-49	29.4
Haiti	AMRO	Low	2	-	32.3**	100	-	-	*Current tobacco smoking*	15-49	-
Honduras	AMRO	Middle	9	7	29.6**	217	-	-	*Current cigarette smoking*	15-49	-
Hungary	EURO	High	30	18	43.0	1,518	42.7	42.7	*Current tobacco smoking*	18+	42.5
Iceland	EURO	High	16	20	-	477	27.4	27.4	*Daily tobacco smoking*	15-89	20.1
India	SEARO	Middle	12	1	26.6	96	10.7	26.2	*Current tobacco smoking*	15+	24.3
Indonesia	SEARO	Middle	20	12	64.7	1,085	57.2	61.3	*Daily tobacco smoking*	10+	46.8
Iran (Islamic Republic of)	EMRO	Middle	7	-	35.4	657	20.7	25.8	*Current tobacco smoking*	15-64	22.1
Iraq	EMRO	Middle	-	-	32.3**	864	25.8	30.8	*Current tobacco smoking*	12+	26.5
Ireland	EURO	High	22	22	-	1,006	31.0	-	*Current cigarette smoking*	18+	31.0
Israel	EURO	High	14	8	-	1,037	28.6	28.6	*Current cigarette smoking*	20+	28.4
Italy	EURO	High	24	7	48.5	1,475	32.8	32.8	*Current tobacco smoking*	11+	29.5
Jamaica	AMRO	Middle	12	6	32.5	283	20.5	-	*Current tobacco smoking*	15-74	22.9
Japan	WPRO	High	22	12	-	1,841	38.2	41.8	*Current tobacco smoking*	20+	38.2
Jordan	EMRO	Middle	18	2	66.0	1,372	41.8	46.9	*Daily tobacco smoking*	18+	49.6
Kazakhstan	EURO	Middle	35	12	67.1	1,934	40.2	40.2	*Current tobacco smoking*	18+	52.2
Kenya	AFRO	Low	3	-	24.7	144	22.5	25.5	*Current tobacco smoking*	18+	-
Kiribati	WPRO	Middle	8	2	68.3	22	71.0	71.0	*Current tobacco smoking*	15-64	74.1
Korea (Democratic People's Republic of)	SEARO	Low	13	11	-	650	-	-	*Current tobacco smoking*	16+	52.3
Korea (Republic of)	WPRO	High	26	15	37.6	1,958	49.3	49.3	*Current cigarette smoking*	-	47.7
Kuwait	EMRO	High	4	2	44.4	1,812	29.9	35.1	*Current tobacco smoking*	20-64	42.3
Kyrgyzstan	EURO	Low	22	5	72.5	942	44.8	44.8	*Current cigarette smoking*	15+	41.7
Lao People's Democratic Republic	WPRO	Middle	18	14	43.2**	435	46.8	51.4	*Current tobacco smoking*	25-64	43.2
Latvia	EURO	Middle	27	4	51.1	785	50.1	50.1	*Current tobacco smoking*	15-64	48.9
Lebanon	EMRO	Middle	-	-	-	2,138	45.6	46.4	*Current cigarette smoking*	25-64	46.8
Lesotho	AFRO	Middle	4	-	36.9	62	-	-	*Current tobacco smoking*	15+	47.9

FEMALE TOBACCO USE					TOTAL (MALE AND FEMALE) CRUDE TOBACCO USE			BOYS' & GIRLS' TOBACCO USE			COUNTRY
Current Cigarette Use	Currently Smoking ANY Tobacco Product	Type of Tobacco Use	Age Group	Crude Female Prevalence	Type of Tobacco Use	Age Group	Crude Male and Female Prevalence	Boys' Current Cigarette Use	Girls' Current Cigarette Use	Total Current Cigarette Use	
% 2009, Female Age Standardized (or country-specific data)		*Female Crude, Latest Available*	*years*	*%*	*Total Crude, Latest Available*	*years*	*% Total*	*% Ages 13–15*			
3.4	3.5	*Current tobacco smoking*	15-64	3.2	*Current tobacco smoking*	15-64	10.2	11.8	9.6	11.5	Dominica
10.8	13.0	*Current tobacco smoking*	18+	12.5	*Current tobacco smoking*	18+	14.9	7.3	5.8	6.6	Dominican Republic
5.8	-	*Current cigarette smoking*	18+	8.2	*Current cigarette smoking*	18+	22.7	23.2**	18.1**	20.5**	Ecuador
<1	<1	*Current tobacco smoking*	15+	0.5	*Current tobacco smoking*	15+	19.4	5.9	1.4	4.0	Egypt
-	-	*Current tobacco use*	12-64	3.4	*Current tobacco use*	12-64	11.7	18.4	10.9	14.0	El Salvador
-	-	-	-	-	-	-	-	9.9	3.4	7.0	Equatorial Guinea
<1	1.8	*Current tobacco smoking*	15-64	-	*Current tobacco smoking*	15-64	8.0	2.0	0.6	1.6	Eritrea
22.8	22.8	*Current tobacco smoking*	15+	25.3	*Current tobacco smoking*	15+	34.1	28.2	26.2	27.2	Estonia
<1	<1	*Current tobacco smoking*	18+	0.5	*Current tobacco smoking*	18+	3.3	2.5**	0.7**	1.9**	Ethiopia
3.0	3.0	*Daily tobacco smoking*	15-85	3.9	*Daily tobacco smoking*	15-85	-	16.2	7.4	11.7	Fiji
21.5	21.5	*Current tobacco smoking*	15-64	21.4	*Current tobacco smoking*	15-64	25.1	-	-	-	Finland
27.4	27.4	*Current tobacco smoking*	12-75	26.5	*Current tobacco smoking*	12-75	29.9	19.1	20.2	19.6	France
1.8	3.3	*Current tobacco smoking*	15-64	4.6	*Current tobacco smoking*	15-64	-	-	-	-	Gabon
<1	2.7	*Current tobacco smoking*	25-64	1.0	*Current tobacco smoking*	25-64	15.6	12.7	8.6	10.8	Gambia
5.7	5.7	*Current tobacco smoking*	18-64	4.8	*Current tobacco smoking*	18-64	30.3	15.2	2.8	8.6	Georgia
27.3	24.8	*Current tobacco smoking*	15+	21.2	*Current tobacco smoking*	15+	25.7	14.0	12.0	12.9	Germany
<1	2.6	*Daily cigarette smoking*	15-49	0.2	*Daily cigarette smoking*	*see †*	-	10.1	7.4	8.9	Ghana
41.4	41.4	*Current cigarette smoking*	18-89	39.0	*Current cigarette smoking*	18-89	-	11.3	9.0	10.4	Greece
-	-	-	-	-	-	-	-	7.0	3.0	4.7	Grenada
3.9	3.9	*Current tobacco smoking*	18+	3.4	*Current tobacco smoking*	18+	11.2	13.7	9.1	11.4	Guatemala
<1	1.9	*Current tobacco smoking*	15-64	2.0	*Current tobacco smoking*	15-64	12.8	11.6	1.6	7.1	Guinea
-	-	-	-	-	-	-	-	7.2**	3.0**	5.1**	Guinea–Bissau
5.3	5.6	*Current cigarette smoking*	15-49	3.2	*Current cigarette smoking*	15-49	-	11.0	5.4	8.1	Guyana
-	-	*Current tobacco smoking*	15-49	4.4	*Current tobacco smoking*	15-49	-	17.2**	17.7**	17.6**	Haiti
3.4	3.4	*Current cigarette smoking*	15-49	2.3	*Current cigarette smoking*	15-49	-	14.4**	14.1**	14.2**	Honduras
33.5	33.5	*Current tobacco smoking*	18+	31.3	*Current tobacco smoking*	18+	36.5	21.5	23.6	23.2	Hungary
20.8	20.8	*Daily tobacco smoking*	15-89	15.0	*Daily tobacco smoking*	15-89	17.6	-	-	-	Iceland
1.1	3.6	*Current tobacco smoking*	15+	2.9	*Current tobacco smoking*	15+	14.0	5.4	1.6	3.8	India
3.7	5.1	*Daily tobacco smoking*	10+	3.1	*Daily tobacco smoking*	10+	24.2	23.9	1.9	11.8	Indonesia
<1	1.7	*Current tobacco smoking*	15-64	1.3	*Current tobacco smoking*	15-64	11.8	5.1	0.9	3.0	Iran (Islamic Republic of)
3.0	4.5	*Current tobacco smoking*	12+	2.9	*Current tobacco smoking*	12+	14.8	3.3**	2.7**	3.2**	Iraq
26.0	-	*Current cigarette smoking*	18+	27.0	*Current cigarette smoking*	18+	29.0	-	-	-	Ireland
12.7	12.7	*Current cigarette smoking*	20+	12.6	*Current cigarette smoking*	20+	20.9	-	-	-	Israel
19.2	19.2	*Current tobacco smoking*	11+	17.0	*Current tobacco smoking*	11+	23.0	19.4	21.6	20.7	Italy
9.2	-	*Current tobacco smoking*	15-74	7.5	*Current tobacco smoking*	15-74	15.1	20.6	10.9	15.4	Jamaica
10.9	12.4	*Current tobacco smoking*	20+	10.9	*Current tobacco smoking*	20+	23.4	12.1	8.5	10.3	Japan
3.4	5.5	*Daily tobacco smoking*	18+	5.7	*Daily tobacco smoking*	18+	29.0	13.2	7.1	10.3	Jordan
8.6	8.6	*Current tobacco smoking*	18+	9.6	*Current tobacco smoking*	18+	29.9	12.7	6.6	9.4	Kazakhstan
<1	1.5	*Current tobacco smoking*	18+	1.9	*Current tobacco smoking*	18+	-	11.2	5.2	8.2	Kenya
42.9	42.9	*Current tobacco smoking*	15-64	43.1	*Current tobacco smoking*	15-64	58.0	-	-	-	Kiribati
-	-	*Current tobacco smoking*	16+	-	*Current tobacco smoking*	16+	-	-	-	-	Korea (Democratic People's Republic of)
6.6	6.6	*Current cigarette smoking*	-	7.3	*Current cigarette smoking*	-	27.7	10.8	6.3	8.8	Korea (Republic of)
1.7	3.5	*Current tobacco smoking*	20-64	4.4	*Current tobacco smoking*	20-64	23.6	23.7	7.5	15.9	Kuwait
1.9	1.9	*Current cigarette smoking*	15+	1.5	*Current cigarette smoking*	15+	20.2	6.8	2.2	4.4	Kyrgyzstan
2.9	3.8	*Current tobacco smoking*	25-64	2.0	*Current tobacco smoking*	25-64	19.0	10.2**	0.7**	5.5**	Lao People's Democratic Republic
22.3	22.3	*Current tobacco smoking*	15-64	20.4	*Current tobacco smoking*	15-64	32.4	36.3	30.2	32.9	Latvia
30.7	30.7	*Current cigarette smoking*	25-64	31.5	*Current cigarette smoking*	25-64	38.5	11.8	5.6	8.6	Lebanon
-	-	*Current tobacco smoking*	15+	34.2	*Current tobacco smoking*	15+	39.3	11.8	7.5	10.1	Lesotho

*** Subnational data used ^ Countries classified as 'middle low income' or 'middle high income' by World Bank are classified here as 'middle' † See male/female crude data for age range*

COUNTRY			HARM: DEATHS		SECONDHAND SMOKE	PRODUCTS & THEIR USE: CIGARETTE CONSUMPTION	MALE TOBACCO USE				
	WHO REGION	World Bank Income Group^	Male Deaths	Female Deaths	Youth Exposed to Secondhand Smoke in Home	Per Capita Consumption	Current Cigarette Use	Currently Smoking ANY Tobacco Product	Type of Tobacco Use	Age Group	Crude Male Prevalence
			% 2004, Due to Tobacco (Estimates)		% Ages 13–15	Cigarettes Per Person	% 2009, Male Age Standardized (or country-specific data)		Male Crude, Latest Available	years	%
Liberia	AFRO	Low	4	-	23.6**	113	10.9	14.4	Current cigarette smoking	15-49	15.2
Libyan Arab Jamahiriya	EMRO	Middle	11	0	37.8	818	41.6	47.2	Current tobacco smoking	25-64	49.6
Lithuania	EURO	Middle	25	3	43.1	804	49.9	49.9	Current tobacco smoking	20-64	41.0
Luxembourg	EURO	High	25	10	-	928	38.8	-	Current tobacco smoking	15+	28.0
Macedonia (The former Yugoslav Republic of)	EURO	Middle	24	5	67.5	1,934	-	-	-	-	-
Madagascar	AFRO	Low	4	0	49.5	260	-	-	Current tobacco smoking	25-64	-
Malawi	AFRO	Low	2	-	10.4	48	22.8	26.0	Current tobacco smoking	25-64	25.9
Malaysia	WPRO	Middle	22	15	11.5	539	45.6	50.3	Current tobacco smoking	18+	46.4
Maldives	SEARO	Middle	29	25	48.3	170	36.1	43.4	Current tobacco smoking	25-64	37.5
Mali	AFRO	Low	3	-	48.5	127	22.2	28.5	Current tobacco smoking	15-64	30.8
Malta	EURO	High	22	1	-	1,378	30.1	30.1	Current tobacco smoking	15-79	31.0
Marshall Islands	WPRO	Middle	13	13	52.1	-	35.8	35.8	Occasional tobacco smoking	15-64	4.9
Mauritania	AFRO	Middle	4	-	42.7	86	23.6	29.4	Occasional tobacco smoking	15-64	1.4
Mauritius	AFRO	Middle	11	4	36.1	787	30.5	30.5	Current tobacco smoking	20-74	35.9
Mexico	AMRO	Middle	7	6	46.2**	371	23.9	24.3	Current tobacco smoking	15+	24.8
Micronesia (Federated States of)	WPRO	Middle	0		60.7	-	29.9	29.9	Current tobacco smoking	25-64	42.0
Moldova (Republic of)	EURO	Middle	19	5	20.3	2,479	43.0	43.0	Current tobacco smoking	15-59	51.1
Monaco	EURO	High	21	4	-	1,038	-	-	-	-	-
Mongolia	WPRO	Middle	27	18	54.4	555	48.2	48.2	Current tobacco smoking	15-64	48.0
Montenegro	EURO	Middle	-	-	76.8	2,157	-	-	-	-	-
Morocco	EMRO	Middle	14	-	27.1	500	28.4	32.7	Daily tobacco smoking	18+	30.3
Mozambique	AFRO	Low	0	0	22.5**	200	16.5	18.2	Current tobacco smoking	25-64	36.0
Myanmar	SEARO	Low	19	18	34.1	189	35.5	40.2	Current tobacco smoking	15-64	44.7
Namibia	AFRO	Middle	6	-	40.3	534	27.5	30.5	Current cigarette smoking	15-49	20.9
Nauru	WPRO	Middle	5	17	-	626	48.6	48.6	Current tobacco smoking	15-64	49.7
Nepal	SEARO	Low	15	2	35.3	420	30.4	35.9	Current tobacco smoking	15-64	34.5
Netherlands	EURO	High	28	14	-	801	28.1	31.4	Current tobacco smoking	15+	29.5
New Zealand	WPRO	High	18	16	36.0	579	26.8	26.8	Current tobacco smoking	15+	21.1
Nicaragua	AMRO	Middle	7	3	43.7**	377	-	-	Current tobacco smoking	15-49	-
Niger	AFRO	Low	8	-	30.3	52	7.2	8.9	Current tobacco smoking	15-64	8.7
Nigeria	AFRO	Middle	2	-	21.7**	116	8.0	10.5	Current cigarette smoking	15-59	9.0
Niue	WPRO	Middle	6	5	34.9	-	37.5	-	-	-	-
Norway	EURO	High	17	13	-	534	31.2	31.2	Current tobacco smoking	16-74	31.0
Oman	EMRO	High	-	-	13.9	852	9.1	11.7	Current tobacco smoking	20+	13.4
Pakistan	EMRO	Middle	15	1	16.1**	468	27.7	34.5	Current tobacco smoking	18+	32.4
Palau	WPRO	Middle	8	9	-	-	37.2	37.2	Current tobacco smoking	35-64	60.3
Panama	AMRO	Middle	8	3	21.9	197	-	17.4	Current tobacco smoking	15+	17.4
Papua New Guinea	WPRO	Middle	1	-	73.9	670	57.7	57.7	Current tobacco smoking	15-64	60.3
Paraguay	AMRO	Middle	13	1	32.5	619	29.4	30.1	Current tobacco smoking	18+	41.6
Peru	AMRO	Middle	4	4	25.5	137	42.6	-	Current cigarette smoking	15-49	-
Philippines	WPRO	Middle	22	8	54.5	838	46.8	47.4	Current tobacco smoking	15+	47.6
Poland	EURO	High	31	12	86.7	1,586	36.2	36.4	Current tobacco smoking	15+	36.9
Portugal	EURO	High	17	3	-	1,114	31.8	31.8	Daily tobacco smoking	15+	27.6
Qatar	EMRO	High	-	-	35.7	281	19.9	-	Daily tobacco use	18+	19.9
Romania	EURO	Middle	24	6	90.4	1,404	45.5	45.5	Current tobacco smoking	15+	40.3
Russian Federation	EURO	Middle	28	4	76.4	2,786	58.6	59.4	Current tobacco smoking	15+	60.2
Rwanda	AFRO	Low	1	0	19.2	94	-	-	Current cigarette smoking	15-49	-

FEMALE TOBACCO USE

PRODUCTS & THEIR USE

Current Cigarette Use	Currently Smoking ANY Tobacco Product	Type of Tobacco Use	Age Group	Crude Female Prevalence	TOTAL (MALE AND FEMALE) CRUDE TOBACCO USE: Type of Tobacco Use	Age Group	Crude Male and Female Prevalence	BOYS' & GIRLS' TOBACCO USE: Boys' Current Cigarette Use	Girls' Current Cigarette Use	Total Current Cigarette Use	COUNTRY
% 2009, Female Age Standardized (or country-specific data)		*Female Crude, Latest Available*	*years*	*%*	*Total Crude, Latest Available*	*years*	*% Total*	*% Ages 13–15*			
-	-	*Current cigarette smoking*	15-49	-	*Current cigarette smoking*	15-49	-	2.0**	1.2**	2.1**	Liberia
<1	<1	*Current tobacco smoking*	25-64	0.8	*Current tobacco smoking*	25-64	25.1	7.7	0.9	4.6	Libyan Arab Jamahiriya
22.0	22.0	*Current tobacco smoking*	20-64	17.4	*Current tobacco smoking*	20-64	27.7	33.8	25.9	29.6	Lithuania
30.4	-	*Current tobacco smoking*	15+	21.0	*Current tobacco smoking*	15+	24.0	-	-	-	Luxembourg
-	-	-	-	-	-	-	-	9.7	9.8	9.8	Macedonia (The former Yugoslav Republic of)
-	-	*Current tobacco smoking*	25-64	-	*Current tobacco smoking*	25-64	17.6	30.7	10.2	19.3	Madagascar
1.7	3.7	*Current tobacco smoking*	25-64	2.9	*Current tobacco smoking*	25-64	14.1	5.9	3.8	4.9	Malawi
1.9	2.4	*Current tobacco smoking*	18+	1.6	*Current tobacco smoking*	18+	21.5	36.3	4.2	20.2	Malaysia
6.6	11.5	*Current tobacco smoking*	25-64	11.8	*Current tobacco smoking*	25-64	-	15.0	3.6	9.1	Maldives
<1	2.2	*Current tobacco smoking*	15-64	2.0	*Current tobacco smoking*	15-64	13.5	17.4	2.5	10.4	Mali
21.1	21.1	*Current tobacco smoking*	15-79	21.4	*Current tobacco smoking*	15-79	25.7	-	-	-	Malta
7.0	7.0	*Occasional tobacco smoking*	15-64	1.8	*Occasional tobacco smoking*	15-64	3.3	-	-	-	Marshall Islands
<1	4.1	*Occasional tobacco smoking*	15-64	0.9	*Occasional tobacco smoking*	15-64	1.1	17.2	16.8	17.0	Mauritania
1.6	1.6	*Current tobacco smoking*	20-74	5.1	*Current cigarette smoking*	20-74	18.0	20.3	7.7	13.7	Mauritius
7.4	7.7	*Current tobacco smoking*	15+	7.8	*Current tobacco smoking*	15+	15.9	26.3**	27.1**	27.1**	Mexico
17.7	17.7	*Current tobacco smoking*	25-64	21.0	*Current tobacco smoking*	25-64	31.6	36.9	19.8	28.3	Micronesia (Federated States of)
5.2	5.2	*Current tobacco smoking*	15-49	7.1	*Current tobacco smoking*	see †	28.0	18.5	5.6	11.3	Moldova (Republic of)
-	-	-	-	-	-	-	-	-	-	-	Monaco
5.9	5.9	*Current tobacco smoking*	15-64	6.9	*Current tobacco smoking*	15-64	27.7	9.2	2.0	5.4	Mongolia
-	-	-	-	-	-	-	-	5.7	4.4	5.1	Montenegro
2.0	2.4	*Daily tobacco smoking*	18+	0.2	*Daily tobacco smoking*	18+	15.1	7.4	2.3	5.2	Morocco
1.1	2.3	*Current tobacco smoking*	25-64	6.4	*Current tobacco smoking*	25-64	18.7	4.5**	1.2**	2.7**	Mozambique
5.5	8.0	*Current tobacco smoking*	15-64	7.8	*Current tobacco smoking*	15-64	21.9	8.5	1.3	4.9	Myanmar
7.8	9.1	*Current cigarette smoking*	15-49	5.3	*Current cigarette smoking*	15-49	-	21.9	16.1	18.8	Namibia
50.0	50.0	*Current tobacco smoking*	15-64	56.0	*Current tobacco smoking*	15-64	52.9	-	-	-	Nauru
28.4	28.6	*Current tobacco smoking*	15-64	15.9	*Current tobacco smoking*	15-64	26.3	5.7	1.9	3.9	Nepal
22.1	26.2	*Current tobacco smoking*	15+	25.9	*Current tobacco smoking*	15+	-	19.1	20.8	20.0	Netherlands
23.7	23.7	*Current tobacco smoking*	15+	18.8	*Current tobacco smoking*	15+	19.9	14.5	20.6	17.6	New Zealand
5.3	-	*Current tobacco smoking*	15-49	5.3	*Current tobacco smoking*	15-49	-	25.6**	17.4**	21.2**	Nicaragua
<1	<1	*Current tobacco smoking*	15-64	1.0	*Current tobacco smoking*	15-64	-	11.7	1.1	6.3	Niger
<1	2.6	*Current cigarette smoking*	15-49	0.2	*Current cigarette smoking*	see †	-	5.6**	1.3**	3.5**	Nigeria
14.5	-	-	-	-	-	-	-	-	-	10.5	Niue
28.4	28.4	*Current tobacco smoking*	16-74	28.0	*Current tobacco smoking*	16-74	30.0	-	-	-	Norway
<1	<1	*Current tobacco smoking*	20+	0.5	*Current tobacco smoking*	20+	7.0	3.5	1.2	2.3	Oman
2.8	6.2	*Current tobacco smoking*	18+	5.7	*Current tobacco smoking*	18+	19.1	9.9	1.0	6.3	Pakistan
9.5	9.5	*Current tobacco smoking*	35-64	27.0	*Current tobacco smoking*	35-64	44.0	31.0	22.6	26.7	Palau
-	3.6	*Current tobacco smoking*	15+	4.0	*Current tobacco smoking*	15+	9.4	5.9	2.8	4.3	Panama
30.8	30.8	*Current tobacco smoking*	15-64	27.0	*Current tobacco smoking*	15-64	44.0	52.1	35.8	43.8	Papua New Guinea
12.6	13.9	*Current tobacco smoking*	18+	13.3	*Current tobacco smoking*	18+	27.3	11.3	5.5	8.3	Paraguay
8.8	9.1	*Current cigarette smoking*	15-49	6.9	*Current cigarette smoking*	15-49	-	22.9	11.9	17.3	Peru
9.9	10.2	*Current tobacco smoking*	15+	9.0	*Current tobacco smoking*	15+	28.3	16.0	6.4	11.0	Philippines
25.1	25.3	*Current tobacco smoking*	15+	24.4	*Current tobacco smoking*	15+	30.3	19.6	17.1	18.6	Poland
15.8	15.8	*Daily tobacco smoking*	15+	10.6	*Daily tobacco smoking*	15+	18.7	-	-	-	Portugal
2.2	-	*Daily tobacco use*	18+	2.2	*Daily tobacco use*	18+	11.1	13.4	2.3	6.5	Qatar
24.1	24.1	*Current tobacco smoking*	15+	25.1	*Current tobacco smoking*	15+	32.4	21.5	14.3	17.6	Romania
23.9	24.3	*Current tobacco smoking*	15+	21.7	*Current tobacco smoking*	15+	39.1	26.9	23.9	25.4	Russian Federation
0.3	-	*Current cigarette smoking*	15-49	0.3	*Current cigarette smoking*	15-49	-	3.0	0.9	1.8	Rwanda

*** Subnational data used ^ Countries classified as 'middle low income' or 'middle high income' by World Bank are classified here as 'middle' † See male/female crude data for age range*

COUNTRY			HARM			PRODUCTS & THEIR USE					
			DEATHS		SECONDHAND SMOKE	CIGARETTE CONSUMPTION	MALE TOBACCO USE				
	WHO REGION	World Bank Income Group^	Male Deaths	Female Deaths	Youth Exposed to Secondhand Smoke in Home	Per Capita Consumption	Current Cigarette Use	Currently Smoking ANY Tobacco Product	Type of Tobacco Use	Age Group	Crude Male Prevalence
			% 2004, Due to Tobacco (Estimates)		*% Ages 13–15*	*Cigarettes Per Person*	*% 2009, Male Age Standardized (or country-specific data)*		*Male Crude, Latest Available*	*years*	*%*
Saint Kitts and Nevis	AMRO	Middle	4	0	16.5	287	12.0	12.4	Current tobacco smoking	25-64	16.2
Saint Lucia	AMRO	Middle	4	2	25.2	249	24.3	27.7	Current cigarette smoking	25+	37.3
Saint Vincent and the Grenadines	AMRO	Middle	10	8	31.5	351	18.3	18.3	Current cigarette smoking	19+	26.4
Samoa	WPRO	Middle	4	1	59.1	34	58.0	58.0	Current tobacco smoking	25-64	56.9
San Marino	EURO	High	24	7	32.9	-	-	-	-	-	-
Sao Tome and Principe	AFRO	Middle	16	10	-	69	8.2	9.3	Current tobacco smoking	25-64	9.7
Saudi Arabia	EMRO	High	-	-	29.5	809	19.2	23.6	Current tobacco smoking	15-64	20.2
Senegal	AFRO	Middle	3	-	47.6	398	12.0	15.6	Current tobacco smoking	18+	22.2
Serbia	EURO	Middle	-	-	76.9	2,861	37.6	37.6	Daily tobacco smoking	20+	32.5
Seychelles	AFRO	Middle	7	2	42.3	565	21.1	24.3	Daily cigarette smoking	25-64	30.8
Sierra Leone	AFRO	Low	7	-	43.9**	177	30.3	38.6	Current tobacco smoking	25-64	43.1
Singapore	WPRO	High	24	18	35.1	547	33.2	35.2	Current cigarette smoking	18+	25.2
Slovakia	EURO	High	26	6	44.9	1,403	38.6	38.6	Current tobacco smoking	18+	40.8
Slovenia	EURO	High	27	11	62.8	2,369	29.8	29.8	Daily tobacco smoking	18+	23.1
Solomon Islands	WPRO	Middle	4	-	-	18	45.8	45.8	Current tobacco smoking	15-64	56.1
Somalia	EMRO	Low	7	1	29.1**	67	-	-	-	-	-
South Africa	AFRO	Middle	11	5	32.1	459	21.2	23.6	Current tobacco smoking	15+	35.1
Spain	EURO	High	25	2	-	1,757	36.2	36.2	Current tobacco smoking	16+	35.4
Sri Lanka	SEARO	Middle	13	0	35.4	195	21.2	26.9	Current tobacco smoking	15-64	29.9
Sudan	EMRO	Middle	1	0	27.5	75	20.5	23.8	Current tobacco smoking	25-64	29.1
Suriname	AMRO	Middle	9	4	49.7	57	17.0	-	Current cigarette smoking	12-65	38.4
Swaziland	AFRO	Middle	4	-	23.0	303	13.7	15.7	Current tobacco smoking	25-64	12.9
Sweden	EURO	High	10	9	-	715	12.8	-	Current tobacco smoking	16-84	25.0
Switzerland	EURO	High	17	8	-	1,722	30.5	30.5	Current tobacco smoking	14-65	31.0
Syrian Arab Republic	EMRO	Middle	-	-	60.1	1,013	35.5	41.5	Current cigarette smoking	18-65	62.0
Tajikistan	EURO	Low	4	3	51.5	1,046	-	-	-	-	-
Tanzania (United Republic of)	AFRO	Low	4	-	19.4**	132	17.4	21.4	Daily cigarette smoking	25-64	23.0
Thailand	SEARO	Middle	16	11	49.0	560	45.0	45.1	Current tobacco smoking	15+	45.6
Timor-Leste	SEARO	Middle	17	8	63.2	-	-	-	Current cigarette smoking	-	30.5
Togo	AFRO	Low	3	-	20.2	307	-	-	-	-	-
Tonga	WPRO	Middle	7	8	56.9	48	43.7	43.7	Current tobacco smoking	15-64	45.8
Trinidad and Tobago	AMRO	High	10	1	40.1	1,106	25.3	27.4	Current tobacco smoking	15+	29.8
Tunisia	EMRO	Middle	12	-	51.9	1,628	52.7	58.4	Daily tobacco smoking	35-70	53.1
Turkey	EURO	Middle	38	6	89.3	1,399	46.4	46.6	Current tobacco smoking	15+	47.9
Turkmenistan	EURO	Middle	19	3	-	135	-	-	-	-	-
Tuvalu	WPRO	Middle	16	12	76.6	29	50.8	50.8	Daily tobacco smoking	15+	54.6
Uganda	AFRO	Low	2	0	20.0	24	15.0	16.2	Current tobacco smoking	15-54	25.2
Ukraine	EURO	Middle	24	2	70.1	2,401	50.0	50.3	Current tobacco smoking	15+	50.0
United Arab Emirates	EMRO	High	-	-	25.3	583	14.9	18.7	Current tobacco smoking	18+	28.1
United Kingdom	EURO	High	22	20	44.9**	750	22.0	24.8	Current cigarette smoking	16-100	22.0
United States of America	AMRO	High	23	23	12.0	1,028	21.6	32.8	Current tobacco smoking	15+	31.2
Uruguay	AMRO	Middle	24	5	50.5	770	30.9	31.3	Current tobacco smoking	15+	30.7
Uzbekistan	EURO	Middle	10	3	17.3**	449	22.3	22.3	Current cigarette smoking	15+	20.0
Vanuatu	WPRO	Middle	9	7	59.3	43	41.7	43.0	Current tobacco smoking	15-64	46.5
Venezuela (Bolivarian Republic of)	AMRO	Middle	11	11	43.5	496	31.6	-	Current tobacco smoking	15+	22.6
Viet Nam	WPRO	Middle	-	-	58.5	1,001	40.0	48.2	Current tobacco smoking	15+	47.4
Yemen	EMRO	Middle	9	1	44.9	402	29.6	35.0	Current tobacco smoking	15+	34.5
Zambia	AFRO	Middle	4	-	23.1**	74	21.9	24.3	Current cigarette smoking	15-49	23.2
Zimbabwe	AFRO	Low	3	1	20.9**	189	24.8	29.8	Current cigarette smoking	15-49	21.3

PRODUCTS & THEIR USE

FEMALE TOBACCO USE					TOTAL (MALE AND FEMALE) CRUDE TOBACCO USE			BOYS' & GIRLS' TOBACCO USE			COUNTRY
Current Cigarette Use	Currently Smoking ANY Tobacco Product	Type of Tobacco Use	Age Group	Crude Female Prevalence	Type of Tobacco Use	Age Group	Crude Male and Female Prevalence	Boys' Current Cigarette Use	Girls' Current Cigarette Use	Total Current Cigarette Use	
% 2009, Female Age Standardized (or country-specific data)		*Female Crude, Latest Available*	*years*	*%*	*Total Crude, Latest Available*	*years*	*% Total*	*% Ages 13–15*			
2.2	2.4	Current tobacco smoking	25-64	1.1	Current tobacco smoking	25-64	-	7.0	1.9	4.6	Saint Kitts and Nevis
9.2	12.1	Current cigarette smoking	25+	5.6	Current cigarette smoking	25+	19.9	17.0	9.6	12.7	Saint Lucia
6.0	6.0	Current cigarette smoking	19+	3.5	Current cigarette smoking	19+	13.5	14.8	9.5	12.0	Saint Vincent and the Grenadines
23.0	23.0	Current tobacco smoking	25-64	21.8	Current tobacco smoking	25-64	-	16.0	12.7	15.2	Samoa
-	-	-	-	-	-	-	-	-	-	-	San Marino
<1	1.5	Current tobacco smoking	25-64	1.7	Current tobacco smoking	25-64	5.5	-	-	-	Sao Tome and Principe
<1	1.3	Current tobacco smoking	15-64	1.4	Current tobacco smoking	15-64	-	13.0	5.0	8.9	Saudi Arabia
<1	<1	Current tobacco smoking	18+	1.7	Current tobacco smoking	18+	11.6	12.1	2.7	7.5	Senegal
27.2	27.2	Daily tobacco smoking	20+	23.7	Daily tobacco smoking	20+	27.7	9.3	8.9	9.3	Serbia
2.0	4.6	Daily cigarette smoking	25-64	3.9	Daily cigarette smoking	25-64	17.4	23.2	20.0	21.5	Seychelles
1.1	8.2	Current tobacco smoking	25-64	10.5	Current tobacco smoking	25-64	25.8	6.3**	4.6**	5.4**	Sierra Leone
5.3	5.9	Current cigarette smoking	18+	4.2	Current cigarette smoking	18+	14.5	10.5	7.5	9.1	Singapore
19.1	19.1	Current tobacco smoking	18+	23.0	Current tobacco smoking	18+	30.5	26.5	23.4	25.0	Slovakia
21.7	21.7	Daily tobacco smoking	18+	15.9	Daily tobacco smoking	18+	19.4	15.2	23.0	20.3	Slovenia
18.9	18.9	Current tobacco smoking	15-64	26.1	Current tobacco smoking	15-64	41.4	28.3	18.4	24.0	Solomon Islands
-	-	-	-	-	-	-	-	4.9**	4.5**	5.8**	Somalia
7.2	8.4	Current tobacco smoking	15+	10.2	Current tobacco smoking	15+	-	17.9	10.6	13.6	South Africa
27.2	27.2	Current tobacco smoking	16+	24.6	Current tobacco smoking	16+	29.9	17.0	20.8	18.9	Spain
<1	<1	Current tobacco smoking	15-64	0.4	Current tobacco smoking	15-64	15.0	1.6	0.9	1.2	Sri Lanka
1.2	2.1	Current tobacco smoking	25-64	3.5	Current tobacco smoking	25-64	14.0	10.2	2.1	6.0	Sudan
2.8	-	Current cigarette smoking	12-65	9.9	Current cigarette smoking	12-65	-	12.5	8.6	10.4	Suriname
1.6	1.8	Current tobacco smoking	25-64	2.2	Current tobacco smoking	25-64	7.1	8.9	3.2	5.6	Swaziland
15.7	-	Current tobacco smoking	16-84	23.0	Current tobacco smoking	16-84	24.0	5.0	13.0	9.0	Sweden
20.6	20.6	Current tobacco smoking	14-65	23.0	Current tobacco smoking	14-65	27.0	35.7	29.6	32.7	Switzerland
-	-	Current cigarette smoking	18-65	21.0	Current cigarette smoking	18-65	-	16.2	4.8	10.6	Syrian Arab Republic
-	-	-	-	-	-	-	-	1.1	0.6	0.9	Tajikistan
1.2	2.9	Daily cigarette smoking	25-64	1.3	Daily cigarette smoking	25-64	-	4.6**	0.7**	2.6**	Tanzania (United Republic of)
2.7	3.0	Current tobacco smoking	15+	3.1	Current tobacco smoking	15+	23.7	15.8	2.4	8.8	Thailand
-	-	Current cigarette smoking	-	1.3	Current cigarette smoking	-	23.4	50.6	17.3	32.4	Timor-Leste
-	-	-	-	-	-	-	-	9.1	1.7	6.2	Togo
12.9	12.9	Current tobacco smoking	15-64	12.0	Current tobacco smoking	15-64	28.7	37.5	21.1	31.1	Tonga
10.0	11.2	Current tobacco smoking	15+	5.1	Current tobacco smoking	15+	21.1	14.7	10.3	12.9	Trinidad and Tobago
3.6	5.3	Daily tobacco smoking	35-70	6.6	Daily tobacco smoking	35-70	29.6	12.7	2.7	7.5	Tunisia
14.5	14.5	Current tobacco smoking	15+	15.2	Current tobacco smoking	15+	31.2	9.4	3.5	6.9	Turkey
19.5	-	-	-	-	-	-	-	-	-	-	Turkmenistan
20.1	20.1	Daily tobacco smoking	15+	22.7	Daily tobacco smoking	15+	37.9	33.2	22.1	26.6	Tuvalu
1.4	2.9	Current tobacco smoking	15-49	3.3	Current tobacco smoking	see †	-	6.6	4.0	5.5	Uganda
13.1	13.2	Current tobacco smoking	15+	11.3	Current tobacco smoking	15+	28.8	27.6	20.6	24.0	Ukraine
<1	1.7	Current tobacco smoking	18+	2.4	Current tobacco smoking	18+	20.5	15.6	5.8	9.8	United Arab Emirates
21.0	23.4	Current cigarette smoking	16-100	21.0	Current cigarette smoking	16-100	21.0	4.0	6.0	5.0	United Kingdom
17.4	24.7	Current tobacco smoking	15+	23.0	Current tobacco smoking	15+	27.0	9.7	7.9	8.8	United States of America
21.9	21.9	Current tobacco smoking	15+	19.8	Current tobacco smoking	15+	25.0	16.4	22.9	20.2	Uruguay
3.5	3.5	Current cigarette smoking	15+	1.1	Current cigarette smoking	15+	10.0	2.4**	1.2**	1.8**	Uzbekistan
6.3	7.6	Current tobacco smoking	15-64	10.1	Current tobacco smoking	15-64	26.2	28.2	11.4	18.2	Vanuatu
26.5	-	Current tobacco smoking	15+	13.6	Current tobacco smoking	15+	18.0	6.0	8.4	7.4	Venezuela (Bolivarian Republic of)
1.3	1.5	Current tobacco smoking	15+	1.4	Current tobacco smoking	15+	23.8	5.9	1.2	3.3	Viet Nam
10.2	10.8	Current tobacco smoking	15+	12.8	Current tobacco smoking	15+	23.7	4.2	1.6	3.9	Yemen
1.8	3.8	Current cigarette smoking	15-49	0.7	Current cigarette smoking	15-49	-	6.7**	6.8**	6.8**	Zambia
2.0	4.3	Current cigarette smoking	15-49	0.4	Current cigarette smoking	15-49	-	4.8**	1.5**	3.2**	Zimbabwe

*** Subnational data used* *^ Countries classified as "middle low income" or "middle high income" by World Bank are classified here as "middle"* *† See male/female crude data for age range*

COUNTRY	SMOKELESS TOBACCO	HEALTH PROFESSIONALS		CIGARETTE PRICES	AFFORDABILITY OF CIGARETTES	MANUFACTURING CIGARETTES	ILLICIT CIGARETTES	TOBACCO TAXES	GROWING TOBACCO
	PRODUCTS & THEIR USE			PRICES		TOBACCO INDUSTRY			
	Adult Smokeless Tobacco Use	Smoking Prevalence of Health Professional Students	Student Type	Cigarette Prices	Relative Income Price	Production	Illicit Share of the Total Cigarette Market	Excise Tax as % of Cigarette Price	Tobacco Area Harvested
	%	%		*per pack in USD*	*2010*	*in billion pieces*	%	%	*hectares, 2000*
Afghanistan	-	18.3**	Medical	2.25	8.46	-		0.0	-
Albania	0.9	10.2	Dental	1.91	2.35	0.10	23.0	33.3	5,700
Algeria	5.7	9.0	Medical	4.15	2.58	30.12	14.6	40.2	6,450
Andorra	-	-	-	3.13	-	-	-	2.5	-
Angola	-	-	-	2.68	-	3.90	-	16.0	3,473
Antigua and Barbuda	-	-	-	2.31	1.87	-	-	0.0	-
Argentina	-	35.5	Medical	1.67	1.47	39.67	4.6	68.8	59,612
Armenia	1.3	45.6	Medical	1.42	5.17	3.30	15.6	18.1	2,528
Australia	0.6	-	-	12.14	1.73	24.46	3.4	54.7	3,185
Austria	0.2	-	-	6.20	1.09	10.00	13.6	58.9	111
Azerbaijan	0.1	-	-	1.88	1.45	2.19	7.9	9.3	8,177
Bahamas	-	2.6	Nursing	5.49	1.23	-	-	31.2	-
Bahrain	-	10.9	Medical	1.84	0.91	-	-	0.0	-
Bangladesh	27.2	19.5	Medical	1.68	10.06	23.68	4.4	53.0	31,161
Barbados	0.3	2.0	Nursing	6.00	3.84	-	5.9	34.2	-
Belarus	-	-	-	0.84	1.44	25.10	1.4	10.0	-
Belgium	-	-	-	6.97	1.42	-	5.0	59.5	400
Belize	-	15.2	Nursing	2.50	6.01	0.01	2.6	10.0	
Benin	9.2	-	-	1.98	14.68	-	-	25.4	1,007
Bhutan	19.4	-	-	-	-	-	-	-	110
Bolivia (Plurinational State of)	-	41.2	Medical	1.56	4.64	1.97	45.0	29.0	1,060
Bosnia and Herzegovina	-	47.0	Medical	2.66	3.61	5.68	7.9	55.2	3,204
Botswana	-	-	-	2.52	3.48	-	-	39.1	-
Brazil	0.4	16.9**	Medical	2.73	2.10	96.97	16.0	26.3	309,989
Brunei Darussalam	-	-	-	2.36	0.47	-	-	63.2	-
Bulgaria	0.0	45.0	Medical	3.29	2.56	17.25	34.0	68.9	28,523
Burkina Faso	-	-	-	1.39	24.03	0.73	19.0	6.9	1,000
Burundi	-	-	-	3.25	36.09	0.47	-	36.3	705
Cambodia	7.3	6.4	Medical	1.03	4.06	4.50	5.0	10.7	9,669
Cameroon	-	-	-	2.03	25.73	1.22	15.2	9.2	3,400
Canada	1.3	6.0	Medical	10.51	1.60	23.38	14.0	58.0	23,800
Cape Verde	4.6	-	-	2.95	7.62	-	-	4.9	-
Central African Republic	-	-	-	3.84	14.48	-	-	13.3	750
Chad	1.2	-	-	1.98	13.17	-	-	13.5	145
Chile	-	28.4	Medical	3.80	1.82	20.19	1.6	60.4	3,508
China	0.5	11.9	Medical	2.25	2.93	2356.27	7.6	26.2	1,441,537
Colombia	-	-	-	1.75	1.60	17.25	17.6	40.3	14,692
Comoros	-	-	-	2.64	16.56	0.00	-	54.4	-
Congo	-	-	-	1.98	3.39	0.01	1.0	16.3	600
Congo (Democratic Republic of)	9.1	-	-	3.33	59.19	6.50	-	24.9	7,958
Cook Islands	-	-	-	8.80	-	0.00	-	0.0	-
Costa Rica	0.5	32.8	Medical	1.53	1.94	1.69	47.5	44.2	117
Côte d'Ivoire	-	1.9	Medical	2.13	15.62	3.60	15.0	21.4	20,000
Croatia	0.4	36.6**	Medical	3.95	2.39	12.50	17.6	53.0	5,678
Cuba	-	29.5**	Medical	3.11	-	14.40	-	87.1	45,323
Cyprus	-	-	-	6.13	1.33	0.97	5.0	64.5	76
Czech Republic	2.1	21.6	Medical	4.33	1.86	27.80	10.0	62.0	-
Denmark	2.0	-	-	6.94	1.17	12.00	1.0	60.9	-
Djibouti	-	-	-	1.13	8.14	-	-	30.7	-

TOBACCO INDUSTRY						TOBACCO MARKETING				COUNTRY
Tobacco Area Harvested	Percent Change in Tobacco Area Harvested	Tobacco Production	Tobacco Production	Percent Change in Tobacco Production	Agricultural Land on Which Tobacco Is Grown	Youth Who Have an Object With a Tobacco Logo on It			Population	
hectares, 2009	*2000–2009*	*tonnes, 2000*	*tonnes, 2009*	*2000–2009*	*2008, % of total agricultural land*	*% Boys, Ages 13–15*	*% Girls, Ages 13–15*	*% Youth, Ages 13–15*	*as of 2009, in thousands*	
-	-	-	-	-	-	11.7**	9.4**	11.4**	28,150	Afghanistan
1,200	-78.9	6,200	1,600	-74.2	0.09	19.4	16.2	17.7	3,155	Albania
4,594	-28.8	7,153	7,668	7.2	0.01	10.6**	8.8**	9.8**	34,895	Algeria
-	-	-	-	-	-	-	-	-	86	Andorra
4,170	20.1	3,300	5,805	75.9	0.01	-	-	-	18,498	Angola
-	-	-	-	-	-	10.7	11.9	11.8	88	Antigua and Barbuda
74,546	25.1	114,509	159,495	39.3	0.07	13.6	10.7	12.1	40,276	Argentina
297	-88.3	4,577	1,055	-76.9	0.01	17.5	14.2	15.6	3,083	Armenia
0	-100.0	7,762	4,315	-44.4	0.00	-	-	-	21,293	Australia
0	-100.0	230	0	-100.0	-	-	-	-	8,364	Austria
1,200	-85.3	17,258	2,609	-84.9	0.02	-	-	-	8,832	Azerbaijan
-	-	-	-	-	-	16.2	14.3	15.6	342	Bahamas
-	-	-	-	-	-	24.8	21.7	23.3	791	Bahrain
29,869	-4.1	35,000	40,265	15.0	0.31	15.3	10.9	12.8	162,221	Bangladesh
-	-	-	-	-	-	19.4	12.3	15.7	256	Barbados
-	-	-	-	-	-	17.2	9.8	13.5	9,634	Belarus
64	-84.0	1,200	153	-87.3	0.00	-	-	-	10,647	Belgium
-	-	-	-	-	-	8.7	10.4	9.6	307	Belize
143	-85.8	679	93	-86.3	0.02	19.1**	20.8**	20.0**	8,935	Benin
97	-11.8	144	128	-11.1	0.02	11.9	9.2	10.5	697	Bhutan
916	-13.6	975	1,284	31.7	0.00	15.9**	14.5**	15.3**	9,863	Bolivia (Plurinational State of)
1,614	-49.6	3,277	2,424	-26.0	0.09	22.1	15.9	18.9	3,767	Bosnia and Herzegovina
-	-	-	-	-	-	12.3	9.6	10.7	1,950	Botswana
442,397	42.7	578,451	863,079	49.2	0.16	6.9**	5.4**	6.2**	193,734	Brazil
-	-	-	-	-	-	-	-	-	400	Brunei Darussalam
27,870	-2.3	32,296	51,322	58.9	0.49	17.2	15.4	16.4	7,545	Bulgaria
1,098	9.8	500	791	58.2	0.01	22.1**	23.6**	23.0**	15,757	Burkina Faso
1,497	112.3	762	1,209	58.7	0.04	17.6	13.0	15.3	8,303	Burundi
9,269	-4.1	7,665	18,599	142.6	0.17	16.3**	11.7**	13.8**	14,805	Cambodia
4,173	22.7	4,700	7,112	51.3	0.04	14.4**	12.6**	13.5**	19,522	Cameroon
16,414	-31.0	53,010	45,991	-13.2	0.02	-	-	-	33,573	Canada
-	-	-	-	-	-	15.7	10.2	12.5	506	Cape Verde
715	-4.7	652	759	16.4	0.01	15.8**	32.8**	24.3**	4,422	Central African Republic
221	52.4	184	237	28.8	0.00	28.9	33.7	30.3	11,206	Chad
1,652	-52.9	10,521	5,626	-46.5	0.01	9.9**	8.6**	9.3**	16,970	Chile
1,391,703	-3.5	2,563,850	3,067,928	19.7	0.25	10.8**	8.3**	9.5**	1,353,311	China
12,768	-13.1	27,767	21,048	-24.2	0.03	11.9**	9.4**	10.5**	45,660	Colombia
-	-	-	-	-	-	22.2	18.1	20.1	676	Comoros
1,029	71.5	200	460	130.0	0.01	24.3	18.8	21.7	3,683	Congo
7,800	-2.0	4,210	5,628	33.7	0.04	19.8**	23.8**	21.9**	66,020	Congo (Democratic Republic of)
-	-	-	-	-	-	14.2	18.0	16.2	20	Cook Islands
44	-62.4	187	62	-66.8	0.00	11.4	7.3	9.3	4,579	Costa Rica
17,799	-11.0	10,200	10,171	-0.3	0.10	15.6	11.4	13.7	21,075	Côte d'Ivoire
6,062	6.8	9,714	13,348	37.4	0.46	15.2	13.3	14.3	4,416	Croatia
24,861	-45.1	32,237	25,200	-21.8	0.35	9.1	10.8	10.0	11,204	Cuba
10	-86.8	374	323	-13.6	0.09	18.3	8.2	13.0	871	Cyprus
-	-	-	-	-	-	17.1	16.6	16.9	10,369	Czech Republic
-	-	-	-	-	-	-	-	-	5,470	Denmark
-	-	-	-	-	-	23.9	27.4	25.5	864	Djibouti

*** Subnational data used*

COUNTRY	SMOKELESS TOBACCO	HEALTH PROFESSIONALS		CIGARETTE PRICES	AFFORDABILITY OF CIGARETTES	MANUFACTURING CIGARETTES	ILLICIT CIGARETTES	TOBACCO TAXES	GROWING TOBACCO
	PRODUCTS & THEIR USE			PRICES		TOBACCO INDUSTRY			
	Adult Smokeless Tobacco Use	Smoking Prevalence of Health Professional Students	Student Type	Cigarette Prices	Relative Income Price	Production	Illicit Share of the Total Cigarette Market	Excise Tax as % of Cigarette Price	Tobacco Area Harvested
	%	*%*		*per pack in USD*	*2010*	*in billion pieces*	*%*	*%*	*hectares, 2000*
Dominica	-	-	-	3.83	2.51	-	-	12.6	-
Dominican Republic	0.8	-	-	3.24	6.23	1.95	29.5	43.3	13,250
Ecuador	-	-	-	2.50	5.02	3.10	14.8	53.6	4,174
Egypt	2.6	7.9	Medical	1.69	2.92	82.00	0.3	73.8	-
El Salvador	-	-	-	2.25	4.73	0.00	11.7	43.3	580
Equatorial Guinea	-	-	-	2.12	-	-	-	19.4	-
Eritrea	2.9	-	-	3.90	98.12	-	-	44.6	-
Estonia	-	-	-	3.33	1.88	0.00	36.2	67.8	-
Ethiopia	1.3	-	-	1.57	15.48	3.40	38.0	43.0	4,700
Fiji	-	11.3	Medical	2.70	-	0.04	4.7	76.9	300
Finland	2.0	-	-	7.61	1.49	0.00	5.8	60.1	-
France	1.4	34.6	Medical	8.31	1.68	18.42	12.8	64.3	9,282
Gabon	1.0	-	-	1.99	2.31	-	-	6.6	-
Gambia	1.1	-	-	1.05	5.93	-	14.0	30.0	-
Georgia	0.6	17.1	Medical	2.71	2.74	2.55	9.0	46.2	1,801
Germany	-	27.5	Medical	6.86	1.53	225.00	8.4	60.7	4,576
Ghana	0.8	4.3	Medical	2.78	10.66	1.50	10.0	14.0	3,950
Greece	0.6	28.8	Medical	5.21	1.46	31.25	7.0	65.0	61,000
Grenada	-	2.5	Nursing	4.14	4.33	-	-	34.0	-
Guatemala	-	73.0	Medical	1.89	5.54	3.77	13.9	46.0	8,374
Guinea	1.4	-	-	0.98	7.75	-	-	11.1	3,470
Guinea-Bissau	-	-	-	1.00	11.93	-	85.0	16.1	-
Guyana	2.5	3.8	Medical	3.16	5.13	-	1.8	16.3	91
Haiti	1.3	-	-	1.66	-	-	-	-	400
Honduras	-	-	-	1.59	7.06	6.18	-	25.9	11,214
Hungary	0.6	-	-	3.56	1.82	5.99	12.4	60.6	5,764
Iceland	2.9	-	-	8.23	1.66	0.00	-	36.1	-
India	25.9	13.4	Medical	2.03	13.22	100.00	10.0	27.7	433,400
Indonesia	1.3	8.6	Medical	1.40	4.56	180.50	8.1	45.7	168,300
Iran (Islamic Republic of)	-	5.6	Medical	2.03	1.56	28.00	28.7	0.0	19,685
Iraq	0.9	19.2	Medical	2.56	2.50	4.40	22.9	0.0	2,400
Ireland	1.3	12.0	Dental	10.92	2.25	-	33.2	61.6	-
Israel	-	-	-	5.26	1.28	1.59	2.8	68.0	0
Italy	0.6	20.0	Medical	6.48	1.48	13.29	2.4	58.3	38,788
Jamaica	-	6.7	Medical	8.73	13.21	-	7.7	36.2	1,163
Japan	-	38.0	Nursing	5.34	0.80	158.50	0.1	58.3	23,991
Jordan	-	43.9	Nursing	2.39	4.07	16.09	11.0	61.2	3,069
Kazakhstan	-	-	-	1.09	0.65	24.26	1.1	16.0	8,900
Kenya	1.7	9.8	Medical	3.01	28.10	15.24	12.0	50.0	14,160
Kiribati	-	16.7	Nursing	7.19	48.33	-	-	0.0	-
Korea (Democratic People's Republic of)	0.0	-	-	-	-	15.50	-	-	44,000
Korea (Republic of)	-	17.5	Medical	2.24	1.05	124.63	0.4	52.9	24,300
Kuwait	-	5.3	Medical	1.79	0.45	0.00	0.9	0.0	-
Kyrgyzstan	3.4	36.6	Medical	0.74	6.04	3.60	31.8	7.6	14,465
Lao People's Democratic Republic	7.9	6.0	Medical	1.40	6.00	2.73	8.8	20.4	6,700
Latvia	0.8	40.3	Medical	3.33	2.68	0.02	35.3	63.2	-
Lebanon	-	28.2	Medical	1.50	1.49	0.56	22.5	36.6	8,726
Lesotho	5.4	-	-	3.82	45.65	-	-	27.5	-

TOBACCO INDUSTRY						TOBACCO MARKETING				COUNTRY
Tobacco Area Harvested	Percent Change in Tobacco Area Harvested	Tobacco Production	Tobacco Production	Percent Change in Tobacco Production	Agricultural Land on Which Tobacco Is Grown	Youth Who Have an Object With a Tobacco Logo on It			Population	
hectares, 2009	*2000–2009*	*tonnes, 2000*	*tonnes, 2009*	*2000–2009*	*2008, % of total agricultural land*	*% Boys, Ages 13–15*	*% Girls, Ages 13–15*	*% Youth, Ages 13–15*	*as of 2009, in thousands*	
-	-	-	-	-	-	15.9	14.6	16.0	67	Dominica
11,000	-17.0	17,229	11,800	-31.5	0.36	11.4	9.5	10.7	10,090	Dominican Republic
3,903	-6.5	5,080	8,087	59.2	0.06	16.9**	8.7**	12.6**	13,625	Ecuador
-	-	-	-	-	-	15.2	10.0	13.2	82,999	Egypt
781	34.7	1,050	1,496	42.5	0.04	11.0	7.9	9.1	6,163	El Salvador
-	-	-	-	-	-	11.2	9.8	10.6	676	Equatorial Guinea
-	-	-	-	-	-	19.1	16.5	18.1	5,073	Eritrea
-	-	-	-	-	-	18.1	16.7	17.3	1,340	Estonia
6,224	32.4	3,300	4,820	46.1	0.01	15.2**	10.2**	12.6**	82,825	Ethiopia
650	116.7	313	343	9.6	0.12	12.0	14.3	13.1	849	Fiji
-	-	-	-	-	-	-	-	-	5,326	Finland
6,707	-27.8	25,252	17,838	-29.4	0.02	-	-	-	62,343	France
-	-	-	-	-	-	-	-	-	1,475	Gabon
-	-	-	-	-	-	28.4	31.9	31.4	1,705	Gambia
700	-61.0	1,855	100	-94.6	0.03	18.4	11.2	14.6	4,260	Georgia
3,091	-32.5	10,985	8,223	-25.1	0.02	-	-	-	82,167	Germany
6,015	52.3	1,350	4,069	201.4	0.04	17.4	13.2	15.4	23,837	Ghana
15,700	-74.3	136,593	27,501	-79.9	0.35	23.0	15.8	19.6	11,161	Greece
-	-	-	-	-	-	16.6	7.9	11.6	104	Grenada
8,376	0.0	18,630	20,158	8.2	0.23	-	-	-	14,027	Guatemala
2,196	-36.7	3,851	2,863	-25.7	0.02	30.1	25.6	28.6	10,069	Guinea
-	-	-	-	-	-	20.0**	19.0**	19.5**	1,611	Guinea–Bissau
115	26.4	90	119	32.2	0.01	14.1	11.4	13.0	762	Guyana
518	29.5	550	605	10.0	0.03	17.6**	14.9**	15.9**	10,033	Haiti
4,189	-62.6	5,035	6,098	21.1	0.14	11.8**	13.6**	12.8**	7,466	Honduras
5,918	2.7	10,485	6,679	-36.3	0.10	15.9	15.1	15.8	9,993	Hungary
-	-	-	-	-	-	-	-	-	323	Iceland
390,000	-10.0	520,000	620,000	19.2	0.21	-	-	-	1,198,003	India
232,160	37.9	146,100	181,319	24.1	0.41	14.3	6.8	10.3	229,965	Indonesia
7,993	-59.4	20,980	8,826	-57.9	0.02	9.9	8.8	9.3	74,196	Iran (Islamic Republic of)
2,320	-3.3	2,250	2,156	-4.2	0.03	15.0**	10.8**	13.2**	30,747	Iraq
-	-	-	-	-	-	-	-	-	4,515	Ireland
0	-	0	0	-	-	-	-	-	7,170	Israel
30,743	-20.7	129,937	119,119	-8.3	0.24	15.4	11.0	13.2	59,870	Italy
1,305	12.2	1,920	1,893	-1.4	0.26	15.4	11.9	14.0	2,719	Jamaica
15,800	-34.1	60,803	36,600	-39.8	0.36	-	-	-	127,156	Japan
2,667	-13.1	2,668	1,961	-26.5	0.30	17.2	18.9	18.6	6,316	Jordan
4,000	-55.0	16,160	9,000	-44.3	0.00	15.8	9.7	12.6	15,637	Kazakhstan
17,000	20.1	17,960	13,605	-24.2	0.05	17.1	17.2	17.6	39,802	Kenya
-	-	-	-	-	-	28.3	21.0	24.2	98	Kiribati
48,795	10.9	63,000	80,324	27.5	1.53	-	-	-	23,906	Korea (Democratic People's Republic of)
13,222	-45.6	68,198	42,075	-38.3	0.83	8.1	6.6	7.4	48,333	Korea (Republic of)
-	-	-	-	-	-	17.7	14.3	16.0	2,985	Kuwait
4,850	-66.5	34,613	12,005	-65.3	0.05	17.2	19.1	18.2	5,482	Kyrgyzstan
5,513	-17.7	39,926	25,966	-35.0	0.25	15.6**	14.4**	15.0**	6,320	Lao People's Democratic Republic
-	-	-	-	-	-	31.2**	24.9**	27.8	2,249	Latvia
8,217	-5.8	10,800	9,010	-16.6	1.24	-	-	-	4,224	Lebanon
-	-	-	-	-	-	16.7	14.3	16.3	2,067	Lesotho

*** Subnational data used*

COUNTRY	SMOKELESS TOBACCO	HEALTH PROFESSIONALS		CIGARETTE PRICES	AFFORDABILITY OF CIGARETTES	MANUFACTURING CIGARETTES	ILLICIT CIGARETTES	TOBACCO TAXES	GROWING TOBACCO
	PRODUCTS & THEIR USE			PRICES		TOBACCO INDUSTRY			
	Adult Smokeless Tobacco Use	Smoking Prevalence of Health Professional Students	Student Type	Cigarette Prices	Relative Income Price	Production	Illicit Share of the Total Cigarette Market	Excise Tax as % of Cigarette Price	Tobacco Area Harvested
	%	*%*		*per pack in USD*	*2010*	*in billion pieces*	*%*	*%*	*hectares, 2000*
Liberia	2.4	-	-	1.04	30.52	-	23.0	6.8	-
Libyan Arab Jamahiriya	1.2	10.1	Medical	1.97	0.71	4.30	80.0	2.0	666
Lithuania	-	67.7	Medical	3.35	2.64	18.10	25.0	60.4	-
Luxembourg	-	-	-	6.20	0.43	4.25	-	57.2	-
Macedonia (The former Yugoslav Republic of)	-	72.5	Medical	2.87	2.42	6.89	7.7	39.0	22,785
Madagascar	22.1	-	-	2.30	23.73	5.36	4.4	59.6	2,807
Malawi	3.5	-	-	-	-	-	1.9	37.3	118,752
Malaysia	0.6	-	-	3.30	2.88	52.10	39.9	47.5	9,129
Maldives	6.8	-	-	1.56	2.54	0.00	-	0.0	-
Mali	2.7	-	-	0.99	20.47	-	40.0	5.9	372
Malta	-	15.3	Medical	3.08	2.69	0.00	6.0	61.9	-
Marshall Islands	65.1	-	-	3.50	-	-	-	0.0	-
Mauritania	9.0	-	-	1.51	12.14	-	6.0	0.0	-
Mauritius	-	-	-	3.31	3.21	-	-	58.7	397
Mexico	0.3	35.3	Medical	2.50	1.74	43.70	6.1	48.9	22,674
Micronesia (Federated States of)	11.4	-	-	2.25	-	0.00	-	25.0	-
Moldova (Republic of)	0.0	23.0	Nursing	1.38	1.46	1.96	3.9	13.5	23,537
Monaco	-	-	-	7.30	-	-	-	0.0	-
Mongolia	1.7	19.9	Medical	1.18	5.00	0.00	0.0	21.7	-
Montenegro	-	-	-	2.29	-	0.24	5.5	50.4	-
Morocco	-	8.7	Medical	3.98	3.95	13.70	11.8	50.6	4,570
Mozambique	6.9	3.4	Medical	2.05	9.88	2.01	10.4	45.8	9,000
Myanmar	29.6	13.4	Medical	-	11.00	9.47	7.0	50.0	33,185
Namibia	2.1	-	-	3.95	6.51	-	-	33.2	-
Nauru	-	-	-	4.46	-	-	-	0.0	-
Nepal	18.6	23.7	Medical	1.21	16.68	13.10	-	17.2	4,283
Netherlands	-	-	-	7.12	1.35	115.30	9.5	62.7	-
New Zealand	-	-	-	10.35	2.73	0.94	3.2	61.2	0
Nicaragua	-	-	-	1.50	11.62	0.10	10.0	16.1	934
Niger	1.9	37.7	Medical	1.98	26.54	-	-	10.1	6,200
Nigeria	2.1	-	-	1.43	9.66	17.00	6.7	15.9	37,000
Niue	-	-	-	7.21	-	-	-	0.0	-
Norway	10.0	-	-	15.11	1.51	-	4.1	52.3	-
Oman	-	2.3	Nursing	1.67	0.91	-	-	0.0	270
Pakistan	4.9	-	-	1.23	9.09	70.00	27.5	47.9	56,400
Palau	-	-	-	4.50	-	0.00	-	0.0	-
Panama	-	58.8	Medical	3.25	4.28	0.00	28.6	42.4	1,100
Papua New Guinea	-	34.9	Nursing	4.86	-	-	11.6	26.3	-
Paraguay	7.5	25.7**	Medical	1.34	2.26	26.40	5.0	7.4	3,235
Peru	-	34.9**	Medical	2.53	3.07	0.00	18.8	31.1	4,900
Philippines	2.0	20.6	Medical	0.74	2.65	93.81	19.9	52.0	41,051
Poland	0.5	76.8	Medical	3.93	2.55	142.86	8.5	66.1	14,057
Portugal	0.0	-	-	5.35	2.22	25.00	6.3	63.0	2,118
Qatar	4.0	-	-	1.79	0.23	-	1.1	0.0	-
Romania	-	-	-	3.79	4.13	28.54	26.3	62.6	11,300
Russian Federation	0.6	38.9	Medical	1.74	0.93	402.70	0.5	19.7	1,840
Rwanda	2.6	-	-	2.04	15.25	-	-	50.8	3,634

TOBACCO INDUSTRY						TOBACCO MARKETING				COUNTRY
Tobacco Area Harvested	Percent Change in Tobacco Area Harvested	Tobacco Production	Tobacco Production	Percent Change in Tobacco Production	Agricultural Land on Which Tobacco Is Grown	Youth Who Have an Object With a Tobacco Logo on It			Population	
hectares, 2009	*2000–2009*	*tonnes, 2000*	*tonnes, 2009*	*2000–2009*	*2008, % of total agricultural land*	*% Boys, Ages 13–15*	*% Girls, Ages 13–15*	*% Youth, Ages 13–15*	*as of 2009, in thousands*	
-	-	-	-	-	-	16.0**	16.5**	16.3**	3,955	Liberia
598	-10.2	1,500	1,416	-5.6	0.00	13.9	8.6	11.3	6,420	Libyan Arab Jamahiriya
-	-	-	-	-	-	20.7	12.2	16.2	3,287	Lithuania
-	-	-	-	-	-	-	-	-	486	Luxembourg
17,800	-21.9	22,175	24,122	8.8	1.59	26.5	21.5	24.1	2,042	Macedonia (The former Yugoslav Republic of)
2,720	-3.1	2,204	1,952	-11.4	0.00	4.7	7.5	6.2	19,625	Madagascar
183,052	54.1	98,675	208,155	111.0	2.95	20.8	20.5	20.6	15,263	Malawi
14,406	57.8	7,172	14,445	101.4	0.17	18.5	11.0	14.7	27,468	Malaysia
-	-	-	-	-	-	9.6	6.4	8.1	309	Maldives
1,188	219.4	446	1,410	216.1	0.00	15.4	11.8	13.9	13,010	Mali
-	-	-	-	-	-	-	-	-	409	Malta
-	-	-	-	-	-	13.8	20.6	17.6	62	Marshall Islands
-	-	-	-	-	-	30.4	24.8	27.8	3,291	Mauritania
238	-40.1	563	314	-44.2	0.26	-	-	-	1,288	Mauritius
4,312	-81.0	45,164	7,822	-82.7	0.01	23.3**	19.0**	20.9**	109,610	Mexico
-	-	-	-	-	-	28.8	21.7	25.1	111	Micronesia (Federated States of)
2,517	-89.3	25,306	4,400	-82.6	0.11	10.2	6.1	8.0	3,604	Moldova (Republic of)
-	-	-	-	-	-	-	-	-	33	Monaco
-	-	-	-	-	-	12.2	7.9	9.9	2,671	Mongolia
126	-	-	272	-	0.03	22.6	18.0	20.2	624	Montenegro
795	-82.6	5,333	2,000	-62.5	0.01	11.1	7.8	9.7	31,993	Morocco
60,000	566.7	9,470	75,660	698.9	0.07	16.3**	11.9**	14.3**	22,894	Mozambique
12,000	-63.8	50,900	18,000	-64.6	0.17	9.5	7.7	8.6	50,020	Myanmar
-	-	-	-	-	-	16.6	15.2	16.0	2,171	Namibia
-	-	-	-	-	-	-	-	-	10	Nauru
2,542	-40.6	3,809	2,497	-34.4	0.06	12.9	8.0	10.7	29,331	Nepal
-	-	-	-	-	-	-	-	-	16,592	Netherlands
0	-	0	0	-	-	-	-	-	4,266	New Zealand
1,841	97.1	1,479	2,952	99.6	0.04	15.1**	10.1**	12.5**	5,743	Nicaragua
789	-87.3	4,422	913	-79.4	0.00	28.3	31.6	29.9	15,290	Niger
20,358	-45.0	22,000	14,103	-35.9	0.02	18.1**	13.8**	16.1**	154,729	Nigeria
-	-	-	-	-	-	-	-	22.3	1	Niue
-	-	-	-	-	-	-	-	-	4,812	Norway
268	-0.7	1,300	1,314	1.1	0.02	11.9	12.5	12.4	2,845	Oman
49,676	-11.9	107,700	104,996	-2.5	0.20	8.9**	14.5**	11.4**	180,808	Pakistan
-	-	-	-	-	-	9.5	9.7	9.6	20	Palau
1,428	29.8	1,800	2,627	45.9	0.07	8.7	4.5	6.4	3,454	Panama
-	-	-	-	-	-	20.3	18.0	18.9	6,732	Papua New Guinea
3,250	0.5	4,486	5,688	26.8	0.01	15.3	8.4	11.8	6,349	Paraguay
521	-89.4	12,249	2,205	-82.0	0.00	7.6	11.1	9.5	29,165	Peru
26,100	-36.4	49,479	36,383	-26.5	0.19	12.4	10.0	11.1	91,983	Philippines
16,900	20.0	29,545	39,293	33.0	0.11	29.5	23.7	26.5	38,074	Poland
600	-71.7	6,135	1,375	-77.6	0.01	-	-	-	10,707	Portugal
-	-	-	-	-	-	18.8	14.5	16.8	1,409	Qatar
850	-92.5	10,900	1,566	-85.6	0.01	22.5	21.2	21.8	21,275	Romania
1	-99.9	1,440	3	-99.8	0.00	18.2	11.1	14.7	140,874	Russian Federation
4,459	22.7	3,800	6,278	65.2	0.15	11.2	7.5	9.6	9,998	Rwanda

*** Subnational data used*

COUNTRY	SMOKELESS TOBACCO	HEALTH PROFESSIONALS		CIGARETTE PRICES	AFFORDABILITY OF CIGARETTES	MANUFACTURING CIGARETTES	ILLICIT CIGARETTES	TOBACCO TAXES	GROWING TOBACCO
	PRODUCTS & THEIR USE			PRICES		TOBACCO INDUSTRY			
	Adult Smokeless Tobacco Use	Smoking Prevalence of Health Professional Students	Student Type	Cigarette Prices	Relative Income Price	Production	Illicit Share of the Total Cigarette Market	Excise Tax as % of Cigarette Price	Tobacco Area Harvested
	%	%		*per pack in USD*	*2010*	*in billion pieces*	%	%	*hectares, 2000*
Saint Kitts and Nevis	0.1	-	-	5.38	2.50	-	-	5.0	-
Saint Lucia	-	-	-	2.21	4.25	-	-	0.0	-
Saint Vincent and the Grenadines	-	-	-	5.00	3.83	-	-	1.7	50
Samoa	0.6	-	-	5.23	-	-	-	48.3	40
San Marino	-	-	-	5.44	-	0.00	-	74.2	-
Sao Tome and Principe	2.8	-	-	2.65	-	-	-	8.7	-
Saudi Arabia	0.8	8.2	Medical	1.57	0.79	0.00	1.2	0.0	-
Senegal	-	10.2	Medical	1.29	9.29	8.25	4.4	26.3	-
Serbia	-	34.7	Medical	2.03	2.19	22.06	5.1	56.9	-
Seychelles	0.1	-	-	5.43	5.74	0.04	-	67.6	-
Sierra Leone	7.8	-	-	1.03	12.32	-	18.0	18.3	40
Singapore	-	-	-	9.29	1.82	7.50	5.7	60.7	0
Slovakia	-	26.0	Medical	3.66	1.98	5.05	15.0	65.0	1,134
Slovenia	-	21.0	Medical	3.91	1.40	0.00	8.1	60.6	-
Solomon Islands	-	-	-	-	-	-	-	-	100
Somalia	-	5.6**	Medical	0.85	-	-	-	0.0	250
South Africa	6.6	-	-	4.14	4.87	19.67	9.0	40.7	15,600
Spain	2.5	21.1	Medical	5.99	1.49	2.95	1.0	64.6	14,078
Sri Lanka	15.8	4.2	Medical	3.62	13.80	4.16	9.0	59.2	4,480
Sudan	12.2	45.8	Medical	2.40	7.41	5.00	25.0	58.9	-
Suriname	-	17.4	Nursing	3.65	3.13	-	-	40.8	-
Swaziland	1.6	-	-	3.47	11.90	-	15.0	32.5	194
Sweden	17.0	-	-	7.74	1.36	-	15.4	56.5	-
Switzerland	0.1	-	-	8.28	0.97	69.12	5.0	55.4	681
Syrian Arab Republic	0.0	66.3	Medical	2.36	2.24	14.19	8.0	33.0	18,100
Tajikistan	-	-	-	1.81	9.25	-	-	3.2	3,702
Tanzania (United Republic of)	1.4	-	-	2.90	34.09	5.68	-	10.9	44,000
Thailand	3.9	2.1	Medical	2.56	3.67	27.63	2.6	62.2	31,363
Timor-Leste	2.2	-	-	1.50	21.24	-	-	-	-
Togo	-	-	-	1.98	24.26	0.00	16.8	15.0	4,000
Tonga	-	-	-	4.93	10.51	0.00	-	54.8	-
Trinidad and Tobago	-	5.7	Nursing	2.82	-	4.86	1.6	20.7	60
Tunisia	5.4	17.6	Medical	2.95	2.83	12.15	3.9	49.6	3,231
Turkey	-	17.9	Medical	4.38	2.88	94.00	15.7	63.0	236,569
Turkmenistan	12.0	-	-	1.89	3.03	0.00	-	31.4	1,600
Tuvalu	-	-	-	5.39	-	0.00	-	14.3	-
Uganda	3.3	2.8	Medical	1.76	14.76	-	2.4	29.3	13,712
Ukraine	0.2	33.1	Medical	1.26	5.84	101.78	1.5	53.6	3,600
United Arab Emirates	-	-	-	1.91	0.23	0.04	45.1	0.0	52
United Kingdom	1.1	-	-	10.99	2.56	65.00	11.0	73.5	-
United States of America	3.5	3.3	Medical	6.36	1.32	338.23	6.4	39.9	189,970
Uruguay	0.0	32.3	Medical	3.61	2.58	4.97	22.6	54.3	830
Uzbekistan	11.3	-	-	1.20	3.65	10.23	8.8	13.0	6,700
Vanuatu	-	-	-	8.03	23.60	-	-	12.3	-
Venezuela (Bolivarian Republic of)	-	-	-	4.66	4.66	28.50	14.0	67.6	5,362
Viet Nam	1.3	11.2	Medical	1.66	5.61	116.50	15.2	32.5	24,400
Yemen	10.7	10.9	Medical	1.25	6.40	13.80	14.5	53.5	5,347
Zambia	0.6	5.5	Nursing	1.83	13.62	0.00	25.0	30.9	9,000
Zimbabwe	1.2	-	-	1.80	6.73	6.00	2.3	38.6	90,769

TOBACCO INDUSTRY

Tobacco Area Harvested	Percent Change in Tobacco Area Harvested	Tobacco Production	Tobacco Production	Percent Change in Tobacco Production	Agricultural Land on Which Tobacco Is Grown	TOBACCO MARKETING: Youth Who Have an Object With a Tobacco Logo on It			Population	COUNTRY
hectares, 2009	2000–2009	tonnes, 2000	tonnes, 2009	2000–2009	2008, % of total agricultural land	% Boys, Ages 13–15	% Girls, Ages 13–15	% Youth, Ages 13–15	as of 2009, in thousands	
-	-	-	-	-	-	20.5	15.6	17.6	52	Saint Kitts and Nevis
-	-	-	-	-	-	19.0	9.1	13.1	172	Saint Lucia
81	62.0	86	109	26.7	0.70	14.9	10.4	12.4	109	Saint Vincent and the Grenadines
50	25.0	140	207	47.9	0.08	26.0	16.9	21.5	179	Samoa
-	-	-	-	-	-	15.3	5.9	10.6	31	San Marino
-	-	-	-	-	-	-	-	-	163	Sao Tome and Principe
-	-	-	-	-	-	11.8	12.0	12.3	25,721	Saudi Arabia
-	-	-	-	-	-	17.4	19.6	18.9	12,534	Senegal
6,103	-	-	9,847	-	0.14	18.4	13.8	16.1	9,850	Serbia
-	-	-	-	-	-	16.8	15.9	16.2	84	Seychelles
48	20.0	20	27	35.0	0.00	20.3**	17.6**	19.5**	5,696	Sierra Leone
0	-	0	0	-	-	-	-	-	4,737	Singapore
19	-98.3	1,870	2	-99.9	0.00	21.1	13.6	17.3	5,406	Slovakia
-	-	-	-	-	-	13.7	11.6	13.3	2,020	Slovenia
100	0.0	85	88	3.5	0.12	21.3	14.4	17.2	523	Solomon Islands
344	37.6	100	173	73.0	0.00	22.4**	13.3**	20.1**	9,133	Somalia
3,562	-77.2	29,700	25,015	-15.8	0.01	20.0	14.4	16.7	50,110	South Africa
10,000	-29.0	42,908	30,400	-29.2	0.04	-	-	-	44,904	Spain
2,210	-50.7	5,400	3,810	-29.4	0.08	6.0	5.5	5.7	20,238	Sri Lanka
-	-	-	-	-	-	18.3	17.8	18.0	42,272	Sudan
-	-	-	-	-	-	22.2	15.2	18.5	520	Suriname
310	59.8	71	130	83.1	0.02	11.4	9.1	10.0	1,185	Swaziland
-	-	-	-	-	-	-	-	-	9,249	Sweden
556	-18.4	1,182	953	-19.4	0.03	-	-	-	7,568	Switzerland
12,674	-30.0	26,112	19,881	-23.9	0.10	15.9	9.8	12.9	21,906	Syrian Arab Republic
130	-96.5	7,186	190	-97.4	0.00	11.1	9.4	10.2	6,952	Tajikistan
41,000	-6.8	26,384	55,400	110.0	0.10	15.1**	12.7**	13.7**	43,739	Tanzania (United Republic of)
30,836	-1.7	74,200	72,229	-2.7	0.20	42.5	41.1	42.0	67,764	Thailand
-	-	-	-	-	-	39.4	29.8	34.3	1,134	Timor-Leste
4,289	7.2	1,800	2,788	54.9	0.11	24.3	26.0	24.8	6,619	Togo
-	-	-	-	-	-	29.4	12.9	23.5	104	Tonga
159	165.0	90	203	125.6	0.24	13.2	10.0	11.8	1,339	Trinidad and Tobago
1,266	-60.8	3,436	1,600	-53.4	0.03	13.9	6.6	10.1	10,272	Tunisia
139,431	-41.1	200,280	85,000	-57.6	0.38	18.6	10.3	15.6	74,816	Turkey
1,297	-18.9	3,220	2,723	-15.4	0.00	-	-	-	5,110	Turkmenistan
-	-	-	-	-	-	30.4	22.7	25.9	10	Tuvalu
14,000	2.1	22,837	18,846	-17.5	0.15	12.4	11.6	12.3	32,710	Uganda
120	-96.7	3,000	110	-96.3	0.00	29.0	23.3	26.0	45,708	Ukraine
40	-23.1	660	811	22.9	0.01	13.7	8.8	11.4	4,599	United Arab Emirates
-	-	-	-	-	-	-	-	-	61,565	United Kingdom
143,275	-24.6	477,753	373,440	-21.8	0.03	13.1	11.6	12.3	314,659	United States of America
789	-4.9	2,800	2,811	0.4	0.01	13.9	8.4	10.7	3,361	Uruguay
5,347	-20.2	19,000	15,402	-18.9	0.02	7.4**	6.1**	6.9**	27,488	Uzbekistan
-	-	-	-	-	-	21.0	15.7	17.8	240	Vanuatu
3,254	-39.3	8,755	5,054	-42.3	0.01	16.6	13.4	14.9	28,583	Venezuela (Bolivarian Republic of)
20,729	-15.0	27,100	38,500	42.1	0.19	13.3	9.5	11.3	88,069	Viet Nam
10,169	90.2	11,613	22,577	94.4	0.04	22.8	20.2	22.1	23,580	Yemen
68,007	655.6	9,533	75,335	690.3	0.20	16.6**	20.0**	18.6**	12,935	Zambia
79,917	-12.0	227,726	96,367	-57.7	0.32	16.6**	13.0**	14.8**	12,523	Zimbabwe

*** Subnational data used*

01 DEATHS

Main Map

SOURCES

World Health Organization. (2012). WHO Global Report: Mortality Attributable to Tobacco. Geneva: World Health Organization. http://www.who.int/tobacco/publications/surveillance/rep_mortality_attibutable/en/index.html. Accessed March 26, 2012.

METHODS

The calculation of tobacco-attributed mortality starts with the number of lung cancer deaths in the country. For countries that had very low lung cancer deaths, the proportion is 0.0%, which indicates low mortality rates rather than no data. Tobacco-attributed mortality data provides estimates that may be influenced by environmental factors. Data excludes deaths caused by secondhand smoke exposure, but this cannot always be controlled for and may be included in the total for some countries.

Symbol

World Health Organization. (2008). The global burden of disease 2004 update.

Projected Deaths by Cause

Mathers C, Loncar D. (2006). Projections of global mortality and burden of disease from 2002 to 2030. *PLoS Medicine, 3*(11): 2011–2024.

One Billion Deaths

Peto R, Lopez A. (2000). The future worldwide health effects of current smoking patterns. Clinical Trial Service Unit & Epidemiological Studies Unit—University of Oxford. http://www.ctsu.ox.ac.uk/pressreleases/2000-08-02/the-future-worldwide-health-effects-of-current-smoking-patterns. Accessed December 3, 2011. Updated via personal communication, June 2011.

Male Cancer Mortality in Poland

Thun M, Peto R, Boreham J, Lopez AD. (2012). Stages of the Cigarette Epidemic on Entering Its Second Century. Supplementary Data page 395.http://tobaccocontrol.bmj.com/content/suppl/2012/02/22/tobaccocontrol-2011-050294.DC1/tobaccocontrol-2011-050294-s1.pdf. Tobacco Control 21(2), 96–101. Accessed April 17, 2012.

China

Yang G, Hu A. (2011). *China tobacco utilization and tobacco control joint report by international experts: Tobacco control and China's future.* Beijing: Economic Daily Press.

European Union

Peto R, Lopez A, Boreham J, Thun M. (2006). Mortality from smoking in developed countries, 2000.

Deaths Among Men and Women

World Health Organization. (2008). The global burden of disease 2004 update.

Quote: N.Y. Campaign Slogan

City pulls no punches with anti-smoking ads. (2011). *Metro New York.* March 8. http://www.metro.us/newyork/local/article/796757-city-pulls-no-punches-with-anti-smoking-ads. Accessed August 2, 2011.

Quote: Vathesatogkit

Treerutkuarkul A. (2011). Tobacco laws to be strengthened as young smokers on rise. *Bangkok Post.* August 27. http://www.bangkokpost.com/news/local/253668/tobacco-laws-to-be-strengthened-as-young-smokers-on-rise. Accessed September 22, 2011.

Text Panel

Basu S, Stuckler D, Bitton A, Glantz S. (2011). Projected effects of tobacco smoking on worldwide tuberculosis control: Mathematical modelling analysis. *British Medical Journal, 343*: d5506.

Ezzati M, Lopez A. (2003). Estimates of global mortality attributable to smoking in 2000. *Lancet, 362*: 847–852.

Jamrozik K, McLaughlin D, McCaul K, Almeida O, Wong K, Vagenas D, Dobson A. (2011). Women who smoke like men die like men who smoke: Findings from two Australian cohort studies. *Tobacco Control, 20*: 258–265.

World Health Organization. (2011). Fact Sheet Number 339: Tobacco. http://www.who.int/mediacentre/factsheets/fs339/en/index.html. Accessed July 28, 2011.

World Health Organization. (2011). News Release: World No Tobacco Day 2011 Celebrates WHO Framework Convention on Tobacco Control. May 30. http://www.who.int/mediacentre/news/releases/2011/wntd_20110530/en/index.html. Accessed July 28, 2011.

World Health Organization. (N.d.). Tobacco Free Initiative: Why tobacco is a public health priority. http://www.who.int/tobacco/health_priority/en/index.html. Accessed July 28, 2011.

02 HARM FROM SMOKING

Main Image: How Tobacco Harms You

Luo J, Margolis K, Wactawski-Wende J, Horn K, Messina C, Stefanick M, Tindle H, Tony E, Rohan T. (2011). Association of active and passive smoking with risk of breast cancer among postmenopausal women: A prospective cohort study. *British Medical Journal, 342*: d1016.

National Institute on Drug Abuse. (2009). *Report Research Series: Tobacco Addiction.* US Department of Health and Human Services. http://www.drugabuse.gov/PDF/TobaccoRRS_v16.pdf. Accessed August 7, 2011.

US Department of Health and Human Services. (2001). *Women and smoking: A report of the Surgeon General.* Rockville, MD: US Department of Health and Human Services, Public Health Service, Office of the Surgeon General.

US Department of Health and Human Services. (2004). *The health consequences of smoking: A report of the Surgeon General.* Rockville, MD: US Department of Health and Human Services, Office of the Surgeon General.

US Department of Health and Human Services. (2010). *How tobacco smoke causes disease: The biology and behavioral basis for smoking-attributable disease: A report of the Surgeon General.* Atlanta: US Department of Health and Human Services, Centers for Disease Control and Prevention, National Center for Chronic Disease Prevention and Health Promotion, Office on Smoking and Health.

World Health Organization. (2011). Tobacco Free Initiative: The smoker's body. http://www.who.int/tobacco/research/smokers_body/en/index.html. Accessed August 7, 2011.

Deadly Chemicals

National Toxicology Program. (2005). *Report on carcinogens.* 11th ed. US Department of Health and Human Services, Public Health Service, National Toxicology Program.

Philip Morris USA. (2011). Tobacco ingredients by brand. http://www.philipmorrisusa.com/en/cms/Products/Cigarettes/Ingredients/Ingredients_by_Brand/default.aspx. Accessed November 15, 2011.

US Department of Health and Human Services. (2006). *The health consequences of involuntary exposure to tobacco smoke: A report of the Surgeon General.* Rockville, MD: US Department of Health and Human Services, Centers for Disease Control and Prevention, Coordinating Center for Health Promotion, National Center for Chronic Disease Prevention and Health Promotion, Office on Smoking and Health.

US Department of Health and Human Services. (2010). *How tobacco smoke causes disease.*

Health Risks of Smoking During Pregnancy

US Department of Health and Human Services. (2001). *Women and smoking.*

US Department of Health and Human Services. (2004). *The health consequences of smoking.*

Tobacco as Only Shared Risk Factor

World Health Organization. (2008). 2008–2013 action plan for the global strategy for the prevention and control of noncommunicable diseases. http://whqlibdoc.who.int/publications/2009/9789241597418_eng.pdf. Accessed August 16, 2011.

Smoking and Tuberculosis

World Health Organization. (2009). Tuberculosis and tobacco. http://www.who.int/tobacco/resources/publications/factsheet_tub_tob.pdf. Accessed August 7, 2011.

Smoking and Diabetes

Rimm E, Chan J, Stampfer M, Colditz G, Willett W. (1995). Prospective study of cigarette smoking, alcohol use, and the risk of diabetes in men. *British Medical Journal, 310*: 555.

Smoking and HIV

Crothers K. (2005). The impact of cigarette smoking on mortality, quality of life, and comorbid illness among HIV-positive veterans. *Journal of General Internal Medicine, 20*(12): 1142–1145.

Quote: Camilleri

Gasp.org. (2011). Excerpts from the PMI 2011 question and answer segment. May 11. http://www.gasp.org/2011TobaccoMeetings.html#PMI2011. Accessed August 12, 2011.

Quote: FDA

Food and Drug Administration. (2011). Tobacco products: Health fraud. US Department of Health and Human Services. http://www.fda.gov/TobaccoProducts/ResourcesforYou/ucm255658.htm. Accessed August 1, 2011.

Text Panel

US Department of Health and Human Services. (2004). *The health consequences of smoking.*

National Institute on Drug Abuse. (2009). *Report Research Series: Tobacco addiction.* US Department of Health and Human Services. http://www.drugabuse.gov/PDF/TobaccoRRS_v16.pdf. Accessed August 7, 2011.

03 SECONDHAND SMOKING

Main Map

SOURCES

Centers for Disease Control and Prevention. (2011). Global Tobacco Surveillance System: Global Youth Tobacco Survey.

World Health Organization. (2011). WHO report on the global tobacco epidemic, 2011: Global Youth Tobacco Survey data.

WHO-GYTS data were used for: **Benin, Cambodia, Guatemala, Honduras, Palau, US.**

ALTERNATE DATA SOURCE

Australia: Australian Institute of Health and Welfare. (2005). National Drug Strategy Household Survey 2004: Detailed findings AIWH cat. no. PHE 66. Canberra: Australian Institute of Health and Welfare.

Mexico: WHO. Mexico – Mexico City (Ages 13-15) Fact Sheet, GYTS. (2006). http://apps.nccd.cdc.gov/gtssdata/Ancillary/DataReports.aspx?CAID=1. Accessed December 27, 2011.

METHODS

When regional Global Youth Tobacco Survey (GYTS) data were used, the country was color-coded using data from the capital city. If data were not available for the capital city, the largest city was selected. The use of regional data is indicated on the map with a circle next to the city whose data were used.

GYTS provided separate data for **West Bank** (2009) and **Gaza Strip** (2008). Data points were averaged together.

Harm Caused by Secondhand Smoke

US Department of Health and Human Services. (2006). *The health consequences of involuntary exposure to tobacco smoke: A report of the Surgeon General.* Atlanta: US Department of Health and Human Services, Centers for Disease Control and Prevention, Coordinating Center for Health Promotion, National Center for Chronic Disease Prevention and Health Promotion, Office on Smoking and Health.

Global SHS Deaths in Men, Women, and Children

Öberg M, Jaakkola M, Woodward A, Peruga A, Prüss-Ustün A. (2011). Worldwide burden of disease from exposure to secondhand smoke: A retrospective analysis of data from 192 countries. *Lancet, 377*: 139–146.

Global SHS Deaths by Region

Öberg M et al. Worldwide burden of disease from exposure to secondhand smoke.

SIDS

Boldo E et al. (2010). Health impact assessment of environmental tobacco smoke in European children: Sudden Infant Death Syndrome and asthma episodes. *Global Health Matters, 125*: 478–487.

Preteens and Nicotine Dependence
Racicot S, McGrath J, O'Loughlin J. (2011). An investigation of social and pharmacological exposure to secondhand tobacco smoke as possible predictors of perceived nicotine dependence, smoking susceptibility, and smoking expectancies among never-smoking youth. *Nicotine and Tobacco Research*, online May 26, 2011. http://ntr.oxfordjournals.org/content/early/2011/05/25/ntr.ntr100.abstract. Accessed August 29, 2011.

Quote: NIH
National Institutes of Health. (2011). How secondhand smoke affects the brain. May 16. http://www.nih.gov/researchmatters/may2011/05162011smoke.htm. Accessed August 29, 2011.

Quote: Roper Organization
The Roper Organization. (1978). A study of public attitudes towards cigarette smoking and the tobacco industry in 1978, vol. 1. In Glantz S, Slade J, Bero L, Hanauer P, Barnes D. (eds.), *The Cigarette Papers*. University of California Press, 1996.

Text Panel
Environmental Policy Administration (1992). The Energy Policy Act—102nd Congress H.R.776.ENR. http://www.afdc.energy.gov/afdc/pdfs/2527.pdf. Accessed December 3, 2011.

National Institute on Drug Abuse. (2009). Research Report Series: Tobacco addiction. http://www.drugabuse.gov/PDF/TobaccoRRS_v16.pdf. Accessed August 29, 2011.

Öberg M et al. Worldwide burden of disease from exposure to secondhand smoke.

US Department of Health and Human Services. (2006). *The health consequences of involuntary exposure to tobacco smoke: A report of the Surgeon General.*

World Health Organization. (2011). News release: World No Tobacco Day 2011 celebrates WHO Framework Convention on Tobacco Control. May 30, 2011. http://www.who.int/mediacentre/news/releases/2011/wntd_20110530/en/index.html. Accessed August 29, 2011.

04 TYPES OF TOBACCO USE

Boffetta P, Hecht S, Gray N, Gupta P, Straif K. (2008). Smokeless tobacco and cancer. *Lancet Oncology, 9*(7): 667–675.

Connolly GN. Submission on Dissolvable Tobacco Products to Office of Science, Center for Tobacco Products, Food and Drug Administration. http://www.fda.gov/AdvisoryCommittees/CommitteesMeetingMaterials/TobaccoProductsScientificAdvisoryCommittee/ucm265295.htm. Accessed October 18, 2008.

Maziak W, Ward KD, Afifi Soweid RA, Eissenberg T. (2004). Tobacco smoking using a waterpipe: A re-emerging strain in a global epidemic. *Tobacco Control, 13*(4): 327–333.

National Cancer Institute. (N.d.). Smokeless tobacco and cancer. http://www.cancer.gov/cancertopics/smokeless-tobacco. Accessed August 19, 2008.

National Cancer Institute, Centers for Disease Control, and Stockholm Center of Public Health. (2002). Smokeless tobacco fact sheets. http://cancercontrol.cancer.gov/tcrb/stfact_sheet_combined10-23-02.pdf. Accessed August 19, 2008.

Prignot J, Sasco A, Poulet E, Gupta P, Aditama T. (2008). Alternative forms of tobacco use. *International Journal of Tuberculosis and Lung Disease, 12*(7): 718–727.

World Health Organization. (1997). Tobacco or health: A global status report. Geneva: WHO.

World Health Organization. (1998). Guidelines for controlling and monitoring the tobacco epidemic. Geneva: WHO.

05 NICOTINE DELIVERY SYSTEMS

Pershagan
Hundley T. (2007). Snuffing out smokes. *Chicago Tribune*. September 16. http://articles.chicagotribune.com/2007-09-16/business/0709150068_1_snus-smokeless-tobacco-tobacco-product/2. Accessed August 2, 2011.

Amount of Nicotine in Cigarettes
American Cancer Society. (2011). Learn about cancer: Cigarette smoking. http://www.cancer.org/Cancer/CancerCauses/TobaccoCancer/CigaretteSmoking/cigarette-smoking-tobacco. Accessed July 28, 2011.

Market for Cessation Aids
Jacobs R. (2011). Pursuit of a safer cigarette gathers pace: BAT subsidiary Nicoventures signs contract to market new nicotine inhalation technology. *Financial Times Online*. June 1. http://www.ft.com/intl/cms/s/0/4ceee0e6-8c7a-11e0-883f-00144feab49a.html#axzz1OoX7f5YO. Accessed July 28, 2011.

DOJ Proposed Statement
Wilson D. (2011). US presses tobacco firms to admit to falsehoods about light cigarettes and nicotine addiction. *New York Times*. February 23. http://www.nytimes.com/2011/02/24/health/24tobacco.html?_r=2. Accessed August 2, 2011.

Quote: Connolly
Wilson D. (2010). Flavored tobacco pellets are denounced as a lure to young users. *New York Times*. April 19. http://www.nytimes.com/2010/04/19/business/19smoke.html. Accessed December 1, 2011.

Text Panel
Breland A, Kleykam B, Eissenber T. (2006). Clinical laboratory evaluation of potential reduced exposure products for smokers. *Nicotine and Tobacco Research, 8*(6): 727–738.

Henningfield J, Zaatari G. (2010). Electronic nicotine delivery systems: Emerging science foundation for policy. *Tobacco Control, 19*: 89–90.

06 CIGARETTE CONSUMPTION

Main Map
ERC. (2010). World Cigarette Reports 2010. Suffolk, UK: ERC Group Ltd.

Euromonitor International. (2011). Cigarette consumption sticks per capita: 2010. Hong Kong.

Symbol
Data derived from ERC. (2010). World Cigarette Reports 2010.

Global Cigarette Consumption
ERC. (2010). World Cigarette Reports 2010.

Top 5 Cigarette-Consuming Countries
ERC. (2010). World Cigarette Reports 2010.

World Cigarette Consumption by Region
Data derived from ERC. (2010). World Cigarette Reports 2010.

2009 Global Cigarette Consumption
Date derived from ERC. (2010). World Cigarette Reports 2010.

Data derived from Population Reference Bureau. (2009). 2009 World Population Data Sheet. http://www.prb.org/pdf09/09wpds_eng.pdf. Accessed August 24, 2011.

2009 China Cigarette Consumption
Data derived from ERC. (2010). World Cigarette Reports 2010.

Quote: WHO, EMRO
World Health Organization. (N.d). Tobacco Free Initiative — Facts and FAQs. Regional Office for the Eastern Mediterranean. http://www.emro.who.int/tfi/facts.htm. Accessed December 11, 2011.

Quote: Camilleri
Bloomberg Businessweek. (2005). Indonesia: As growth heats up, buyouts are smokin'. March 28. http://www.businessweek.com/magazine/content/05_13/b3926070.htm. Accessed August 25, 2011.

Text Panel
SOURCES
ERC. (2010). World Cigarette Reports 2010.

Population Reference Bureau. (2009). 2009 World Population Data Sheet.

Tobacco Journal International. (2011). Asia gain props up PMI shipment volume. July 12. http://www.tobaccojournal.com/Asia_gain_props_up_PMI_shipment_volume.50643.0.html. Accessed August 25, 2011.

METHODS
The fact that nearly 20% of the world's population smokes is based on 1.2 billion smokers and a 2009 world population of more than 6.8 billion with data derived from ERC (2010) and Population Reference Bureau (2009).

07 MALE TOBACCO USE

Main Map
SOURCES
World Health Organization. (2011). *WHO report on the global tobacco epidemic, 2011: Warning about the dangers of tobacco.* Geneva: World Health Organization.

ALTERNATE DATA SOURCES
Algeria, Cuba, Ecuador, Jamaica, Luxembourg, Suriname, Venezuela World Health Organization. (2010). World health statistics 2010. http://www.who.int/whosis/whostat/EN_WHS10_Full.pdf. Accessed November 2, 2011. Prevalence of smoking any tobacco product among adults age 15+, 2006.

Australia Australian Institute of Health and Welfare. (2011). 2010 National Drug Strategy Household Survey Report. http://tobacco.health.usyd.edu.au/assets/pdfs/2010-NDSHS-Report.pdf. Accessed November 2, 2011. Data reflect a combination of daily and weekly and less than weekly smoking status of adults age 14+, 2010.

Bhutan Royal Government of Bhutan Ministry of Health. (2009). Report on 2007 STEPS Survey for risk factors and prevalence of noncommunicable diseases in Thimphu. http://www.health.gov.bt/reports/2007NCDreport.pdf. Accessed November 8, 2011.

Brazil Ministry of Health. (2010). Global Adult Tobacco Survey, Brazil report. http://new.paho.org/hq/dmdocuments/2010/GATS%202010%20Brazil%20Report%20en.pdf. Accessed November 2, 2011. Current smokers age 15+, 2008.

Germany Federal Ministry of Health. (2011). Drugs and addiction report: May 2011. https://www.bundesgesundheitsministerium.de/fileadmin/dateien/Publikationen/Drogen_Sucht/Broschueren/Drogen_und_Suchtbericht_2011_110517_Drogenbeauftragte.pdf. Accessed October 10, 2011. Prevalence of smoking among adults age 18–64, 2010.

Hong Kong Tobacco Control Office—Department of Health. (2007). Pattern of smoking in Hong Kong. http://www.tco.gov.hk/textonly/english/infostation/infostation_sta_01.html#a1. Accessed November 8, 2011.

Japan World Health Organization. (2011). WHO Report on the Global Tobacco Epidemic, 2011, cites Japan National Health and Nutrition Survey, 2009. Considers current tobacco smoking among users age 20+.

Niue World Health Organization. (2011). WHO Global Infobase: Tobacco use prevalence, Niue. https://apps.who.int/infobase/Indicators.aspx. Accessed November 8, 2011. Current cigarette users age 15–100, 2002.

Peru World Health Organization. (2011). WHO Global Infobase: Tobacco use prevalence, Peru. Current smoking tobacco users age 12–64, 2005.

Qatar World Health Organization. (2010). Country profile: Qatar. Smoking prevalence among adults age 15+, 2006. http://www.emro.who.int/emrinfo/index.aspx?Ctry=qat. Accessed November 2, 2011.

Sweden National Board of Health and Welfare. (2009). Open comparisons 2009: Public health (including the indicator: Smoking habits). http://www.fhi.se/PageFiles/9183/open-comparisons-2009.pdf. Accessed November 8, 2011. Daily smokers age 18–80, 2008.

UK World Health Organization. (2011). WHO Report on the Global Tobacco Epidemic, 2011, cites National Health Service General Lifestyle Survey. Current cigarette users age 16–100, 2009.

US Centers for Disease Control and Prevention. (2011). Current smoking, adults, early release. http://www.cdc.gov/nchs/data/nhis/earlyrelease/201106_08.pdf. Accessed November 2, 2011. Current smokers 18+, 2010.

West Bank and Gaza Strip (Palestine) World Health Organization. (2010). Country profile: Palestine. Smoking prevalence among adults age 15+, 2007. http://www.emro.who.int/emrinfo/index.aspx?Ctry=pal. Accessed November 2, 2011.

METHODS
WHO Report on the Global Tobacco Epidemic (RGTE) age-standardized prevalence data were the primary data source for 2009 male smoking prevalence for all countries unless otherwise listed above.

Symbol

World Health Organization. (2011). *WHO report on the global tobacco epidemic, 2011: Warning about the dangers of tobacco.* Geneva: World Health Organization.

Smoking Trends

SOURCES

Japan and UK World Health Organization. (2011). *WHO report on the global tobacco epidemic, 2011.*

US Centers for Disease Control and Prevention. (2011). National Health Interview Survey, 2010: Early release of selected estimates. http://www.cdc.gov/nchs/data/nhis/earlyrelease/201106_08.pdf. Accessed August 25, 2011.

METHODS
National data sources were used for the 2010 estimate for the US and for the 2009 estimates of Japan and UK.

Average Smoking Prevalence Along Tobacco Epidemic Continuum

SOURCES
Hong Kong population: US Department of State. (2011). Background note: Hong Kong. http://www.state.gov/r/pa/ei/bgn/2747.htm. Accessed August 20, 2011.

Lopez A, Collishaw N, Piha T. (1994). A descriptive model of the cigarette epidemic in developed countries. *Tobacco Control 3*: 242–247.

Data derived from World Health Organization. (2011). *WHO report on the global tobacco epidemic, 2011. Warning about the dangers of tobacco.* Geneva: World Health Organization.

METHODS
This is an estimate of the average smoking prevalance among males. Countries with prevalence data from the WHO RGTE 2011 were used for this analysis. Population estimates came from 2010 World Bank estimates. An average smoking prevalance was used for countries without prevalence data. The percentages provided represent a weighted average of the prevalence rates for adult male smokers in low-, middle-, and high-income countries.

Low Daily Smoking Rates

Australia Australian Institute of Health and Welfare. (2011). 2010 National Drug Strategy Household Survey Report. http://tobacco.health.usyd.edu.au/assets/pdfs/2010-NDSHS-Report.pdf. Accessed October 5, 2011.

Canada Health Canada. (2011). Canadian Tobacco Use Monitoring Survey: Summary of annual results for 2010. http://www.hc-sc.gc.ca/hc-ps/tobac-tabac/research-recherche/stat/_ctums-esutc_2010/ann_summary-sommaire-eng.php. Accessed October 5, 2011.

Hong Kong Susan Mercado, World Health Organization: Western Pacific Region Office. (2011). Personal communication.

Iceland Organization for Economic Co-Operation and Development. (2011). OECD health data 2011: Frequently requested data. http://www.oecd.org/document/16/0,3746,en_2649_37407_2085200_1_1_1_37407,00.html. Accessed November 29, 2011.

Singapore Ministry of Health, Singapore. (2010). National Health Survey 2010, Singapore. Epidemiology and Disease Control Division, Ministry of Health, Singapore.http://www.moh.gov.sg/content/dam/moh_web/Publications/Reports/2011/NHS2010%20-%20low%20res.pdf. Accessed April 9, 2012.

Sweden Organization for Economic Co-Operation and Development. (2011). Stat extracts: Health status. http://stats.oecd.org/index.aspx?DataSetCode=HEALTH_STAT. Accessed October 5, 2011.

US Centers for Disease Control and Prevention. (2011). Current smoking, adults, early release. http://www.cdc.gov/nchs/data/nhis/earlyrelease/201106_08.pdf. Accessed November 2, 2011. Current smokers 18+, 2010.

Low- and Middle-Income Countries With High Prevalence

World Health Organization. (2011). WHO Report on the Global Tobacco Epidemic, 2011: Warning about the dangers of tobacco.

Quote: Mizuno

Kageyama Y. (2009). Japan's smoking habit runs into court challenge. *Japan Times.* August 7. http://search.japantimes.co.jp/cgi-bin/nn20090807f3.html. Accessed August 25, 2011.

Quote: Weissman

Martin D. (2009). George Weissman, leader at Philip Morris and in the arts in New York, dies at 90. *New York Times.* July 28. http://www.nytimes.com/2009/07/28/business/28weissman.html?scp=4&sq=smoking&st=nyt. Accessed August 28, 2011.

Text Panel

Lopez A, Collishaw N, Piha T. (1994). A descriptive model of the cigarette epidemic in developed countries.

Mathers C. (2011). Personal communication.

World Health Organization. (2011). *WHO report on the global tobacco epidemic, 2011.*

8 FEMALE TOBACCO USE

Main Map

SOURCES
World Health Organization. (2011). *WHO report on the global tobacco epidemic, 2011: Warning about the dangers of tobacco.* Geneva: World Health Organization.

ALTERNATE DATA SOURCES
Algeria, Azerbaijan, Cuba, Ecuador, Jamaica, Luxembourg, Suriname, Turkmenistan, Venezuela World Health Organization. (2010). World health statistics 2010. http://www.who.int/whosis/whostat/EN_WHS10_Full.pdf. Accessed November 2, 2011. Prevalence of smoking any tobacco product among adults age 15+, 2006.

Australia Australian Institute of Health and Welfare. (2011). 2010 National Drug Strategy Household Survey Report. http://tobacco.health.usyd.edu.au/assets/pdfs/2010-NDSHS-Report.pdf. Accessed November 2, 2011. Data reflect a combination of daily and weekly, and less than weekly smoking status of adults age 14+, 2010.

Bhutan Royal Government of Bhutan Ministry of Health. (2009). Report on 2007 STEPS Survey for risk factors and prevalence of noncommunicable diseases in Thimphu. http://www.health.gov.bt/reports/2007NCDreport.pdf. Accessed November 8, 2011.

Brazil Ministry of Health. (2010). Global Adult Tobacco Survey, Brazil report. http://new.paho.org/hq/dmdocuments/2010/GATS%202010%20Brazil%20Report%20en.pdf. Accessed November 2, 2011. Current smokers age 15+, 2008.

Germany Federal Ministry of Health. (2011). Drugs and addiction report: May 2011. https://www.bundesgesundheitsministerium.de/fileadmin/dateien/Publikationen/Drogen_Sucht/Broschueren/Drogen_und_Suchtbericht_2011_110517_Drogenbeauftragte.pdf. Accessed October 10, 2011. Prevalence of smoking among adults age 18–64, 2010.

Hong Kong Tobacco Control Office—Department of Health. (2007). Pattern of smoking in Hong Kong. http://www.tco.gov.hk/textonly/english/infostation/infostation_sta_01.html#a1. Accessed November 8, 2011.

Japan World Health Organization (2011). *WHO report on the global tobacco epidemic, 2011*, cites Japan National Health and Nutrition Survey, 2009. Considers current tobacco smoking among users age 20+.

Nicaragua World Health Organization (2011). WHO Global Infobase: Tobacco use prevalence, Nicaragua. https://apps.who.int/infobase/Indicators.aspx. Accessed November 8, 2011. Smoking tobacco, age 15–49, 2001.

Niue World Health Organization (2011). WHO Global Infobase: Tobacco use prevalence, Niue. Current cigarette users age 15–100, 2002.

Qatar World Health Organization. (2010). Country profile: Qatar. Smoking prevalence among adults age 15+, 2006. http://www.emro.who.int/emrinfo/index.aspx?Ctry=qat. Accessed November 2, 2011.

Rwanda World Health Organization. (2011). WHO Global Infobase: Tobacco use prevalence, Rwanda. Current cigarette users age 15–49, 2005.

Sweden National Board of Health and Welfare. (2009). Open comparisons 2009: Public health (including the indicator: Smoking habits). http://www.fhi.se/PageFiles/9183/open-comparisons-2009.pdf. Accessed November 8, 2011. Daily smokers age 18–80, 2008.

UK World Health Organization (2011). *WHO report on the global tobacco epidemic*, 2011, cites National Health Service General Lifestyle Survey. Current cigarette users age 16–100, 2009.

US Centers for Disease Control and Prevention. (2011). Current smoking, adults, early release. http://www.cdc.gov/nchs/data/nhis/earlyrelease/201106_08.pdf. Accessed November 2, 2011. Current smokers 18+, 2010.

West Bank and Gaza Strip (Palestine) World Health Organization. (2010). Country profile: Palestine. Smoking prevalence among adults age 15+, 2007. http://www.emro.who.int/emrinfo/index.aspx?Ctry=pal. Accessed November 2, 2011.

METHODS
WHO report on the global tobacco epidemic (RGTE) age-standardized prevalence data were the primary data source for 2009 female smoking prevalence for all countries unless otherwise listed above.

Symbol

Swedish National Institute of Public Health. (2009). Public health 2009: Open comparisons.

World Health Organization. (2011). *WHO report on the global tobacco epidemic, 2011.*

Smoking Trends

Japan and UK World Health Organization. (2011). *WHO report on the global tobacco epidemic, 2011.*

US Centers for Disease Control and Prevention. (2011). National Health Interview Survey, 2010: Early release of selected estimates. http://www.cdc.gov/nchs/data/nhis/earlyrelease/201106_08.pdf. Accessed August 25, 2011.

METHODS
National data sources were used for the 2010 estimate for the US and for the 2009 estimates of Japan and UK.

Average Smoking Prevalence Along Tobacco Epidemic Continuum

Source: Data derived from World Health Organization. (2011). *WHO report on the global tobacco epidemic, 2011.*

METHODS
This is an estimate of the average smoking prevalence rate among females. Countries with prevalence data from the WHO RGTE 2011 were used for this analysis. Population estimates came from 2010 World Bank estimates. An average smoking prevalence was used for countries without prevalence data. The percentages provided represent a weighted average of the prevalence rates for adult female smokers in low-, middle-, and high-income countries.

Cambodian Women

Singh P, Yel D, Sin S, Khieng S, Lopez J, Job J, Ferry L, Knutsen S. (2009). *Bulletin of the World Health Organization 2009, 87*: 905–912. http://www.who.int/bulletin/volumes/87/12/08-058917/en/index.html. Accessed August 25, 2011.

Half of Countries Have Less Than 10% Prevalence

World Health Organization. (2011). *WHO report on the global tobacco epidemic, 2011.*

Carotid Arterial Walls

European Society of Cardiology. (2011). Cigarette smoking causes more arterial damage in women than in men. August 29. http://www.escardio.org/about/press/press-releases/esc11-paris/Pages/tobacco-smoke-social-class-athersclerosis.aspx. Accessed October 5, 2011.

Quote: Curtis

Curtis A. (2002). Century of the self. http://www.archive.org/details/AdaCurtisCenturyoftheSelf_0. Accessed November 10, 2011.

American Tobacco Company

American Tobacco Company. (N.d.). Silva Thins cigarettes: Magazine sales message. http://legacy.library.ucsf.edu/documentStore/w/c/f/wcf51a00/Swcf51a00.pdf. Accessed October 5, 2011.

Text Panel

US Department of Health and Human Services. (2001). *Women and smoking: A report of the Surgeon General.* Washington, DC: Public Health Service, Office of the Surgeon General, 2001. http://www.cdc.gov/tobacco/data_statistics/sgr/sgr_2001/index.htm.

US Department of Health and Human Services. (2004). *The health consequences of smoking: A report of the Surgeon General.* Atlanta: Centers for Disease Control and Prevention, National Center for Chronic Disease Prevention and Health Promotion, Office on Smoking and Health.

Lopez A, Collishaw N, Piha T. (1994). A descriptive model of the cigarette epidemic in developed countries. *Tobacco Control, 3:* 242–247.

Museum of Public Relations. (2011). 1929 Torches of Freedom. http://www.prmuseum.com/bernays/bernays_1929.html. Accessed July 31, 2011.

Singh P, Yel D, Sin S, Khieng S, Lopez J, Job J, Ferry L, Knutsen S. (2009). *Bulletin of the World Health Organization 2009, 87:* 905–912. http://www.who.int/bulletin/volumes/87/12/08-058917/en/index.html. Accessed August 25, 2011.

Thun M, Peto R, Boreham J, Lopez AD. (2012). Stages of the Cigarette Epidemic on Entering Its Second Century. Tobacco Control 21(2), 96–101.

World Health Organization. (2011). *WHO report on the global tobacco epidemic, 2011.*

09 BOYS' TOBACCO USE

Main Map

SOURCES

Centers for Disease Control and Prevention. (2011). Global Tobacco Surveillance System: Global Youth Tobacco Survey.

Centers for Disease Control and Prevention and World Health Organization. (2011). Global School Based Student Health Survey. http://www.who.int/chp/gshs/en/. Accessed April 26, 2012.

ALTERNATE DATA SOURCES

Australia Australian Institute of Health and Welfare. (2011). 2010 National Drug Strategy Household Survey Report. http://tobacco.health.usyd.edu.au/assets/pdfs/2010-NDSHS-Report.pdf. Accessed November 2, 2011. Considers daily, weekly, and less than weekly smokers age 12–17.

Canada Health Canada. (2010). Canadian Tobacco Use Monitoring Survey. http://www.hc-sc.gc.ca/hc-ps/tobac-tabac/research-recherche/stat/_ctums-esutc_2010/w-p-1_sum-som-eng.php. Accessed October 10, 2011. Considers current smokers age 15–19.

Denmark Health Behavior in School-age Children. (2011). School Children Survey 2010. http://www.hbsc.dk/rapport.php?file=HBSC-Rapport-2010.pdf. Accessed October 10, 2011. Considers daily smokers age 15.

France Godeau E, Vignes C, Navarro F, Monéger M-L. (2004). Consumptions of cannabis, tobacco and alcohol by French 15-year-olds: Results of the international HBSC survey. *Courrier des addictions, 6*(3): 117–120. http://www.hbsc.org/countries/downloads_countries/France/Godeau_Focus2004.pdf. Accessed October 10, 2011. Considers daily smokers age 15.

Germany Federal Ministry of Health. (2011). Drugs and addiction report: May 2011. https://www.bundesgesundheitsministerium.de/fileadmin/dateien/Publikationen/Drogen_Sucht/Broschueren/Drogen_und_Suchtbericht_2011_110517_Drogenbeauftragte.pdf. Accessed October 10, 2011. Considers current smokers age 12–17.

Hong Kong Tobacco Control Office Department of Health. (2010). Infostation: Statistics. http://www.tco.gov.hk/textonly/english/infostation/infostation_sta_01.html. Considers daily smokers age 15–19.

Japan Osaki Y, Tanihata T, Ohida T, Kanda H, Kaneita Y, Minowa M, Suzuki K, Wada K, Hayashi K. (2008). Decrease in the prevalence of smoking among Japanese adolescents and its possible causes: Periodic nationwide cross-sectional surveys. *Environmental Health Prevention Medicine, 13:* 219–226. http://www.ncbi.nlm.nih.gov/pmc/articles/PMC2698236/pdf/12199_2008_Article_33.pdf. Accessed October 11, 2011. Considers current smokers in 8th and 9th grades.

Netherlands Health Behavior in School-age Children. (2011). School Children Survey 2009. http://www.hbsc-nederland.nl/uploads/publicaties/openbaar/HBSC_Rapport_2010.pdf. Accessed October 10, 2011. Considers daily smokers age 13–15.

Spain Health Behavior in School-age Children. (2011). School Children Survey 2006. http://www.msps.es/profesionales/saludPublica/prevPromocion/promocion/saludJovenes/docs/Divulgativo_completo_HBSC2006.pdf. Accessed October 10, 2011. Considers daily and weekly smokers age 11–18.

Sweden National Institute of Public Health, Sweden. (2004). Reduced use of tobacco: How far have we come? Statistics, December 2004. http://www.fhi.se/PageFiles/3137/reduceduseoftobacco0412.pdf. Accessed October 10, 2011. Considers everyday / almost everyday smokers age 15–16.

Switzerland Health Behavior in School-age Children. (2011). School Children Survey 2010. http://www.hbsc.ch/pdf/hbsc_bibliographie_197.pdf. Accessed October 10, 2011. Considers daily and weekly smokers ages 13–15.

UK National Health Service. (2011). Smoking, drinking and drug use among young people in England in 2010. http://www.ic.nhs.uk/webfiles/publications/003_Health_Lifestyles/Smoking%20drinking%20drug%20use%202010/Smoking_drinking_and_drug_use_among_young_people_in_England_2010_Full_report.pdf. Accessed October 10, 2011. Considers regular smokers (at least one time per week) age 11–15.

US Centers for Disease Control and Prevention. (2010). National Youth Tobacco Survey. Data provided by CDC, December 2011 and reanalyzed for current smokers ages 13–15 to correspond with GYTS data.

METHODS

Centers for Disease Control and Prevention's Global Youth Tobacco Survey (GYTS) data were the primary data source for Boys' smoking prevalence for all countries (unless otherwise noted above).

Data from the Centers for Disease Control and Prevention's Global School-based Health Survey (GSHS) were used when it provided more recent data or national-level data, or when GYTS data were not available. Both surveys consider youth age 13–15.

GSHS data were used for:

Algeria, Antigua and Barbuda, Benin, Cook Islands, Costa Rica, Djibouti, Fiji, Grenada, Jamaica, Kuwait, Malawi, Maldives, Mauritania, Mongolia, Morocco, Pakistan, Peru, Philippines, Solomon Islands, Suriname, Syrian Arab Republic, Tajikistan, Thailand, Tunisia, United Arab Emirates, and West Bank and Gaza Strip.

When only subnational data were available, the capital city was selected. If the capital city was not available, the most populated city was used. The use of subnational data is indicated on the map with a circle next to the city whose data were used.

Countries With the Highest Smoking Rates Among Boys

Centers for Disease Control and Prevention. (2011). Global Tobacco Surveillance System: Global School-based Health Survey.

Centers for Disease Control and Prevention. (2011). Global Tobacco Surveillance System: Global Youth Tobacco Survey.

Percentage of Boys Susceptible to Smoking

Warren C, Jones N, Eriksen M, Asma S. (2006). Patterns of global tobacco use in young people and implications for future chronic disease burden in adults. *Lancet, 367:* 749–753.

Youth Death

Doll R, Peto R, Boreham J, Sutherland I. (2004). Mortality in relation to smoking: 50 years' observations on male British doctors. BMJ, doi:10.1136/bmj.38142.554479.AE (published 22 June 2004).

Madagascar Smokers

WHO. Madagascar (ages 13–15) Fact Sheet, GYTS. 2008. http://apps.nccd.gov/gtssdata/Ancillary/DataReports.aspx?CAID=1. Accessed December 27, 2011.

Quote: Racicot

Concordia University. (2011). Preteens surrounded by smokers get hooked on nicotine, study suggests. *Science Daily.* http://www.sciencedaily.com/releases/2011/06/110613103948.htm. Accessed October 6, 2011.

Quote: Philip Morris USA

Johnston M. (1981). PM USA Research Center: Young smokers prevalence, trends, implications and related demographic trends. http://legacy.library.ucsf.edu/documentStore/f/t/s/fts84a00/Sfts84a00.pdf. Accessed October 6, 2011.

Text Panel

Arday D, Giovino G, Schulman J, Nelson D, et al. (1995). Cigarette smoking and self-reported health problems among US high school seniors, 1982–1989. *American Journal of Health Promotion, 10*(2): 111–116.

Centers for Disease Control and Prevention. (2011). Global Youth Tobacco Survey. Personal communication.

Johnston M. (1981). PM USA Research Center: Young smokers prevalence, trends, implications and related demographic trends.

R.J. Reynolds Tobacco Company. (1984). RJR report—Young adult smokers: Strategies and opportunities. http://legacy.library.ucsf.edu/tid/fet29d00/pdf. Accessed October 6, 2011.

US Department of Health and Human Services. (1994). *Youth and tobacco: Preventing tobacco use among young people: A report of the Surgeon General.* Rockville, MD: US Department of Health and Human Services, Office of the Surgeon General.

US Department of Health and Human Services. (2004). *The health consequences of smoking: A report of the Surgeon General.* Rockville, MD: US Department of Health and Human Services, Office of the Surgeon General.

Warren C. (2006). Patterns of global tobacco use in young people and implications for future chronic disease burden in adults. *Lancet, 367:* 749–753.

10 GIRLS' TOBACCO USE

Main Map

SOURCES

Centers for Disease Control and Prevention. (2011). Global Tobacco Surveillance System: Global Youth Tobacco Survey.

Centers for Disease Control and Prevention and World Health Organization. (2011). Global School Based Student Health Survey. http://www.who.int/chp/gshs/en/. Accessed April 26, 2012.

ALTERNATE DATA SOURCES

Australia Australian Institute of Health and Welfare. (2011). 2010 National Drug Strategy Household Survey Report. http://tobacco.health.usyd.edu.au/assets/pdfs/2010-NDSHS-Report.pdf. Accessed November 2, 2011. Considers daily, weekly, and less-than-weekly smokers age 12–17.

Canada Health Canada. (2010). Canadian Tobacco Use Monitoring Survey. http://www.hc-sc.gc.ca/hc-ps/tobac-tabac/research-recherche/stat/_ctums-esutc_2010/w-p-1_sum-som-eng.php. Accessed October 10, 2011. Considers current smokers age 15–19.

Denmark Health Behavior in School-age Children. (2011). School Children Survey 2010. http://www.hbsc.dk/rapport.php?file=HBSC-Rapport-2010.pdf. Accessed October 10, 2011. Considers daily smokers age 13–15.

France Godeau E, Vignes C, Navarro F, Monéger M-L. (2004). Consumptions of cannabis, tobacco and alcohol by French 15-year-olds: Results of the international HBSC survey. *Courrier des addictions, 6*(3): 117–120. http://www.hbsc.org/countries/downloads_countries/France/Godeau_Focus2004.pdf. Accessed October 10, 2011. Considers daily smokers age 15.

Germany Federal Ministry of Health. (2011). Drugs and addiction report: May 2011. https://www.bundesgesundheitsministerium.de/fileadmin/dateien/Publikationen/Drogen_Sucht/Broschueren/Drogen_und_Suchtbericht_2011_110517_Drogenbeauftragte.pdf. Accessed October 10, 2011. Considers current smokers age 12–17.

Hong Kong Tobacco Control Office Department of Health. (2010). Infostation: Statistics. http://www.tco.gov.hk/textonly/english/infostation/infostation_sta_01.html. Considers daily smokers age 15–19.

Japan Osaki Y, Tanihata T, Ohida T, Kanda H, Kaneita Y, Minowa M, Suzuki K, Wada K, Hayashi K. (2008). Decrease in the prevalence of smoking among Japanese adolescents and its possible causes: Periodic nationwide cross-sectional surveys. *Environmental Health Prevention Medicine, 13*: 219–226. http://www.ncbi.nlm.nih.gov/pmc/articles/PMC2698236/pdf/12199_2008_Article_33.pdf. Accessed October 11, 2011. Considers current smokers in 8th and 9th grades.

Netherlands Health Behavior in School-age Children. (2011). School Children Survey 2009. http://www.hbsc-nederland.nl/uploads/publicaties/openbaar/HBSC_Rapport_2010.pdf. Accessed October 10, 2011. Considers daily smokers age 13–15.

Spain Health Behavior in School-age Children. (2011). School Children Survey 2006. http://www.msps.es/profesionales/saludPublica/prevPromocion/promocion/saludJovenes/docs/Divulgativo_completo_HBSC2006.pdf. Accessed October 10, 2011. Considers daily and weekly smokers age 11–18.

Sweden National Institute of Public Health, Sweden. (2004). Reduced use of tobacco: How far have we come? Statistics, December 2004. http://www.fhi.se/PageFiles/3137/reduceduseoftobacco0412.pdf. Accessed October 10, 2011. Considers everyday and almost-everyday smokers age 15–16.

Switzerland Health Behavior in School-age Children. (2011). School Children Survey 2010. http://www.hbsc.ch/pdf/hbsc_bibliographie_197.pdf. Accessed October 10, 2011. Considers daily and weekly smokers age 13–15.

UK National Health Service. (2011). Smoking, drinking and drug use among young people in England in 2010. http://www.ic.nhs.uk/webfiles/publications/003_Health_Lifestyles/Smoking%20drinking%20drug%20use%202010/Smoking_drinking_and_drug_use_among_young_people_in_England_2010_Full_report.pdf. Accessed October 10, 2011. Considers regular smokers (at least one time per week) age 11–15.

US Centers for Disease Control and Prevention. (2010). National Youth Tobacco Survey. Data provided by CDC, December 2011 and reanalyzed for current smokers ages 13–15 to correspond with GYTS data.

METHODS

Centers for Disease Control and Prevention's Global Youth Tobacco Survey (GYTS) data were the primary data source for girls' smoking prevalence for all countries (unless otherwise noted above).

Data from the Global School-based Health Survey (GSHS) were used when it provided more recent data or national-level data, or when GYTS data were not available. Both surveys consider youth age 13–15.

GSHS data were used for: **Algeria, Antigua and Barbuda, Benin, Cook Islands, Costa Rica, Djibouti, Fiji, Grenada, Jamaica, Kuwait, Malawi, Maldives, Mauritania, Mongolia, Morocco, Pakistan, Peru, Philippines, Solomon Islands, Suriname, Syrian Arab Republic, Tajikistan, Thailand, Tunisia, United Arab Emirates, and West Bank and Gaza Strip.**

When only subnational data were available, the capital city was selected. If the capital city was not available, the most populated city was used. The use of subnational data is indicated on the map with a circle next to the city whose data were used.

Countries Where More Girls Than Boys Smoke

Data derived from sources listed in the Main Map.

Percentage of Girls Susceptible to Smoking

Warren C, Jones N, Eriksen M, Asma S. (2006). Patterns of global tobacco use in young people and implications for future chronic disease burden in adults. *Lancet, 367*: 749–753.

Common Reasons Young Women Start Smoking

US Department of Health and Human Services. (2001). *Women and smoking: A Report of the Surgeon General.* Rockville, MD: US Department of Health and Human Services, Public Health Service, Office of the Surgeon General.

Madagascar Smokers

WHO. Madagascar (ages 13–15) Fact Sheet, GYTS. 2008. http://apps.nccd.cdc.gov/gtssdata/Ancillary/DataReports.aspx?CAID=1. Accessed December 27, 2011.

Quote: Pierce

UC San Diego Health Systems. (2005). On-screen smoking by movie stars leads young teens to smoke, says Moores UCSD Cancer Center Study. November 14. Press release. http://health.ucsd.edu/news/2005/Pages/06_29_Pierce.aspx. Accessed October 5, 2011.

Quote: Pilote

Louise Pilote, McGill University, Canada, 2006.

Kiss Advertisement Slogan

Okorokova L. (2011). Teenage cigarette scandal. *Moscow News.* August 25. http://themoscownews.com/society/20110825/188961025.html. Accessed August 28, 2011.

Text Panel

Centers for Disease Control and Prevention. (2011). Global Youth Tobacco Survey. Personal communication.

RJ Reynolds Tobacco Company. (1982). Project planning premises and positioning hypotheses. October 21. http://legacy.library.ucsf.edu/tid/cnx18c00/pdf?search=%22natural%20appetite%20suppressant%22. Accessed October 6, 2011.

Warren C. (2006). Patterns of global tobacco use in young people and implications for future chronic disease burden in adults. *Lancet, 367*: 749–753.

World Health Organization. (2011). *WHO report on the global tobacco epidemic, 2011: Warning about the dangers of tobacco.* Geneva: World Health Organization.

11 SMOKELESS TOBACCO

Main Map

Albania Institute of Statistics, Institute of Public Health [Albania], and ICF Macro. (2010). Albania Demographic and Health Survey 2008–09. Tirana, Albania: Institute of Statistics, Institute of Public Health and ICF Macro.

Algeria Tarfani Y. (2011). Algeria: Second (Five-Year) Implementation Report. Framework Convention on Tobacco Control, World Health Organization. February 22. http://www.who.int/fctc/reporting/Algeriareport.pdf. Accessed June 28, 2011.

Armenia National Statistical Service [Armenia], Ministry of Health [Armenia], and ORC Macro. (2006). Armenia Demographic and Health Survey 2005. Calverton, MD: National Statistical Service, Ministry of Health, and ORC Macro.

Australia Australian Institute of Health and Welfare. (2005) *National drug strategy household survey: Detailed findings.* Canberra: Australian Institute of Health and Welfare.

Austria, Bulgaria, Croatia, Czech Republic, Finland, France, Greece, Hungary, Ireland, Italy, Latvia, Portugal, Spain, UK Gallus S, Lugo A, La Vecchia C, Boffetta P, Chaloupka FJ, Colombo P, Currie L, Fernandez E, Fischbacher C, Gilmore A, Godfrey F, Joossens L, Leon ME, Levy DT, Rosenqvist G, Ross H, Townsend J, Clancy L. (2012). PPACTE, WP2: *European survey on smoking.* Dublin: PPACTE Consortium.

Azerbaijan State Statistical Committee (SSC) [Azerbaijan] and Macro International Inc. (2008). Azerbaijan Demographic and Health Survey 2006. Calverton, MD: State Statistical Committee and Macro International Inc.

Bangladesh, Egypt, India, Mexico, Philippines, Poland, Russian Federation, Thailand, Ukraine, Uruguay Centers for Disease Control and Prevention. (2011). Global Adult Tobacco Survey. www.cdc.gov/tobacco/global/gtss/. Accessed September 1, 2011.

Barbados, Benin, Bhutan, Cape Verde, Chad, Gambia, Georgia, Guinea, Libyan Arab Jamahiriya, Malawi, Mali, Micronesia (Federated States of), Mongolia, Myanmar, Saint Kitts and Nevis, Sao Tome and Principe, Saudi Arabia, Sri Lanka, Swaziland STEPwise Approach to Surveillance via WHO. (2011). *WHO report on the global tobacco epidemic, 2011. The MPOWER package.* Geneva: World Health Organization.

Brazil Centers for Disease Control and Prevention. (2011). Global Adult Tobacco Survey.

Cambodia Sokrin K., Sovann S. (2011). Cambodia: Second (Five-Year) Implementation Report, Framework Convention on Tobacco Control, World Health Organization. February 13. http://www.who.int.proxy.library.emory.edu/fctc/reporting/Cambodiarep.pdf. Accessed December 12, 2011.

Centers for Disease Control and Prevention. (2011). Global Adult Tobacco Survey.

Canada Sabiston C. (2010). Canada: Second (Five-Year) Implementation Report. Framework Convention on Tobacco Control, World Health Organization. March 10. http://www.who.int/fctc/reporting/Canada_5y_report_v2_final.pdf. Accessed September 1, 2011.

China, Viet Nam Global Adult Tobacco Survey via WHO. (2011). *WHO report on the global tobacco epidemic, 2011.*

Congo (Democratic Republic of) Longo-Mbenza. (2006). STEPS Survey Report: Democratic Republic of the Congo, Selon l'approche STEPS de l'OMS. Kinshasa: DRC Ministry of Health, November. http://www.who.int.proxy.library.emory.edu/chp/steps/STEPS_DRC_Final.pdf. Accessed July 7, 2011.

Costa Rica Ávila Aguero M, Córdoba R, Barrantes O. (2011). Costa Rica: First (Two-Year) Implementation Report. Framework Convention on Tobacco Control, World Health Organization. March 10. http://www.who.int.proxy.library.emory.edu/fctc/reporting/party_reports/Costa_Rica_2y_report.pdf. Accessed October 9, 2011.

Denmark Monitorering af danskernes rygevaner via WHO, *WHO report on the global tobacco epidemic*, 2011.

Dominican Republic Centro de Estudios Sociales y Demográficos (CESDEM) y Macro International Inc. (2008). Encuesta Demográfica y de Salud 2007. Santo Domingo, DR: CESDEM y Macro International Inc.

Eritrea Mebrahtu G, Usman A. (2004). STEPS Survey Report: Eritrea. Eritrea Ministry of Health. http://www.who.int.proxy.library.emory.edu/chp/steps/STEPS_Eritrea_Data.pdf. Accessed July 7, 2011.

Ethiopia Central Statistical Agency [Ethiopia] and ORC Macro. (2006). Ethiopia Demographic and Health Survey 2005. Addis Ababa: Central Statistical Agency and ORC Macro.

Gabon Comlan P. (2009). STEPS Survey Report: Gabon. Libreville: Gabon Ministry of Public Health and Hygiene, June 23. http://www.who.int.proxy.library.emory.edu/chp/steps/2009_STEPS_Report_Gabon.pdf. Accessed July 8, 2011.

Ghana Ghana Statistical Service, Ghana Health Service, and ICF Macro. (2009). Ghana Demographic and Health Survey 2008. Accra: GSS, GHS, and ICF Macro.

Guyana Yussuf S. (2010). Guyana: Second (Five-Year) Implementation Report. Framework Convention on Tobacco Control, World Health Organization. December 21. http://www.who.int.proxy.library.emory.edu/fctc/Guyana_5y_report.pdf. Accessed October 19, 2011.

Haiti Cayemittes M, Placide M, Mariko S, Barrère B, Sévère B, Canez A. (2007). *Enquête mortalité, morbidité et utilisation des services, Haïti, 2005–2006.* Calverton, MD: Ministère de la Santé Publique et de la Population, Institut Haïtien de l'Enfance et Macro International Inc.

Iceland, Malaysia, Mauritania, Nepal, Tunisia, Uzbekistan, Yemen World Health Organization, WHO Report on the Global Tobacco Epidemic. (2009). Implementing smoke-free environments. http://www.who.int/tobacco/mpower/en/. Accessed October 1, 2011.

Indonesia Statistics Indonesia (Badan Pusat Statistik) and Macro International. (2008). Indonesia Demographic and Health Survey 2007. Calverton, MD: BPS and Macro International.

Iraq World Health Organization. (2006). STEPS Survey Report: Iraq. http://www.who.int.proxy.library.emory.edu/chp/steps/IraqSTEPSReport2006.pdf. Accessed July 8, 2011.

Kenya Kenya National Bureau of Statistics and ICF Macro. (2010). Kenya Demographic and Health Survey 2008–09. Calverton, MD: KNBS and ICF Macro.

Korea (Democratic People's Republic of) Nagi. (2007). STEPS Survey Report: DPRK. http://www.who.int.proxy.library.emory.edu/chp/steps/DPRK_STEPS_Report_2007.pdf. Accessed July 8, 2011.

Kyrgyzstan National Epidemiological Study of Tobacco Use Prevalence in Kyrgyzstan via WHO. (2011). *WHO Report on the Global Tobacco Epidemic, 2011.* http://www.who.int/fctc/reporting/Kyrgyzstan_annex1_prevalence_data_2006.pdf. Accessed October 1, 2011.

Lao People's Democratic Republic Vongvichith E, Phounsavath S. (2010). STEPS Survey Report: Laos PDR. January. http://www.who.int.proxy.library.emory.edu/chp/steps/2008_STEPS_Report_Laos.pdf. Accessed July 8, 2011.

Lesotho Ministry of Health and Social Welfare (Lesotho) and ICF Macro. (2010). Lesotho Demographic and Health Survey 2009. Maseru, Lesotho: MOHSW and ICF Macro.

Liberia Liberia Institute of Statistics and Geo-Information Services (Liberia), Ministry of Health and Social Welfare (Liberia), National AIDS Control Program (Liberia), and Macro International Inc. (2008). Liberia Demographic and Health Survey 2007. Monrovia.

Madagascar Institut National de la Statistique (INSTAT) et ICF Macro. (2010). *Enquête Démographique et de Santé de Madagascar 2008–2009.* Antananarivo, Madagascar: INSTAT et ICF Macro.

Maldives Ministry of Health and Family (Maldives) and ICF Macro. (2010). *Maldives Demographic and Health Survey 2009.* Calverton, MD: MOHF and ICF Macro.

Marshall Islands Edward R, Langdrik J. (2010). Marshall Islands: Second (Five-Year) Implementation Report. Framework Convention on Tobacco Control, World Health Organization. March 8. http://www.who.int/fctc/reportingMarshallislands report.pdf. Accessed June 8, 2011.

Moldova (Republic of) National Scientific and Applied Center for Preventive Medicine (Moldova) and ORC Macro. (2006). *Moldova Demographic and Health Survey 2005.* Calverton, MD: National Scientific and Applied Center for Preventive Medicine of the Ministry of Health of Moldova.

Mozambique Araújo C et al. Manufactured and hand-rolled cigarettes and smokeless tobacco consumption in Mozambique: Regional differences at early stages of the tobacco epidemic. In *Drug and Alcohol Dependence.* http://www.sciencedirect.com/science/article/pii/S0376871611002572. Accessed November 5, 2011.

Namibia Ministry of Health and Social Services (Namibia) and Macro International Inc. (2008). *Namibia Demographic and Health Survey 2006–07.* Windhoek, Namibia: MoHSS and Macro International Inc.

Nepal World Health Organization. (2009). *WHO Report on the Global Tobacco Epidemic, 2009: Implementing smoke-free environments.* http://www.who.int/tobacco/mpower/en/. Accessed May 1, 2011.

Niger Niger Ministry of Public Health. (2008). STEPS Survey Report: Niger. December. http://www.who.int.proxy.library.emory.edu/chp/steps/2007_STEPS_Report_Niger.pdf. Accessed July 8, 2011.

Nigeria National Population Commission (Nigeria) and ICF Macro. (2009). *Nigeria Demographic and Health Survey 2008.* Abuja, Nigeria: National Population Commission and ICF Macro.

Norway Statistisk sentralbyrås Reise—og ferieundersøkelse via WHO. (2011). *WHO report on the global tobacco epidemic, 2011.*

Pakistan World Health Organization. (2008). STEPS Survey Report: Pakistan. December. http://www.who.int.proxy.library.emory.edu/chp/steps/Pakistan_Book_chapter.pdf. Accessed July 8, 2011.

Paraguay ERC Group. (2010). World cigarettes: Americas. Suffolk, UK. February.

Qatar World Health Survey Qatar. (2010). Qatar: Second (Five-Year) Implementation Report. Framework Convention on Tobacco Control, World Health Organization. July 27. http://www.who.int.proxy.library.emory.edu/fctc/reporting/Qatar_5y_report.pdf. Accessed December 1, 2011.

Rwanda Institut National de la Statistique du Rwanda and ORC Macro. (2006). *Rwanda Demographic and Health Survey 2005.* Calverton, MD: INSR and ORC Macro.

Samoa Ministry of Health (Samoa), Bureau of Statistics (Samoa), and ICF Macro. (2010). *Samoa Demographic and Health Survey 2009.* Apia, Samoa: Ministry of Health, Samoa.

Seychelles Bovet P, Julita W. (2007). STEPS Survey Report: Seychelles. Victoria: Seychelles Ministry of Health and Social Development. July 7. http://www.who.int.proxy.library.emory.edu/chp/steps/2004_STEPS_Report_Seychelles.pdf. Accessed July 8, 2011.

Sierra Leone Sierra Leone Ministry of Health. (2009). STEPS Survey Report: Sierra Leone. http://www.who.int.proxy.library.emory.edu/chp/steps/2009_STEPS_Report_SierraLeone.pdf.

South Africa South Africa Demographic and Health Survey. (2003). http://whqlibdoc.who.int/publications/2009/9789241563918_eng_full.pdf. Accessed July 8, 2011.

Sudan Elzein M. (2005). STEPS Survey Report: Sudan, Selon l'approche STEPS de l'OMS. Kinshasa: Sudan Ministry of Health. http://www.who.int.proxy.library.emory.edu/chp/steps/STEPS_Report_Sudan2005.pdf. Accessed July 8, 2011.

Sweden The National Survey on Public Health via WHO. (2011). *WHO report on the global tobacco epidemic, 2011.*

Switzerland Tabakmonitoring: Schweizerische Umfrage zum Tabakkonsum via WHO. (2011). *WHO report on the global tobacco epidemic, 2011.*

Syrian Arab Republic World Health Organization. (2010). Syria: Second (Five-Year) Implementation Report. Framework Convention on Tobacco Control, World Health Organization. February 28. http://www.who.int.proxy.library.emory.edu/fctc/reporting/Syria_5y_report.pdf. Accessed July 7, 2011.

Tanzania (United Republic of) National Bureau of Statistics (Tanzania) and ICF Macro. (2011). *Tanzania Demographic and Health Survey 2010.* Dar es Salaam: NBS and ICF Macro.

Timor-Leste National Statistics Directorate (Timor-Leste), Ministry of Finance (Timor-Leste), and ICF Macro. (2010). *Timor-Leste Demographic and Health Survey 2009–10.* Dili, Timor-Leste: NSD and ICF Macro.

Turkmenistan ERC Group. (2007). World cigarettes: Central & Eastern Europe. Suffolk, UK. February.

Uganda Uganda Bureau of Statistics (UBOS) and Macro International Inc. (2007). *Uganda Demographic and Health Survey 2006.* Calverton, MD: UBOS and Macro International Inc.

US Centers for Disease Control and Prevention, Office on Smoking and Health. (2009). Smoking and tobacco use: Fact sheets on smoking and tobacco use. http://www.cdc.gov/tobacco/data_statistics/fact_sheets/smokeless/smokeless_facts/index.htm#use. Accessed June 14, 2011.

Zambia World Health Organization. (2008). STEPS Survey Report: Zambia. Zambia Ministry of Public Health and World Health Organization. November. http://www.who.int.proxy.library.emory.edu/chp/steps/2008_STEPS_Report_Zambia.pdf. Accessed July 8, 2011.

Zimbabwe Central Statistical Office (Zimbabwe) and Macro International Inc. (2007). *Zimbabwe Demographic and Health Survey 2005–06.* Calverton, MD: CSO and Macro International Inc.

METHODS

If male and female prevalence were reported separately, a weighted average prevalence was calculated based on adult gender distribution (age 15–64) using data from:

Central Intelligence Agency. (2011). CIA: The world factbook. https://www.cia.gov/library/publications/the-world-factbook/geos/bg.html. Accessed July 13, 2011.

Symbol

Countries with a full or partial ban on the manufacture, sale, or import of smokeless tobacco products:

Australia Chapman S, Wakefield M. (2001). Tobacco control advocacy in Australia: Reflections on 30 years of progress. *Health Education and Behavior, 28*: 274–289.

Austria, Belgium, Bulgaria, Cyprus, Czech Republic, Denmark, Estonia, Finland, France, Germany, Greece, Hungary, Hong Kong, Ireland, Italy, Latvia, Lithuania, Luxembourg, Malta, Netherlands, Poland, Portugal, Romania, Slovakia, Slovenia, Spain, UK Council Directive 92/41/EEC of 15 May 1992 amending Directive 89/622/EEC on the approximation of the laws, regulations and administrative provisions of the Member States concerning the labelling of tobacco products (European Economic and Social Committee, May 15, 1992), http://www.estoc.org/regulation/background. Accessed June 24, 2011.

Bahrain *Time Out Bahrain* Staff. (2009). Smoking ban in Bahrain. http://www.timeoutbahrain.com/knowledge/features/8573-smoking-ban-in-bahrain. Accessed July 7, 2011.

Bhutan Norbu U. (2010). Bhutan: Second (Five-Year) Implementation Report. Framework Convention on Tobacco Control, World Health Organization. November 15. http://www.who.int/fctc/reporting/Bhutan_5y_report.pdf. Accessed July 7, 2011.

Israel, Japan, Kuwait, Saudi Arabia, Singapore, Thailand, Turkey WHO International Agency for Research in Cancer. (2007). Smokeless tobacco and some tobacco-specific n-nitrosamines. IARC Monographs 89. Lyon, France: IARC.

New Zealand World Health Organization. (1997). *Tobacco or health: A global status report.* Geneva: WHO.

United Arab Emirates J. Bowman. (2008). Chewing tobacco outlawed. Arabian Business Publishing. May. http://www.arabianbusiness.com/chewing-tobacco-outlawed-49783.html. Accessed July 13, 2011.

Tanzania (United Republic of) Kaduri P, Kitua H, Mbatia J, Kitua AY, Mbwambo J. (2008). Smokeless tobacco use among adolescents in Ilala Municipality, Tanzania. *Tanzania Journal of Health Research, 10*(1): 28–33.

Global Smokeless Tobacco Sales Volume

Smokeless tobacco sales volumes (historical and projected): Euromonitor International. (2011). *Passport Database.* Accessed October 1, 2011.

Tonnes of smokeless tobacco were converted to shipping containers according to:

Maersk Line. (2011). Maersk Line equipment guide. http://www.maerskline.com/globalfile/?path=/pdf/containerDimensions. Accessed December 23, 2011.

Patterns of Smokeless and Smoking Tobacco Use

Centers for Disease Control and Prevention. (2011). Global Adult Tobacco Survey. www.cdc.gov/tobacco/global/gtss/. Accessed October 1, 2011.

Snuff and Cigarettes Sold in Sweden

1990–2006 SALES FIGURES

Forey B, Hamling J, Hamling J, Lee P. (2009). International smoking statistics: Sweden. Web edition. Sutton, UK: P N Lee Statistics & Computing Ltd. July 24. http://www.pnlee.co.uk/Downloads/ISS/ISS-Sweden_090724.pdf. Accessed May 4, 2011.

2007–2010 SALES FIGURES AND COMMENT ON ST TAX INCREASE
Euromonitor International. (2011). Smokeless tobacco in Sweden. August 18. Passport Database. Accessed October 1, 2011.

Butler: Butler D. (2008). A path forward in tobacco harm reduction. Speech presented at the 93rd Annual TMA Industry Conference, May 19.

WHO Study Group on Smokeless Tobacco Control
World Health Organization. (1988). Smokeless tobacco control: Report of a WHO study group. Geneva: World Health Organization.

Quote
Title track from the Bollywood movie *Wanted*. (2009). Dir. Deva.

Text Panel
IARC. (2009). IARC handbooks of cancer prevention, tobacco control, Vol. 13: Evaluating the effectiveness of smoke-free policies. Lyon, France.

Conference of the Parties to the WHO Framework Convention on Tobacco Control. (2010). Control and prevention of smokeless tobacco products and electronic cigarettes. Punta del Este, Uruguay, September 15. http://apps.who.int/gb/fctc/PDF/cop4/FCTC_COP4_12-en.pdf. Accessed July 13, 2011.

Chassin L, Presson C, Sherman S, McLaughlin L, Gioia D. (1985). Psychosocial correlates of adolescent smokeless tobacco use. *Addictive Behaviors, 10*(4): 431–435. doi:10.1016/0306-4603(85)90041-3.

Critchley JA, Unal B. (2003). Health effects associated with smokeless tobacco: A systematic review. *Thorax, 58*(5): 435–443. doi:10.1136/thorax.58.5.435.

Mejia A, Ling P. (2010). Tobacco industry consumer research on smokeless tobacco users and product development. *American Journal of Public Health, 100*(1): 78–87. doi: 10.2105/AJPH.2008.152603.

Mejia A, Ling P, Glantz S. (2010). Quantifying the effects of promoting smokeless tobacco as a harm reduction strategy in the USA. *Tobacco Control, 19*(4): 297–305. doi:10.1136/tc.2009.031427.

Steyn K, De Wet T, Saloojee Y, Nel H, Yach D. (2006). The influence of maternal cigarette smoking, snuff use and passive smoking on pregnancy outcomes: The Birth to Ten Study. *Pediatric and Perinatal Epidemiology, 20*(2): 90–99. doi:10.1111/j.1365-3016.2006.00707.x.

Warnakulasuriya S, Dietrich T, Bornstein M, Casals Peidró E, Preshaw P, Walter C, Wennström J, Bergström J. (2010). Oral health risks of tobacco use and effects of cessation. *International Dental Journal, 60*(1): 7–30.

12 HEALTH PROFESSIONALS

Main Map
SOURCES

Centers for Disease Control and Prevention. (2011). Global Tobacco Surveillance System: Global Health Professions Student Survey.

ALTERNATE DATA SOURCES
Canada Thakore S, Zahinoor I, Jarvis S, Payne E, Keetbaas S, Payne R, Rothenburg L. (2009). The perceptions and habits of alcohol consumption and smoking among Canadian medical students. *Academic Psychiatry, 33*: 193–197.

China Ma X. (2011). The report on the baseline survey of CMB: China medical tobacco control initiative. Presented at the China Tobacco Control Research Symposium, Yunan, China. October.

France Josseran L, Raffin J, Dautzenberg B, Brücker G. (2003). Knowledge, opinions and tobacco consumption in a French faculty of medicine. *La Presse Médicale, 32*(40): 1883–1886.

Germany Kusma B, Quarcoo D, Vitzthum K, Welte T, Mache S, Meyer-Falcke A, Groneberg D, Raupach T. (2010). Berlin's medical students' smoking habits, knowledge about smoking and attitudes toward smoking cessation counseling. *Journal of Occupational Medicine and Toxicology, 5*(9). Note: Study only includes medical students in Berlin.

Ireland McCartan B, McCreary C, Healy C. (2008). Attitudes of Irish dental, dental hygiene and dental nursing students and newly qualified practitioners to tobacco use cessation: A national survey. *European Journal of Dental Education, 12*: 17–22.

Japan Suzuki K, Ohida T, Yokoyama E, Kaneita Y, Takemura S. (2005). Smoking among Japanese nursing students: Nationwide survey. *Journal of Advanced Nursing, 49*(3): 268–275. Note: Study only includes female nursing students.

US Patkar A, Hill K, Batra V, Vergare M, Leone F. (2003). A comparison of smoking habits among medical and nursing students. *CHEST 124*(4): 1415–1420.

METHODS
Centers for Disease Control and Prevention Global Health Professions Student Survey (GHPSS) data were the primary data source for current smoking rates among health professions students for all countries unless otherwise noted.

When only subnational data were available, the capital city was selected. If the capital city was not available, the most populated city was used. The use of subnational data is indicated on the map with a circle next to the city whose data were used.

Data were used for medical students when available. If medical student data were not available, nursing student data, and then dental student data were used. Nursing student data were used instead of medical student data in the following countries due to a substantially larger sample size among the nursing student survey: **Oman, Papua New Guinea, Suriname, Trinidad and Tobago, West Bank** (not including Gaza Strip), **Zambia.**

Percent of Countries With Smoke-Free Health-Care Facilities
World Health Organization. (2011). *WHO report on the global tobacco epidemic, 2011: Warning about the dangers of tobacco.* Geneva: World Health Organization.

METHODS:
West Bank and Gaza Strip classified in the Eastern Mediterranean Region for the purposes of this inset.

Countries Providing Cessation Support Services in the Offices of Health Professionals
World Health Organization. (2011). Data derived from *WHO report on the global tobacco epidemic, 2011: Warning about the dangers of tobacco.*

Even Brief Tobacco Cessation Interventions Are Effective
Fiore M, Bailey W, Cohen S, et al. (2000). *Treating tobacco use and dependence.* Quick Reference Guide for Clinicians. Rockville, MD: US Department of Health and Human Services. Public Health Service. October. http://www.surgeongeneral.gov/tobacco/tobaqrg.htm. Accessed August 10, 2011.

Hong Kong
Lam T, Tse L, Yu I, Griffiths S. (2009). Prevalence of smoking and environmental tobacco smoke exposure, and attitudes and beliefs towards tobacco control among Hong Kong medical students. *Public Health, 123*: 42–46.

Buenos Aires
Warren C, Jones N, Chauvin J, Peruga A. (2008). Tobacco use and cessation counseling: Cross-country data from the Global Health Professions Student Survey (GHPSS), 2005–2007. *Tobacco Control, 17*(4): 238–247.

Uganda
Warren C, Jones N, Chauvin J, Peruga A. (2008). Tobacco use and cessation counseling.

Pfizer
Loo D. (2011). China endorsing tobacco in schools adds to $10 trillion cost. *Bloomberg News.* September 21. http://www.bloomberg.com/news/2011-09-20/china-endorsing-tobacco-in-schools-adds-to-10-trillion-gdp-cost.html. Accessed October 6, 2011.

Quote: WHO
World Health Organization. (N.d.). *MPOWER:* Offer help to quit. http://www.who.int/tobacco/mpower/publications/en_tfi_mpower_brochure_o_page2.pdf. Accessed August 28, 2011.

Quote: American Tobacco Company
Robert Wood Johnson Foundation. (2011). The way we were: Tobacco ads through the years. April. http://www.rwjf.org/files/research/72060.tobaccoads.041511.pdf. Accessed December 15, 2011.

Text Panel
American Cancer Society. (2011). Guide to quitting smoking. http://www.cancer.org/acs/groups/cid/documents/webcontent/002971-pdf.pdf. Accessed August 30, 2011.

Fiore M, Bailey W, Cohen S, et al. (2000). *Treating tobacco use and dependence.*

Lam T, Tse L, Yu I, Griffiths S. (2009). Prevalence of smoking and environmental tobacco smoke exposure.

World Health Organization. (2004). News release: Health professionals to promote a new code of conduct on tobacco. January 30. http://www.who.int/mediacentre/news/releases/2004/pr9/en/. Accessed August 10, 2011.

13 COSTS TO SOCIETY

Main Map and Symbol
SOURCES
Estimates of the direct costs of smoking derived from:

Argentina Cevallos D. (2008). Health-Latin America: Tobacco regulations as solid as smoke. June 4. http://www.ipsnews.net/news.asp?idnews=42657. Accessed June 9, 2011.

Australia Collins D, Lapsley H. (2008). The costs of tobacco, alcohol and illicit drug abuse to Australian society in 2004/05. Department of Health and Ageing at the University of New South Wales.

Bangladesh Bangladesh Ministry of Health & Family Welfare. (2010). Bangladesh: Second (Five-Year) Implementation Report. Framework Convention on Tobacco Control, World Health Organization. February 25. http://www.who.int/fctc/reporting/Bangladesh_5y_report.pdf. Accessed June 28, 2011.

Barbados Lwegaba A. (2004). Excess health care cost associated with a low smoking prevalence, Barbados. *West Indian Medical Journal, 53*(1): 12–16. (Authors' calculation)

Brazil Pinto M, Alicia Domínguez Ugá M. (2010). The costs of tobacco-related diseases for the National Health System. *Cadernos de Saúde Públicai, 26*(6): 1234–1245. http://www.scielo.br/scielo.php?pid=S0102-311X2010000600016&script=sci_arttext&tlng=en. Accessed February 3, 2011.

Canada Health Canada, Government of Canada. (2010). News release: Harper government to strengthen and enlarge health warnings on cigarette packages. December 30. http://www.hc-sc.gc.ca/ahc-asc/media/nr-cp/_2010/2010_233-eng.php. Accessed February 7, 2011.

Chile Cevallos D. (2008). Health-Latin America.

China Yang L et al. (2011). Economic costs attributable to smoking in China: Update and an 8-year comparison, 2000–2008. *Tobacco Control.* January 21. http://tobaccocontrol.bmj.com/content/early/2011/01/21/tc.2010.042028.abstract.

Czech Republic Ross H. (2004). Critique of the Philip Morris study of the cost of smoking in the Czech Republic. *Nicotine & Tobacco Research: Official Journal of the Society for Research on Nicotine and Tobacco, 6*(1): 181–189.

Denmark Falk J. (2010). Denmark: Second (Five-Year) Implementation Report. Framework Convention on Tobacco Control, World Health Organization. July 13. http://www.who.int/fctc/reporting/Denmark_5y_report.pdf. Accessed June 28, 2011.

Egypt Nassar H. (2003). The economics of tobacco in Egypt: A new analysis of demand. Washington, DC: The International Bank for Reconstruction and Development / The World Bank. March.

Estonia Taal A, Kiivet R, Hu T-W. (2004). The economics of tobacco in Estonia. Washington, DC: The International Bank for Reconstruction and Development / The World Bank. June.

Finland Siukola R, Paaso K. (2010). Finland: Second (Five-Year) Implementation Report. Framework Convention on Tobacco Control, World Health Organization, April 23. http://www.who.int/fctc/reporting/Finland_5y_report_version2_final.pdf. Accessed June 28, 2011.

France Tolstoi N. (2010). France: Second (Five-Year) Implementation Report. Framework Convention on Tobacco Control, World Health Organization. June 10. http://www.who.int.proxy.library.emory.edu/fctc/reporting/France_5y_report.pdf. Accessed October 17, 2011.

Germany Neubauer S et al. (2006). Mortality, morbidity and costs attributable to smoking in Germany: Update and a 10-year comparison. *Tobacco Control, 15*(6): 464–471.

Guatemala Center for Tobacco Free Kids. (1998). Central America case study. October. http://www.healthbridge.ca/tcmanual.pdf. Accessed October 1, 2011.

Hong Kong SAR, China McGhee S et al. (2006). Cost of tobacco-related diseases, including passive smoking, in Hong Kong. *Tobacco Control, 15*(2): 125–130.

Hungary Hungarian National Institute for Health Development. (2007). Tobacco Control. http://www.oefi.hu/DOHANYZAS_2007.pdf. Accessed October 1, 2011.

Iceland Sigillum Universitatis Islandiae. (2000). Cost of smoking in Icelandic society 2000: Report to Tobacco Control Task Force. Haskola Islands.

India John R, Sung H-Y, Max W. (2009). Economic cost of tobacco use in India, 2004. *Tobacco Control, 18*(2): 138–143.

Indonesia SEATCA. (2010). ASEAN Tobacco Tax Report Card: Regional comparisons and trends. Southeast Asia Tobacco Control Alliance.

Israel Ginsberg G, Rosen B, Rosenberg E. (2010). Cost-utility analyses of interventions to reduce the smoking-related burden of disease in Israel. Jerusalem: Myers-JDC-Brookdale Institute; Smokler Center for Health Policy Research. February. http://brookdale.jdc.org.il/?CategoryID=192&ArticleID=115. Accessed February 23, 2011.

Japan Tanaka Y. (2007) Comparison of the direct healthcare costs between smokers and non-smokers. Research on the economic impact of smoking.p.9-18 National Institute of Public Health: Saitama.

Korea (Republic of) Kang HY, Kim HJ, Park TK, Jee SH, Nam CM, Park HW. (2003). Economic burden of smoking in Korea. *Tobacco Control, 12*: 37–44.

Lao People's Democratic Republic SEATCA. (2010). ASEAN Tobacco Tax Report Card.

Lebanon Chaaban J, Naamani N, Salti N. (2010). The economics of tobacco in Lebanon: An estimation of the social costs of tobacco consumption. American University in Beirut Tobacco Control Research Group. April. http://www.aub.edu.lb/ifi/public_policy/rapp/rapp_research/Documents/economics_of_tobacco_lebanon/Final_Report/The_Economics_of_Tobacco_in_Lebanon.pdf. Accessed May 25, 2011.

Malaysia Zain Z. (2010). Malaysia: Second (Five-Year) Implementation Report. Framework Convention on Tobacco Control, World Health Organization. December 15. http://www.who.int.proxy.library.emory.edu/fctc/Malaysia_5y_report.pdf. Accessed May 25, 2011.

Mexico Waters H et al. (2010). The economics of tobacco and tobacco taxation in Mexico. Paris: International Union Against Tuberculosis and Lung Disease. http://www.tobaccofreecenter.org/files/pdfs/en/Mexico_tobacco_taxes_report_en.pdf. Accessed August 1, 2011.

Myanmar Kyaing N. (2003). Tobacco economics in Myanmar. Washington DC: The International Bank for Reconstruction and Development / The World Bank.

Nepal Himalayan News Service. (2011). Govt directive on tobacco soon. *Himalayan Times* (Kathmandu). April 14. http://www.thehimalayantimes.com/fullNews.php?headline=Govt+directive+on++tobacco+soon+&NewsID=284019. Accessed May 25, 2011.

Netherlands van der Avert M, van Bolhuis A. (2010). Netherlands: Second (Five-Year) Implementation Report. Framework Convention on Tobacco Control, World Health Organization. April 27. http://www.who.int.proxy.library.emory.edu/fctc/reporting/Netherlands_5y_report_v2_final.pdf. Accessed October 17, 2011.

New Zealand Cancer Society of New Zealand. (2004). What smoking costs. Cancer Society of New Zealand. September.

Nigeria Daramola Z. (2007). FG hailed over move against tobacco costs. *Daily Trust*. November 12.

Panama Roa R, Vergara F. (2010). Panama: Second (Five-Year) Implementation Report. Framework Convention on Tobacco Control, World Health Organization. February 27. http://www.who.int/fctc/reporting/Panama_5y_report_final.pdf. Accessed June 28, 2011.

Philippines Quimbo S, Casorla A, Miguel-Baquilod M, Medalla F. (2007). The economics of tobacco and tobacco taxation (Philippines). UPecon Foundation and Department of Health.

Poland Krzyżanowska A, Głogowski C. (2004). Nikotynizm na świecie: Nastepstwa ekonomiczne (The global nicotine addiction and its economic consequences), *Menedżer Zdrowia, 2*: 98–103. (In Polish)

Singapore Quah E, Tan K, Saw S, Yong J. (2002). The social cost of smoking in Singapore. *Singapore Medical Journal, 43*(7): 340–344.

South Africa Yach D, McIntyre D, Saloojee Y. (1992). Smoking in South Africa: The health and economic impact. *Tobacco Control, 1*(4): 272–280.

Spain Ahn N, Molina J. (2001). Smoking in Spain: Analysis of initiation and cessation. FEDEA. February.

Sweden Johansson A. (2010). Sweden: Second (Five-Year) Implementation Report. Framework Convention on Tobacco Control, World Health Organization, October 5. http://www.who.int/fctc/reporting/swe/en/index.html. Accessed March 1, 2011.

Switzerland Weiser S. (2009). Synthesis report: Economic evaluation of prevention measures in Switzerland. Zurich: Swiss Federal Office of Public Health. December. http://www.health-evaluation.admin.ch. Accessed May 25, 2011.

Thailand Leartsakulpanitch J, Nganthavee W, Salole E. (2007). The economic burden of smoking-related disease in Thailand: A prevalence-based analysis. *Journal of the Medical Association of Thailand-Chotmaihet Thangphaet, 90*(9): 1925–1929.

UK Allender S. et al. (2009). The burden of smoking-related ill health in the UK. *Tobacco Control, 18*(4): 262.

US Centers for Disease Control and Prevention. (2008). Smoking-attributable mortality, years of potential life lost, and productivity losses—United States, 2000–2004. *Morbidity and Mortality Weekly Report, 57*(45): 1226–1228.

Uruguay Amos A. (2006). Tobacco control economy in the countries of Mercosur and Associated States. Organización Panamericana de la Salud. (In Spanish)

Venezuela (Bolivarian Republic of) Pan American Sanitary Bureau. (1998). Cost–benefit analysis of smoking. Caracas: Pan American Health Organization.

Viet Nam Ross H, Trung D, and Phu V. (2007). The costs of smoking in Vietnam: The case of inpatient care. *Tobacco Control, 16*(6): 405–409.

METHODS

If the estimate was provided in currency other than US dollars, the amount was converted to US dollars using average yearly exchange rates: OANDA. (N.d.). Average exchange rates. http://www.oanda.com/currency/average.

The direct cost of smoking as a percentage of countries' GDP was calculated based on data on GDP from International Monetary Fund. (2011). World economic outlook database. April.

Direct vs. Indirect Tobacco-Related Costs

ESTIMATES FROM

Centers for Disease Control and Prevention. (2008). Smoking-attributable mortality, years of potential life lost, and productivity losses—United States, 2000–2004.

Economics of Tobacco Control in Southern Africa. (1998). The economics of tobacco control project. School of Economics, University of Cape Town. Report submitted for the Research for International Tobacco Control (RITC). June 30.

Weiser S. (2009). Synthesis report.

The Opportunity Costs of Smoking

The sources for the estimate of direct costs of smoking are the same as in the main map. The estimates of opportunity costs obtained from:

Badawi H. (2006). The 2007 budget speech. Malaysia Ministry of Finance. September 1. http://www.treasury.gov.my/pdf/budget/bs07.pdf. Accessed October 17, 2011.

Chile Ministry of the Interior. (2008). Project Budget, 2008. http://www.dipres.gob.cl/572/articles-37002_doc_pdf.pdf. Accessed October 17, 2011.

HM Treasury Great Britain. (2010). Spending review 2010. Norwich: Stationery Office.

New Zealand Ministry of Education. (2009). Budget 2009: Education initiatives. http://www.minedu.govt.nz/theMinistry/Budget/Budget2009/EducationInitiatives.aspx. Accessed October 17, 2011.

Thailand Ministry of Finance. (2010). Outlays by function of government. http://dw.mof.go.th/foc/gfs/database/C7_Budgetary.html. Accessed October 17, 2011.

Tobacco Is a Drain on Health-Care Systems

Health-care spending on tobacco-related illnesses:

China Yang L et al. (2011). Economic costs attributable to smoking in China.

Finland Siukola R, Paaso K. (2010). Finland: Second (Five-Year) Implementation Report.

Egypt Nassar H. (2003). The economics of tobacco in Egypt.

Germany Neubauer S et al. (2006). Mortality, morbidity and costs attributable to smoking in Germany.

Mexico Waters H et al. (2010). The economics of tobacco and tobacco taxation in Mexico.

UK Allender S et al. (2009). The burden of smoking-related ill health in the UK, 262.

US Centers for Disease Control and Prevention. (2008). Smoking-attributable mortality, years of potential life lost, and productivity losses—United States, 2000–2004.

TOTAL HEALTH-CARE SPENDING

World Bank. (2011). World databank. http://databank.worldbank.org. Accessed October 17, 2011.

Estimate of Direct Costs

Centers for Disease Control and Prevention. (2008). Smoking-attributable mortality, years of potential life lost, and productivity losses—United States, 2000–2004.

Cigarette Market Value

Euromonitor International. (2011). Passport Database. Accessed October 1, 2011.

Quote: Gruber

Gruber J and Koszegi B. (2008). A modern economic view of tobacco taxation. International Union Against Tuberculosis and Lung Disease. http://www.tobaccofreecenter.org/files/pdfs/en/modern_economic_view_taxation_en.pdf. Accessed December 6, 2011.

Text Panel

Danaei G, Ding E, Mozaffarian D, Taylor B, Rehm J, Murray C, et al. (2009). The preventable causes of death in the United States: Comparative risk assessment of dietary, lifestyle, and metabolic risk factors. *PLoS Medicine, 6*(4): e1000058.

Fenoglio P, Parel V, Kopp P. (2003). The social cost of alcohol, tobacco and illicit drugs in France, 1997. *European Addiction Research, 9*(1): 18–28.

Geist H. (1999). Global assessment of deforestation related to tobacco farming. *Tobacco Control, 8*(1): 18–28.

Geist H, Chang K, Etges V, Abdallah J. (2009). Tobacco growers at the crossroads: Towards a comparison of diversification and ecosystem impacts. *Land Use Policy, 26*(4): 1066–1079.

Jha P. (2000). *Tobacco control in developing countries*. Oxford: Oxford University Press.

Leistikow B, Martin D, Milano C. (2000). Fire injuries, disasters, and costs from cigarettes and cigarette lights: A global overview. *Preventive Medicine, 31*(2 Pt 1): 91–99.

Otañez M, Glantz S. (2011). Social responsibility in tobacco production? Tobacco companies' use of green supply chains to obscure the real costs of tobacco farming. *Tobacco Control*. April 19. http://tobaccocontrol.bmj.com/content/early/2011/04/15/tc.2010.039537.abstract. Accessed May 9, 2011.

Ross H. (2004). Critique of the Philip Morris study of the cost of smoking in the Czech Republic. *Nicotine and Tobacco Research, 6*(1): 181–189.

Warner K. (2000). The economics of tobacco: Myths and realities. *Tobacco Control, 9*(1): 78–89.

Warner K, Hodgson T, Carroll C. (1999). Medical costs of smoking in the United States: Estimates, their validity, and their implications. *Tobacco Control, 8*(3): 290–300.

Yach D, Hawkes C, Gould C, Hofman K. (2004). The global burden of chronic diseases. *JAMA, 291*(21): 2616–2622.

14 CIGARETTE PRICES

Main Map

SOURCES

Data derived from:

Afghanistan, Albania, Andorra, Angola, Antigua and Barbuda, Bahamas, Barbados, Belarus, Belize, Benin, Bolivia (Plurinational State of), Bosnia and Herzegovina, Botswana, Burkina Faso, Burundi, Cape Verde, Central African Republic, Chad, Comoros, Congo, Congo (Democratic Republic of) , Croatia, Cuba, Djibouti, Dominica, Dominican Republic, El Salvador, Equatorial Guinea, Eritrea, Estonia, Ethiopia, Gabon, Gambia, Georgia, Ghana, Grenada, Guinea, Guinea-Bissau, Guyana, Haiti, Honduras, Iraq, Jamaica, Kiribati, Kyrgyzstan, Lesotho, Liberia, Madagascar, Maldives, Mali, Mauritania, Mauritius, Moldova (Republic of), Monaco, Montenegro, Mozambique, Namibia, Nauru, Nicaragua, Niger, Palau, Rwanda, Saint Kitts and Nevis, Saint Lucia, Saint Vincent and the Grenadines, Samoa, Sao Tome and Principe, Senegal, Sierra Leone, Slovenia, Somalia, Suriname, Tajikistan, Tanzania (United Republic of), Timor-Leste, Togo, Tonga, Trinidad and Tobago, Turkmenistan, Tuvalu, Uganda, Vanuatu, Yemen, World Health Organization (2012) Tobacco Control Country Profiles. http://who.int/tobacco/surveillance/policy/country_profile/en/index.html. Accessed April 5, 2012.

Algeria; Argentina; Australia; Austria; Azerbaijan; Bahrain; Bangladesh; Belgium; Brazil; Brunei Darussalam; Bulgaria; Cambodia; Cameroon; Canada; Chile; China; Colombia; Côte d'Ivoire; Czech Republic; Denmark; Ecuador; Egypt; Finland; France; Germany; Greece; Guatemala; Hong Kong SAR, China; Hungary; Iceland; India; Indonesia; Iran (Islamic Republic of); Ireland; Israel; Italy; Japan; Jordan; Kazakhstan; Kenya; Korea (Republic of); Kuwait; Libyan Arab Jamahiriya; Luxembourg; Malaysia; Mexico; Morocco; Nepal; Netherlands; New Zealand; Nigeria; Norway; Oman; Pakistan; Panama; Papua New Guinea; Paraguay; Peru; Philippines; Poland; Portugal; Qatar; Romania; Russian Federation; Saudi Arabia; Serbia; Singapore; Slovakia; South Africa; Spain; Sri Lanka; Sweden; Switzerland; Syrian Arab Republic; Thailand; Tunisia; Turkey; Ukraine; United Arab Emirates; United Kingdom; United States; Uruguay; Uzbekistan; Venezuela (Bolivarian Republic of); Vietnam; Zambia; Zimbabwe Economist Intelligence Unit. (2011). World Cost of Living Survey. London.

Costa Rica, Cyprus, Macedonia (the former Yugoslav Republic of), Malta, Sudan ERC Group. (2010). World cigarettes. Suffolk, UK. February.

Armenia Bazarchyan A. (2010). Armenia: Second (Five-Year) Implementation Report. Framework Convention on Tobacco Control, World Health Organization. June 10. http://www.who.int/fctc/reporting/Armenia_5y_report_FINAL.pdf. Accessed July 7, 2011.

Cook Islands Mataio M, Faireka T. (2010). Cook Islands: First (Two-Year) Implementation Report. Framework Convention on Tobacco Control, World Health Organization. February 28. http://www.who.int/fctc/reporting/Cooislandsreport.pdf. Accessed July 21, 2011.

Fiji Waqatakirewa L, Corerega I. (2007). Fiji: First (Two-Year) Implementation Report. Framework Convention on Tobacco Control, World Health Organization, May 2. http://www.who.int/tobacco/framework/cop/party_reports/fiji_report.pdf. Accessed July 21, 2011.

Lao People's Democratic Republic Insisiengmay S, Phandouangsy K. (2010). Lao PDR: First (Two-Year) Implementation Report. Framework Convention on Tobacco Control, World Health Organization. March 2. http://www.who.int/fctc/LaoPDR_report_final.pdf. Accessed October 28, 2011.

Latvia Martinsone U, Remese I. (2010). Latvia: Second (Five-Year) Implementation Report. Framework Convention on Tobacco Control, World Health Organization. March 10. http://www.who.int/fctc/reporting/Latvia_5y_report_final.pdf. Accessed October 28, 2011.

Lebanon Saade G. (2009). Lebanon: First (Two-Year) Implementation Report. Framework Convention on Tobacco Control, World Health Organization, August 20. http://www.who.int/fctc/secretariat/lebanon_report_version_final.pdf. Accessed October 28, 2011.

Lithuania Suliene D. (2010). Lithuania: Second (Five-Year) Implementation Report. Framework Convention on Tobacco Control, World Health Organization. April 8. http://www.who.int/fctc/reporting/Lithuania_5y_report_v2_final.pdf. Accessed October 28, 2011.

Marshall Islands Edward R, Langdrik J. (2010), Marshall Islands: Second (Five-Year) Implementation Report. Framework Convention on Tobacco Control, World Health Organization. March 8. http://www.who.int/fctc/reporting/Marshallislandsreport.pdf. Accessed June 7, 2011.

Micronesia (Federated States of) Skilling V. (2010). Micronesia: Second (Five-Year) Implementation Report. Framework Convention on Tobacco Control, World Health Organization. September 29. http://www.who.int/fctc/reporting/Micronesia_5y_report.pdf. Accessed June 7, 2011.

Mongolia Tsetsegdary G. (2011). Mongolia: Second (Five-Year) Implementation Report. Framework Convention on Tobacco Control, World Health Organization. January 18. http://www.who.int/fctc/Mongolia_5y_report.pdf. Accessed March 1, 2011.

Niue Nosa, M. (2010). Niue: Second (Five-Year) Implementation Report. Framework Convention on Tobacco Control, World Health Organization. October 10. http://www.who.int.proxy.library.emory.edu/fctc/reporting/Niuereport.pdf. Accessed October 28, 2011.

San Marino Gualtieri A, Fiorini M. (2011). San Marino: Second (Five-Year) Implementation Report. Framework Convention on Tobacco Control, World Health Organization. February 25. http://www.who.int/fctc/reporting/party_reports/sanmarino_5y_report_final.pdf. Accessed July 21, 2011.

Seychelles Viswanathan B, Mellie M, Gedeon J. (2010). Seychelles: Second (Five-Year) Implementation Report. Framework Convention on Tobacco Control, World Health Organization. March 15. http://www.who.int/fctc/reporting/Seychelles_5y_report_final.pdf. Accessed July 21, 2011.

Swaziland Dlamini V. (2009). Swaziland: First (Two-Year) Implementation Report. Framework Convention on Tobacco Control, World Health Organization. September 15. http://www.who.int/fctc/reporting/Swaziland_report.pdf. Accessed June 28, 2011.

METHODS

If the estimate was provided in currency other than US dollars, the price was converted to US dollars using average yearly exchange rates from:

OANDA. (N.d.). Average exchange rates. http://www.oanda.com/currency/average.

If prices were collected in multiple cities in a country, an average of those prices was used.

Symbol

Cigarette Prices: Economist Intelligence Unit. (2011). World Cost of Living Survey.

Inflation: International Monetary Fund. (2011). World economic outlook database. April.

A total of 70 countries with data on both 2000 and 2010 cigarette prices have been investigated: **Argentina, Australia, Austria, Bahrain, Bangladesh, Belgium, Brazil, Cameroon, Canada, Chile, China, Colombia, Cote d'Ivoire, Czech Republic, Denmark, Ecuador, Egypt, Finland, France, Germany, Greece, Guatemala, Hong Kong, Hungary, Iceland, India, Indonesia, Iran (Islamic Republic of), Ireland, Israel, Italy, Japan, Kenya, Kuwait, Luxembourg, Malaysia, Mexico, Morocco, Netherlands, New Zealand, Nigeria, Norway, Oman, Pakistan, Panama, Papua New Guinea, Paraguay, Peru, Philippines, Poland, Portugal, Qatar, Russian Federation, Saudi Arabia, Singapore, South Africa, Spain, Sri Lanka, Sweden, Switzerland, Taiwan Province of China, Thailand, Tunisia, UK, Ukraine, United Arab Emirates, Uruguay, US, Uzbekistan, Viet Nam**

Price of Other Tobacco Products Compared to Cigarettes

CIGARETTE PRICES

Economist Intelligence Unit. (2011). World Cost of Living Survey.

PRICES OF OTHER TOBACCO PRODUCTS

Centers for Disease Control and Prevention. (2011). Global Adult Tobacco Survey. http://www.cdc.gov/tobacco/global/gtss/. Accessed October 1, 2011.

European Commission Directorate General Taxation and Customs Union. (2011). Excise duty tables: Part III: Manufactured tobacco. http://ec.europa.eu/taxation_customs/taxation/excise_duties/tobacco_products/index_en.htm. Accessed June 30, 2011.

Lindbak R, Wilson H. (2010). Norway: Second (Five-Year) Implementation Report. Framework Convention on Tobacco Control, World Health Organization. March 22. http://www.who.int/fctc/reporting/Norway_5y_report_v2_final.pdf. Accessed June 28, 2011.

Nichter M et al. (2009). Reading culture from tobacco advertisements in Indonesia. *Tobacco Control, 18*(2): 98–107.

How Much Rice Can a Pack of Marlboro Buy?

MARLBORO CIGARETTE AND RICE PRICES

Economist Intelligence Unit. (2011). World Cost of Living Survey.

KILOGRAMS OF RICE WERE CONVERTED TO SERVINGS USING: Batres-Marquez SP et al. (2005) Rice consumption in the US: New evidence from food consumption surveys. Center for Agricultural and Rural Development, Iowa State University, Ames, IA.

Price of Local Brand as a Percent of Marlboro Prices

Marlboro cigarette and local cigarette prices: Economist Intelligence Unit. (2011). World Cost of Living Survey.

Quote

Efroymson D, Ahmed S, Townsend J, Alam S, Dey A, Saha R, et al. (2001). Hungry for tobacco: An analysis of the economic impact of tobacco consumption on the poor in Bangladesh. *Tobacco Control, 10*(3): 212–217.

India and Malawi Dugan E. (2011). The unstoppable march of the tobacco giants. *The Independent*. May 29. http://www.independent.co.uk/life-style/health-and-families/health-news/the-unstoppable-march-of-the-tobacco-giants-2290583.html. Accessed October 28, 2011.

Viet Nam PATH Canada, Viet Nam. (2006). Viet Nam: The economics of tobacco use at the household level — tobacco expenditures and their opportunity cost. http://web.idrc.ca/en/ev-84056-201-1-DO_TOPIC.html. Accessed October 28, 2011.

India John R, Sung H, Max W, Ross H. (2011). Counting 15 million more poor in India, thanks to tobacco. *Tobacco Control*. Online. http://tobaccocontrol.bmj.com/content/early/2011/02/03/tc.2010.040089.abstract. Accessed January 3, 2012.

Niger Tobacco Free Initiative. (2004). Tobacco and poverty, A Vicious Circle. http://escholarship.org/uc/item/4n15f79w#page-1. Accessed October 28, 2011.

Cambodia John R, Ross H, Blecher E. (2011) Tobacco expenditures and its implications for household resource allocation in Cambodia. *Tobacco Control*. Online. http://tobaccocontrol.bmj.com/content/early/2011/08/09/tc.2010.042598.abstract. Accessed January 3, 2012

Text Panel

Best C, Sun K, de Pee S, Bloem M, Stallkamp G, Semba RD. (2007). Parental tobacco use is associated with increased risk of child malnutrition in Bangladesh. *Nutrition, 23*(10): 731–738.

Chaloupka F, Cummings K, Morley C, Horan J. (2002). Tax, price and cigarette smoking: Evidence from the tobacco documents and implications for tobacco company marketing strategies. *Tobacco Control, 11*(Suppl 1): i62–72.

Efroymson D, Pham HA, Jones L, Fitzgerald S, Thu LT, Thu Hien LT. (2011). Tobacco and poverty: Evidence from Vietnam. *Tobacco Control*. March 31. http://www.ncbi.nlm.nih.gov/pubmed/21454384. Accessed May 19, 2011.

Esson KM, Leeder SR. (2004). The Millennium Development Goals and tobacco control: An opportunity for global partnership. World Health Organization. http://www.bvsde.paho.org/bvsacd/cd51/mdg-tobacco.pdf. Accessed May 20, 2011.

Gilmore AB, Branston JR, Sweanor D. (2010). The case for OFSMOKE: How tobacco price regulation is needed to promote the health of markets, government revenue and the public. *Tobacco Control, 19*(5): 423–430.

Gupta PC, Ray CS. (2007). Tobacco, education and health. *Indian Journal of Medical Research, 126*(4): 289–299.

Jarvis MJ. (1998). Supermarket cigarettes: The brands that dare not speak their name. *British Medical Journal, 316*(7135): 929–931.

John RM. (2008). Crowding out effect of tobacco expenditure and its implications on household resource allocation in India. *Social Science and Medicine, 66*(6): 1356–1367.

Nonnemaker J, Sur M. (2007). Tobacco expenditures and child health and nutritional outcomes in rural Bangladesh. *Social Science and Medicine, 65*(12): 2517–2526.

World Health Organization. (2010). WHO technical manual on tobacco tax administration. World Health Organization. http://whqlibdoc.who.int/publications/2010/9789241563994_eng.pdf. Accessed March 22, 2011.

Zohrabian A, Philipson TJ. (2010). External costs of risky health behaviors associated with leading actual causes of death in the US: A review of the evidence and implications for future research. *International Journal of Environmental Research and Public Health, 7*(6): 2460–2472.

15 AFFORDABILITY

Main Map

PER CAPITA GDP DERIVED FROM:

International Monetary Fund. (2011). World economic outlook database. April. http://www.imf.org/external/pubs/ft/weo/2011/02/weodata/index.aspx. Accessed May 4, 2011.

CIGARETTE PRICES DERIVED FROM:

Economist Intelligence Unit. (2011). World Cost of Living Survey.

World Health Organization. (2011). *WHO report on the global tobacco epidemic, 2011: Warning about the dangers of tobacco*. http://www.who.int/tobacco/mpower/en/. Accessed August 1, 2011.

METHODS

Relative income price (RIP) calculated as a percentage of annual per capita income, measured by per capita GDP, needed to purchase 100 packs of cheapest cigarettes. Methodology from:

Blecher E, van Walbeek C. (2009). Cigarette affordability trends: An update and some methodological comments. *Tobacco Control, 18*(3): 167–175.

Symbol

Countries with more than a 50% drop in relative income price between 2000 and 2010; a total of 75 countries with data on both 2000 and 2010 RIP have been investigated: **Argentina, Australia, Austria, Azerbaijan, Bahrain, Bangladesh, Belgium, Brazil, Cameroon, Canada, Chile, China, Colombia, Costa Rica, Cote d'Ivoire, Croatia, Czech Republic, Denmark, Ecuador, Egypt (Arab Republic of), Finland, France, Gabon, Germany, Greece, Guatemala, Hungary, Iceland, India, Indonesia, Iran (Islamic Republic of), Ireland, Israel, Italy, Japan, Jordan, Kenya, Korea (Republic of), Kuwait, Libya, Luxembourg, Malaysia, Mexico, Morocco, Netherlands, New Zealand, Nigeria, Norway, Pakistan, Panama, Paraguay, Peru, Philippines, Poland, Portugal, Romania, Russian Federation, Saudi Arabia, Senegal, Singapore, South Africa, Spain, Sri Lanka, Sweden, Switzerland, Thailand, Tunisia, Turkey, UK, United Arab Emirates, Uruguay, US, Venezuela, Viet Nam, Zimbabwe**

Methodology and sources the same as in the main map.

Minutes of Labor

Affordability measured as the percentage of daily wage required to buy a pack of cigarettes. The median net wage calculated based on the lowest-paid half of the occupations surveyed by Union Bank of Switzerland: Union Bank of Switzerland. (N.d.). Prices and earnings: A comparison of purchasing power around the globe. http://www.ubs.com/1/e/ubs_ch/wealth_mgmt_ch/research.html.

CIGARETTE PRICES

Economist Intelligence Unit. (2011). World Cost of Living Survey.

Change in Cigarette Affordability Between 2000 and 2010

Methodology and sources the same as in the main map.

China Affordability

Methodology and sources the same as in the main map.

Quote

World Health Organization. (2011). *WHO report on the global tobacco epidemic, 2011: Warning about the dangers of tobacco.*

Text Panel

Blecher E, van Walbeek C. (2004). An international analysis of cigarette affordability. *Tobacco Control, 13*(4): 339–346.

Guindon G, Tobin S, Yach D. (2002). Trends and affordability of cigarette prices: Ample room for tax increases and related health gains. *Tobacco Control, 11*(1): 35–43.

World Health Organization. (2009). *WHO report on the global tobacco epidemic, 2009: Implementing smoke-free environments.* http://www.who.int/tobacco/mpower/en/. Accessed August 1, 2011.

16 GROWING TOBACCO

Main Map

Food and Agricultural Organization. (2011a). FAOSTAT data, tobacco unmanufactured: Area harvested, 2009. http://faostat.fao.org/site/567/DesktopDefault.aspx?PageID=567#ancor. Accessed October 10, 2011.

Australia Scollo, MM and Winstanley, MH [editors]. *Tobacco in Australia: Facts and Issues*. Third Edition. Melbourne: Cancer Council Victoria; 2008. Available from: http://www.tobaccoinaustralia.org.au. Accessed March 26, 2012.

Symbol

Data derived from Food and Agricultural Organization. (2011b). FAOSTAT data, agricultural area, 2008. http://faostat.fao.org/site/377/DesktopDefault.aspx?PageID=377. Accessed October 10, 2011.

Food and Agricultural Organization. (2011a). FAOSTAT data, tobacco unmanufactured: Area harvested, 2008.

Leading Tobacco Leaf Producers

Data derived from Food and Agricultural Organization. (2011c). FAOSTAT data, tobacco unmanufactured: Production quantity, 2000, 2009. http://faostat.fao.org/site/567/DesktopDefault.aspx?PageID=567#ancor. Accessed October 10, 2011.

Trend in Production

Food and Agricultural Organization. (2011d). FAOSTAT data, tobacco unmanufactured: Production quantity, 1965–2009. http://faostat.fao.org/site/567/DesktopDefault.aspx?PageID=567#ancor. Accessed October 10, 2011.

Top 5 Countries

Data derived from Food and Agricultural Organization. (2011e). FAOSTAT data, tobacco unmanufactured: Area harvested, 2000, 2009. http://faostat.fao.org/site/567/DesktopDefault.aspx?PageID=567. Accessed October 10, 2011.

Brazil vs. Africa Production

Data derived from Food and Agricultural Organization. (2011f). FAOSTAT data, tobacco unmanufactured: Production quantity, 2009. http://faostat.fao.org/site/567/DesktopDefault.aspx?PageID=567#ancor. Accessed May 23, 2011.

China Production

Data derived from Food and Agricultural Organization. (2011f). FAOSTAT data, tobacco unmanufactured: Production quantity, 2009.

Quote: Strosberg

Blackwell T. (2010). Farmers sue tobacco firms for $150M. *National Post*. http://www.parliament.nz/NR/rdonlyres/24E903B3-4D13-4913-BB54-BC02269D9129/145695/49SCMA_EVI_00DBSCH_INQ_9591_1_A55117_Smokefree Coal.pdf. Accessed December 28, 2011.

Zhao Yaqiao

Wan W. (2011). Ban on public smoking has little effect, and that's the way China wants it. *Washington Post*. July 10. http://m.southcoasttoday.com/apps/pbcs.dll/article?AID=/20110710/NEWS02/107100301/-1/WAP06&template=wapart&m_section. Accessed August 2, 2011.

Text Panel

Capehart T. (2004). The changing tobacco user's dollar. US Department of Agriculture. October.

Food and Agricultural Organization. (2011a). FAOSTAT data, tobacco unmanufactured: Area harvested, 2009.

Food and Agricultural Organization. (2011g). FAOSTAT data, tobacco unmanufactured: Production quantity, 2009.

Food and Agricultural Organization. (2011g). Hunger map 2010: Prevalence of undernourishment in developing countries (2005–2007). http://faostat.fao.org/site/563/default.aspx. Accessed April 1, 2011.

Food and Agricultural Organization. (2011h). Hunger statistics: 2005–2007. http://www.fao.org/hunger/en/. Accessed April 1, 2011.

Food and Agricultural Organization. (2011a). FAOSTAT data, tobacco unmanufactured: Area harvested, 2008.

Food and Agricultural Organization. (2011i). FAOSTAT data, tobacco unmanufactured: Production quantity, 2008. http://faostat.fao.org/site/567/DesktopDefault.aspx?PageID=567#ancor. Accessed April 1, 2011.

Food and Agricultural Organization. (2011j). FAOSTAT data, potatoes: Production quantity, 2008. http://faostat.fao.org/site/567/DesktopDefault.aspx?PageID=567#ancor. Accessed April 1, 2011.

Geist H. (1999). Global assessment of deforestation related to tobacco farming. *Tobacco Control, 8*: 18–28.

World Bank. (2011). Prevalence of undernourishment, 2007. http://data.worldbank.org/indicator/SN.ITK.DEFC.ZS. Accessed October 10, 2011.

World Health Organization. (2008). WHO Framework Convention on Tobacco Control: Conference of the Parties to the WHO Framework Convention on Tobacco Control, Third session, Durban, South Africa. http://apps.who.int/gb/fctc/PDF/cop3/FCTC_COP3_11-en.pdf. Accessed January 10, 2012.

World Health Organization. (2004). Tobacco and poverty: A vicious circle. http://www.who.int/tobacco/communications/events/wntd/2004/en/wntd2004_brochure_en.pdf. Accessed April 25, 2011.

World Health Organization. (2010). 2010 Global progress report on the implementation of the WHO Framework Convention on Tobacco Control. http://www.who.int/fctc/reporting/summaryreport.pdf. Accessed April 25, 2011.

METHODS
Top tobacco-producing countries with undernourishment rates between 5% and 27% include **Malawi** (27%), **Pakistan** (25%), **India** (19%), **Indonesia** (13%), **China** (10%), and **Brazil** (6%).

17 MANUFACTURING

Main Map

Albania, Algeria, Angola, Argentina, Armenia, Australia, Austria, Azerbaijan, Bangladesh, Belarus, Bolivia (Plurinational State of), Bosnia and Herzegovina, Brazil, Bulgaria, Cambodia, Cameroon, Canada, Chile, China, Colombia, Congo (Democratic Republic of), Costa Rica, Cote D'Ivoire, Croatia, Cuba, Cyprus, Czech Republic, Denmark, Dominican Republic, Ecuador, Egypt, El Salvador, Estonia, Ethiopia, Finland, France, Georgia, Germany, Ghana, Greece, Guatemala, Honduras, Hong Kong, Hungary, India, Indonesia, Iran (Islamic Republic of), Iraq, Israel, Italy, Japan, Jordan, Kazakhstan, Kenya, Korea (Democratic People's Republic of), Korea (Republic of), Kuwait, Kyrgyzstan, Lao People's Democratic Republic, Latvia, Lebanon, Libyan Arab Jamahiriya, Lithuania, Macedonia (former Yugoslav Republic of), Madagascar, Malaysia, Malta, Mauritius, Mexico, Moldova (Republic of), Morocco, Mozambique, Myanmar, Nepal, Netherlands, New Zealand, Nicaragua, Nigeria, Pakistan, Panama, Paraguay, Peru, Philippines, Poland, Portugal, Romania, Russian Federation, Saudi Arabia, Senegal, Serbia, Singapore, Slovakia, Slovenia, South Africa, Spain, Sri Lanka, Sudan, Switzerland, Syrian Arab Republic, Tanzania (United Republic of), Thailand, Togo, Trinidad and Tobago, Tunisia, Turkey, Turkmenistan, UK, Ukraine, United Arab Emirates, Uruguay, US, Uzbekistan, Venezuela (Bolivarian Republic of), Viet Nam, Yemen, Zambia, Zimbabwe ERC. (2010). World cigarette reports, 2010. Suffolk, UK: ERC Group Ltd.

Belize Goldson E, Polanco J. (2008). Belize: First (Two-Year) Implementation Report. Framework Convention on Tobacco Control, World Health Organization. April 7. http://www.who.int/fctc/reporting/belize_report.pdf. Accessed July 7, 2011.

Burkina Faso Théodore K. (2009). Burkina Faso: Second (Five-Year) Implementation Report. Framework Convention on Tobacco Control, World Health Organization. February 23. http://www.who.int/fctc/reporting/burkina_faso_report.pdf. Accessed June 28, 2011.

Burundi Thierry G. (2008). Burundi: First (Two-Year) Implementation Report. Framework Convention on Tobacco Control, World Health Organization. November 11. http://www.who.int/fctc/reporting/burundi_report.pdf. Accessed July 7, 2011.

Comoros Abdou C, Msaidie M. (2009). Comoros: First (Two-Year) Implementation Report. Framework Convention on Tobacco Control, World Health Organization. April. http://www.who.int/fctc/reporting/Comoros_report.pdf. Accessed July 21, 2011.

Congo Likibi-Boho R, Raoul E. (2008). Congo: First (Two-Year) Implementation Report. Framework Convention on Tobacco Control, World Health Organization. May 21. http://www.who.int/fctc/reporting/congo_report.pdf. Accessed July 7, 2011.

Cook Islands Mataio M, Faireka T. (2010). Cook Islands: First (Two-Year) Implementation Report. Framework Convention on Tobacco Control, World Health Organization. February 28. http://www.who.int/fctc/reporting/Cookislands report.pdf. Accessed July 21, 2011.

Fiji Waqatakirewa L, Corerega I. (2007). Fiji: First (Two-Year) Implementation Report. Framework Convention on Tobacco Control, World Health Organization. May 2. http://www.who.int/tobacco/framework/cop/party_reports/fiji_report.pdf. Accessed July 21, 2011.

Iceland Guðmundsdóttir S, Jensson V. (2009). Iceland: First (Two-Year) Implementation Report. Framework Convention on Tobacco Control, World Health Organization. October 29. http://www.who.int/fctc/reporting/Iceland_report_final.pdf. Accessed July 11, 2011.

Luxembourg Steil S. (2010). Luxembourg: Second (Five-Year) Implementation Report. Framework Convention on Tobacco Control, World Health Organization. October 11. http://www.who.int/fctc/reporting/Luxembourg_5y_report.pdf. Accessed July 21, 2011.

Maldives Afaal A. (2006). Maldives: First (Two-Year) Implementation Report. Framework Convention on Tobacco Control, World Health Organization. October 30. http://www.who.int/tobacco/framework/cop/party_reports/maldives_report.pdf. Accessed July 21, 2011.

Micronesia, Federated States of Skilling V. (2010). Micronesia: Second (Five-Year) Implementation Report. Framework Convention on Tobacco Control, World Health Organization. September 29. http://www.who.int/fctc/reporting/Micronesia_5y_report.pdf. Accessed June 7, 2011.

Mongolia Tsetsegdary G. (2011). Mongolia: Second (Five-Year) Implementation Report. Framework Convention on Tobacco Control, World Health Organization. January 18. http://www.who.int/fctc/Mongolia_5y_report.pdf. Accessed March 1, 2011.

Montenegro Ljaljevic A. (2008). Montenegro: First (Two-Year) Implementation Report. Framework Convention on Tobacco Control, World Health Organization. October 27. http://www.who.int/fctc/reporting/montenegro_report.pdf. Accessed March 1, 2011. (Estimated based on data for eight months.)

Palau Oseked R, Sr. (2010). Palau: Second (Five-Year) Implementation Report. Framework Convention on Tobacco Control, World Health Organization. February 26. http://www.who.int/fctc/reporting/Palaufive.pdf. Accessed July 21, 2011.

San Marino Gualtieri A, Fiorini M. (2011). San Marino: Second (Five-Year) Implementation Report. Framework Convention on Tobacco Control, World Health Organization. February 25. http://www.who.int/fctc/reporting/party_reports/sanmarino_5y_report_final.pdf. Accessed July 21, 2011.

Seychelles Viswanathan B, Mellie M, Gedeon J. (2010). Seychelles: Second (Five-Year) Implementation Report. Framework Convention on Tobacco Control, World Health Organization. March 15. http://www.who.int/fctc/reporting/Seychelles_5y_report_final.pdf. Accessed July 21, 2011.

Tonga Vivili P. (2009). Tonga: First (Two-Year) Implementation Report. Framework Convention on Tobacco Control, World Health Organization. August 28. http://www.who.int/fctc/reporting/Tonga_report.pdf. Accessed June 30, 2011.

Tuvalu Ituaso-Conway N, Homasi-Paelate A, Homasi S. (2009). Tuvalu: First (Two-Year) Implementation Report. Framework Convention on Tobacco Control, World Health Organization. November 13. http://www.who.int/fctc/reporting/tuvreport.pdf. Accessed July 21, 2011.

Symbol

Stanford University. (2011). Cigarette citadels map project. http://www.stanford.edu/group/tobaccoprv/cgi-bin/wordpress/. Accessed October 1, 2011.

Cigarettes Dominate, but Are Not the Only Tobacco Product of the Tobacco Industry

Euromonitor International. (2011). *Passport Database*. Accessed October 1, 2011.

Global Cigarette Production

ERC. (2010). World cigarette reports 2010. Suffolk, UK: ERC Group Ltd.

Parker J. (2011). Intra-EU cigarette trade turned out differently than expected. *Tobacco International:* June 29–35.

Top Cigarette Exporting Countries

ERC. (2010). World cigarette reports 2010.

Who Is Getting the Money Spent on a Cigarette?

Euromonitor International. (2011). *Passport Database*. Accessed October 1, 2011.

China Workers Employment

International Labour Organization. (2009). LABORSTA database. http://laborsta.ilo.org/. Accessed May 23, 2011.

United Nations Industrial Development Organization. (2011). INDSTAT database. http://w3.unece.org/pxweb/Dialog/. Accessed May 23, 2011.

Quote

Proctor R. (2012). *Golden holocaust*. Berkeley: University of California Press.

Text Panel

ERC. (2010). World cigarette reports 2010.

Euromonitor International. (2010). Illicit trade in tobacco products: A world view. July. *Passport Database*. Accessed October 1, 2011.

Facilicom. (2009). Annual report 2009. http://www.facilicom.com/FR/Documents/Rapport%20annuel%202009.pdf. Accessed October 1, 2011.

Proctor R. (2001). Tobacco and the global lung cancer epidemic. *Nature Reviews Cancer, 1*(1): 82–86.

Stanford University. (2011). Cigarette citadels map project.

18 TOBACCO COMPANIES

Main Map

SOURCE
Data derived from ERC. (2010). World cigarette reports 2010. Suffolk, UK: ERC Group Ltd.

METHODS
Myanmar and Lebanon have state-owned tobacco companies, but as of 2008 the state-owned companies were not the leading manufacturers in those countries.

Symbol

Altria Group. (2011). Financial information FAQs. http://investor.altria.com/phoenix.zhtml?c=80855&p=irol-faq_main_fi#. Accessed July 25, 2011.

British American Tobacco. (2011). Contact us. http://www.bat.com/group/sites/uk__3mnfen.nsf/vwPagesWebLive/DO52GC8F?opendocument&SKN=1&TMP=1. Accessed July 25, 2011.

China National Tobacco Import and Export Inc. (2011). *Bloomberg Businessweek*. http://investing.businessweek.com/research/stocks/private/snapshot.asp?privcapId=7940018. Accessed July 25, 2011.

Imperial Tobacco. (2011). Contact us. http://www.imperial-tobacco.com/index.asp?page=46. Accessed July 25, 2011.

Japan Tobacco Inc. (2011). Investor information. http://www.jti.com/page.aspx?pointerid=497a8cbd7c7d454d86d1bcfc1c43dd4a. Accessed July 25, 2011.

Philip Morris International. (2011). Contact us. http://www.pmi.com/marketpages/pages/market_en_ch.aspx. Accessed July 25, 2011.

Global Cigarette Market Share

Data derived from ERC. (2010). World cigarette reports 2010.

Tobacco Company Profits

SOURCES
Altria/Philip Morris USA—Altria Group Inc. (2010). 2010 annual report. http://investor.altria.com/phoenix.zhtml?c=808. Accessed August 9, 2011.

British American Tobacco. (2010). Annual report 2010. http://www.bat.com/servlet/SPMerge?mainurl=%2Fgroup%2Fsites%2Fuk__3mnfen.nsf%2FvwPagesWebLive%2FDO52AK34%3Fopendocument%26amp%3BSKN%3D1. Accessed August 9, 2011.

China National Tobacco Corporation—Wang Ke-an. (2011). Think Tank Beijing. Personal communication.

Imperial Tobacco. (2010). Annual report and accounts 2010. http://www.imperial-tobacco.com/files/financial/reports/ar2010/index.asp?pageid=64. Accessed August 9, 2011.

Japan Tobacco International—Japan Tobacco Inc. (2010). Annual report 2010. http://www.jti.com/documents/annualreports/Annualreport2010.pdf. Accessed August 9, 2011.

Philip Morris International. (2010). Annual report 2010. http://investors.pmi.com/phoenix.zhtml?c=146476&p=irol-reportsannual. Accessed August 9, 2011.

METHODS

BAT income reported in pounds. Converted to US dollars using December 31, 2010, conversion rates: http://www.oanda.com/currency/converter/.

Imperial Tobacco income reported in pounds. Converted to US dollars using September 30, 2010, conversion rates: http://www.oanda.com/currency/converter/.

CNTC income reported in RMB Yuan. Converted to US dollars using December 31, 2010, conversion rates: http://www.oanda.com/currency/converter/.

Tobacco Company CEO Compensation

Bloomberg Businessweek. (2011a). Altria Group Inc.: Louis Camilleri. http://investing.businessweek.com/businessweek/research/stocks/people/person.asp?personId=296312&ticker=MO:US. Accessed August 23, 2011.

Bloomberg Businessweek. (2011b). Altria Group Inc.: Michael Szymanczyk. http://investing.businessweek.com/research/stocks/people/person.asp?personId=296360&ticker=MO:US. Accessed August 23, 2011.

Bloomberg Businessweek. (2011c). British American Tobacco: Nicandro Durante. http://investing.businessweek.com/research/stocks/people/person.asp?personId=8811457&ticker=BTI:US. Accessed August 23, 2011.

China National Tobacco Corporation: State Tobacco Monopoly Administration. (2006). http://www.gov.cn/english/2005-10/03/content_74295.htm. Accessed November 22, 2011.

Imperial Tobacco. (2010). Annual report and accounts 2010.

Combined Profits

Altria Group Inc. (2010). Annual report 2010.

British American Tobacco. (2010). Annual report 2010.

Businessweek. (2010a). McDonalds Corporation: 2010 financials. http://investing.businessweek.com/research/stocks/financials/financials.asp?ticker=MCD:US. Accessed August 9, 2011.

Businessweek. (2010b). Microsoft Corporation: 2010 financials. http://investing.businessweek.com/research/stocks/financials/financials.asp?ticker=MSFT:US. Accessed August 9, 2011.

Businessweek. (2010c). The Coca-Cola Company: 2010 financials. http://investing.businessweek.com/research/stocks/financials/financials.asp?ticker=KO:US. Accessed August 9, 2011.

Imperial Tobacco. (2010). Annual report and accounts 2010.

Japan Tobacco Inc. (2010). Annual report 2010.

Philip Morris International Inc. (2010). Annual report 2010.

Wang K. (2011). Personal communication regarding China National Tobacco Corporation.

PMI

Philip Morris International Inc. (2010). Annual report 2010.

Quote: Gilmore

Dugan E. (2011). The unstoppable march of the tobacco giants. *The Independent*. May 29. http://www.independent.co.uk/life-style/health-and-families/health-news/the-unstoppable-march-of-the-tobacco-giants-2290583.html. Accessed August 9, 2011.

Quote: Altria

Altria. (2011). National impact. http://www.altria.com/en/cms/About_Altria/At_A_Glance/National_Impact/default.aspx?src=top_nav. Accessed August 25, 2011.

Text Panel

SOURCES

British American Tobacco. (2011) News release: British American Tobacco establishes stand-alone company, Nicoventures Limited. April 5. http://www.bat.com/group/sites/uk__3mnfen.nsf/vwPagesWebLive/DO8FLL93?opendocument&SKN=1. Accessed June 21, 2011.

ERC. (2010). World cigarette reports 2010. *Euromonitor International*. (2011). World tobacco market 2011. July 2011 webinar.

Hu TW, Mao Z, Shi J, Chen W. (2010). The role of taxation in tobacco control and its potential economic impact in China. *Tobacco Control*, 19: 58-64.

Kesmodel D, Korn M. (2011). Philip Morris looks to nicotine aerosol. *Wall Street Journal*. May 27. http://online.wsj.com/article/SB10001424052702304066504576347513991162274.html. Accessed June 21, 2011.

World Bank. (2011). Gross domestic product, 2010. http://siteresources.worldbank.org/DATASTATISTICS/Resources/GDP.pdf. Accessed June 21, 2011.

METHODS

Estimates of the total tobacco market value vary greatly between 400 and 500 billion USD annually, depending on at which point in the distribution channel (manufacturer vs. retail) the value is measured.

19 ILLICIT CIGARETTES

Main Map

Estimates of the illicit share of the total cigarettes market:

Albania, Argentina, Bolivia (Plurinational State of), Bosnia and Herzegovina, Brazil, Bulgaria, Costa Rica, Côte d'Ivoire, Cyprus, Czech Republic, Ecuador, El Salvador, Estonia, Ghana, India, Iraq, Jordan, Kenya, Kyrgyzstan, Lebanon, Libyan Arab Jamahiriya, Malta, Morocco, Nicaragua, Nigeria, Pakistan, Paraguay, Russian Federation, Saudi Arabia, Slovakia, Spain, Sri Lanka, Sudan, Sweden, Switzerland, Syrian Arab Republic, Togo, Venezuela (Bolivarian Republic of), Yemen, Zambia ERC. (2010). World cigarette reports 2010. Suffolk, UK: ERC Group Ltd.

Algeria, Australia, Austria, Azerbaijan, Belarus, Belgium, Cameroon, Chile, China, Colombia, Croatia, Denmark, Dominican Republic, Egypt, Finland, France, Macedonia (the former Yugoslav Republic of), Georgia, Germany, Greece, Guatemala, Hong Kong SAR, China, Hungary, Indonesia, Ireland, Iran (Islamic Republic of), Israel, Italy, Japan, Kazakhstan, Malaysia, Mexico, Netherlands, Norway, Peru, Philippines, Portugal, Korea (Republic of), Romania, Serbia, Singapore, Slovenia, Thailand, Tunisia, Turkey, United Arab Emirates, Uruguay, US, Uzbekistan, Viet Nam Euromonitor International. (2011). Passport Database. Accessed October 1, 2011.

Armenia Amirjanyan P. (2006). Tobacco, smuggling in Armenia. Yerevan: Open Society Institute. http://www.policy.hu/amirjanyan/paper.htm. Accessed October 1, 2011.

Bangladesh, Barbados, Belize, Fiji, Guyana, Jamaica, Kuwait, Madagascar, Malawi, Mozambique, Papua New Guinea, Qatar, Moldova (Republic of), Senegal, Trinidad and Tobago, Uganda, Zimbabwe Yurekli A, Sayginsoy O. (2010). Worldwide organized cigarette smuggling: An empirical analysis. *Applied Economics*, *42*(5): 545–561.

Burkina Faso, Gambia, Guinea-Bissau, Liberia, Mauritania, Sierra Leone Legget T. (2009). Transnational trafficking and the rule of law in West Africa: A threat assessment. Vienna, Austria: United Nations Office on Drugs and Crime, 2009. http://www.unodc.org/documents/data-and-analysis/Studies/West_Africa_Report_2009.pdf. Accessed March 1, 2011.

Cambodia National Institute of Statistics. (2011). National Adult Tobacco Survey of Cambodia: Country report. Ministry of Planning, Kingdom of Cambodia.

Canada Luk R et al. (2009). Prevalence and correlates of purchasing contraband cigarettes on First Nations reserves in Ontario, Canada. *Addiction*, *104*(3): 488–495.

Congo Likibi-Boho R. (2008). Congo: First (Two-Year) Implementation Report. Framework Convention on Tobacco Control, World Health Organization. May 21. http://www.who.int/fctc/reporting/congo_report.pdf. Accessed July 7, 2011.

Ethiopia Cochrane P. (2008). Ethiopia's legal tobacco sector grows as counterfeit trade declines. *World Tobacco*, September: 33–35.

Lao People's Democratic Republic Duke University, SEATCA, American Cancer Society. Capacity-building project in illicit trade in tobacco.

Latvia Lukss J. (2011). Tobacco taxation and illicit trade in Latvia. Ministry of Finance of Latvia, Riga.

Lithuania National Tobacco Manufacturers' Association. (2009). Tobacco market development in Latvia, Riga.

Mali Nazoum J. (2009). Mali: First (Two-Year) Implementation Report. Framework Convention on Tobacco Control, World Health Organization. March 17. http://www.who.int/fctc/reporting/Mali_report_rev1.pdf. Accessed March 1, 2011.

Mongolia Tsetsegdary G. (2011). Mongolia: Second (Five-Year) Implementation Report. Framework Convention on Tobacco Control, World Health Organization. January 18. http://www.who.int/fctc/Mongolia_5y_report.pdf. Accessed March 1, 2011.

Montenegro Ljaljevic A. (2008). Montenegro: First (Two-Year) Implementation Report. Framework Convention on Tobacco Control, World Health Organization. October 27. http://www.who.int/fctc/reporting/montenegro_report.pdf. Accessed March 1, 2011.

Myanmar Dasgupta S. (2009). Where There's Smoke... *Business Today*. March 19. http://businesstoday.intoday.in/bt/story/where-there%E2%80%99s-smoke.../1/3903.html. Accessed April 1, 2011.

New Zealand Wilson W et al. (2009). Estimating missed government tax revenue from foreign tobacco: Survey of discarded cigarette packs. *Tobacco Control*, *18*(5): 416–418.

Panama Roa R, Vergara F. (2010). Panama: Second (Five-Year) Implementation Report. Framework Convention on Tobacco Control, World Health Organization. February 27. http://www.who.int/fctc/reporting/Panama_5y_report_final.pdf. Accessed June 28, 2011.

Poland Centers for Disease Control and Prevention and World Health Organization. (2010). Global Adult Tobacco Survey (GATS), Poland 2009–2010. Warsaw.

South Africa Blecher E. (2009). A mountain or a molehill: Is the illicit trade in cigarettes undermining tobacco control policy in South Africa? Atlanta: American Cancer Society. http://www.fctc.org/dmdocuments/INB3_report_illicit_trade_in_South_Africa.pdf, archived by WebCite at http://www.webcitation.org/5pBkDBXWf. Accessed April 21, 2010.

Swaziland Dlamini V. (2009). Swaziland: First (Two-Year) Implementation Report. Framework Convention on Tobacco Control, World Health Organization. September 11. http://www.who.int/fctc/reporting/Swaziland_report.pdf. Accessed June 28, 2011.

UK HM Revenue and Customs. (2010). Measuring tax gaps, 2010. September. http://www.hmrc.gov.uk/stats/measuring-tax-gaps 2010.htm.pdf. Accessed October 17, 2011.

Ukraine Centers for Disease Control and Prevention and World Health Organization. (2010). Global Adult Tobacco Survey (GATS), Ukraine 2010. Kiev, Ukraine.

Symbol
World Customs Organization. (2011). Customs and tobacco report 2010. http://www.wcoomd.org/files/1.%20Public%20files/PDFandDocuments/Enforcement/WCO_Customs_Tobacco_2010_public_en.pdf. Accessed October 17, 2011.

Cigarette Prices and Illicit Cigarette Trade in UK
European Commission Directorate General Taxation and Customs Union. (2011). Excise duty tables: Part III: Manufactured tobacco. http://ec.europa.eu/taxation_customs/taxation/excise_duties/tobacco_products/index_en.htm. Accessed March 3, 2011.

HM Revenue and Customs. (2010). Measuring tax gaps 2010.

The Industry Tends to Exaggerate the Scope of Illicit Trade
INDUSTRY ESTIMATES
ERC (2010). World cigarette reports 2010.

Euromonitor International. (2010). Tobacco in Poland. August 26. *Passport Database*. Accessed October 1, 2011.

Tobacco Institute of South Africa. (2007). Submissions to the Select Committee on Social Services on the Tobacco Products Control Amendment Bill [B 24B: 2006]. http://www.pmg.org.za/docs/2007/070821tisa.htm. Accessed October 17, 2011.

ACADEMIC STUDIES
Blecher E. (2010). A mountain or a molehill: Is the illicit trade in cigarettes undermining tobacco control policy in South Africa? *Trends in Organized Crime, 13*(4): 299–315.

Centers for Disease Control and Prevention. (2011). Global Adult Tobacco Survey in Poland. http://www.cdc.gov/tobacco/global/gtss/. Accessed October 1, 2011.

HM Revenue and Customs. (2010). Measuring tax gaps, 2010.

Illicit Trade Impact
Joossens L, Merriman D, Ross H, Raw M. (2010). The impact of eliminating the global illicit cigarette trade on health and revenue. *Addiction, 105*(9): 1640–1649. doi:10.1111/j.1360-0443.2010.03018.x.

Quote
World Health Organization Western Pacific Regional Office. (2000). Tobacco and smuggling. July. http://www.wpro.who.int/internet/resources.ashx/TFI/tobacco_and_smuggling_brochure.pdf. Accessed December 14, 2011.

Text Panel
Euromonitor International. (2010). Illicit trade in tobacco products: A world view. July 22. http://www.portal.euromonitor.com/Portal/Default.aspx. Accessed October 17, 2011.

Joossens L, Chaloupka F, Merriman D, Yurekli A. (2000). Issues in the smuggling of tobacco products. In *Tobacco control in developing countries*, Ed: Chaloupka F and Jha P. 393–406. New York: Oxford University Press.

Joossens L, Merriman D, Ross H, Raw M. (2010). The impact of eliminating the global illicit cigarette trade on health and revenue.

Joossens L, Raw M. (1998). Cigarette smuggling in Europe: Who really benefits? *Tobacco Control, 7*(1): 66–71.

Joossens L, Raw M. (2008). Progress in combating cigarette smuggling: Controlling the supply chain. *Tobacco Control, 17*(6): 399–404.

Laxminarayan R, Chow J, Shahid-Salles SA. (2006). Intervention cost-effectiveness: Overview of main messages. In *Disease control priorities in developing countries*. Ed: Jamison D. et al. 35–86. New York: Oxford University Press.

Liberman J, Blecher E, Carbajales AR, Fishburn B. (2011). Opportunities and risks of the proposed FCTC protocol on illicit trade. *Tobacco Control*. http://www.ncbi.nlm.nih.gov/pubmed/21821819. Accessed October 17, 2011.

World Health Organization. (2003). Framework Convention on Tobacco Control. http://www.who.int.proxy.library.emory.edu/fctc/en/. Accessed October 17, 2011.

World Health Organization. (2009). *WHO report on the global tobacco epidemic, 2009: Implementing smoke-free environments*. Geneva: World Health Organization.

Zaloshnja E, Ross H, Levy D. (2010). The impact of tobacco control policies in Albania. *Tobacco Control, 19*(6): 463–468.

20 TOBACCO MARKETING

Main Map
Centers for Disease Control and Prevention. (2011). Global Tobacco Surveillance System: Global Youth Tobacco Survey.

US Data derived from National Youth Tobacco Survey. (2006). Centers for Disease Control and Prevention. http://www.cdc.gov/tobacco/data_statistics/surveys/yts/pdfs/yts_2003-2006_revised.pdf. Accessed December 27, 2011. Considers middle and high school students who bought or received anything with tobacco company name or picture on it. Considers individuals who have never used tobacco or are current users.

Symbol: Youth Smoking and Movies
Select references that are illustrative articles of the international evidence:
Arora M, Mathur N, Gupta V, Nazar G, Reddy K, Sargent J. (Accepted for publication). Tobacco use in Bollywood movies, tobacco promotional activities, and their association with tobacco use among Indian adolescents. *Tobacco Control*.

Dalton M, Beach M, Adachi-Mejia A, Longacre M, Matzkin A, Sargent J, Heatherton T, Titus-Ernstoff L. (2009). Early exposure to movie smoking predicts established smoking by older teens and young adults. *Pediatrics, 124*(4): e551–e558.

Goldberg M. (2003). American media and the smoking-related behaviors of Asian adolescents. *Journal of Advertising Research, 42*: 2–11.

Goldberg M, Baumgartner H. (2002). Cross-country attraction as a motivation for product consumption. *Journal of Business Research, 55*(11): 901–906.

Hanewinkel R, Sargent J. (2007). Exposure to smoking in popular contemporary movies and youth smoking in Germany. *American Journal of Preventive Medicine, 32*(6): 466–473.

Hunt K, Henderson M, Wight D, Sargent J. (Accepted for publication). Exposure to smoking in films and own smoking amongst Scottish adolescents: A cross-sectional study. *Thorax*.

Laugesen M, Scragg R, et al. (2007). R-rated film viewing and adolescent smoking. *Preventive Medicine, 45*(6): 454–459.

Morgenstern M, Poelen E, Scholte R, Karlsdottir S, Jonsson S, Mattis F, Faggiano F, Florek E, Sweeting H, Hunt K, Sargent J, Hanewinkel R. (Submitted for publication). Smoking in movies and adolescent smoking: Cross-cultural study in six European countries.

Thrasher J, Jackson C, Arillo-Santillán E, Sargent J. (2008). Exposure to smoking imagery in popular films and adolescent smoking in Mexico. *American Journal of Preventive Medicine, 35*(2): 95–102.

Wagner D, Dal Cin S, Sargent J, Kelley W, Heatherton T. (2011). Spontaneous action representation in smokers when watching movie characters smoke. *Journal of Neuroscience, 31*(3): 894–898.

Waylen A, Leary S, Ness A, Tanski S, Sargent J. (Accepted for publication). Cross-sectional association between smoking depictions in films and adolescent tobacco use nested in a British cohort study. *Thorax*.

Cigarette Marketing Expenditures
Federal Trade Commission. (2011). Cigarette report for 2007 and 2008. http://www.ftc.gov/os/2011/07/110729cigarettereport.pdf. Accessed July 30, 2011.

Cigarette Advertising Among Adults
World Health Organization. Global Adult Tobacco Survey Results (all nation-specific links accessed August 16, 2011):

Bangladesh (2009). http://www.who.int/tobacco/surveillance/fact_sheet_of_gats_bangladesh_2009.pdf. Data updated November 2011 by CDC.

Brazil (2008). http://www.who.int/tobacco/surveillance/gats_factsheet_brazil.pdf. Data updated November 2011 by CDC.

Egypt (2009). http://www.who.int/tobacco/surveillance/gats_egypt_executive_summary_en.pdf.

India (2009/2010). http://whoindia.org/LinkFiles/Tobacco_Free_Initiative_GATS2010_Chapter-08.pdf.

Mexico (2009). http://www.who.int/tobacco/surveillance/gats_rep_mexico.pdf.

Philippines (2009). http://www.who.int/tobacco/surveillance/2009_gats_report_philippines.pdf.

Poland (2009/2010). http://www.who.int/tobacco/surveillance/gats_poland/en/index.html.

Russian Federation (2009). http://www.who.int/tobacco/surveillance/en_tfi_gats_russia_factsheet.pdf.

Thailand (2009). http://www.who.int/tobacco/surveillance/thailand_gats_report_2009.pdf.

Turkey (2008). http://www.who.int/tobacco/surveillance/en_tfi_gats_turkey_2009.pdf.

Ukraine (2010). http://www.who.int/tobacco/surveillance/en_tfi_gats_ukraine_2010.pdf.

Uruguay (2010). http://www.who.int/tobacco/surveillance/fact_sheet_of_gats_uruguay_2010.pdf. Data updated November 2011 by CDC.

Viet Nam. (2010). http://www.who.int/tobacco/surveillance/en_tfi_vietnam_gats_fact_sheet.pdf.

Chinese Gift Giving
Chu A, Jiang N, Glantz S. (2011). Transnational tobacco industry promotion of the cigarette gifting custom in China. *Tobacco Control*. Online. http://tobaccocontrol.bmj.com/content/early/2011/01/30/tc.2010.038349.abstract. Accessed August 28, 2011.

Russian Cigarette Advertisement
Okorokova L. (2011). Teenage cigarette scandal. *Moscow News*. August 25. http://themoscownews.com/society/20110825/188961025.html. Accessed August 28, 2011.

Indonesian Billboard Slogan
Sentinel A. (2011). Smoking ad in Indonesia condemned. Asiancorrespondent.com. August 27. http://asiancorrespondent.com/63568/smoking-ad-in-indonesia-condemned/. Accessed August 28, 2011.

Quote: Arnott
The Australian. (2011). Films that show smoking should have 18+ rating, UK study says. http://www.theaustralian.com.au/news/breaking-news/films-that-show-smoking-should-have-18-rating-uk-study-says/story-fn3dxity-1226141789571. Accessed October 20, 2011.

Quote: Campaign for Tobacco-Free Kids
Campaign for Tobacco-Free Kids. (2011). Tobacco product marketing on the Internet. May 9. http://www.tobaccofreekids.org/research/factsheets/pdf/0081.pdf. Accessed August 12, 2011.

Quote: Reiter
Paynter B. (2003). Burn and crash. *Pitch Weekly*. June 5. http://www.pitch.com/2003-06-05/news/burn-and-crash/. Accessed August 4, 2011.

Text Panel
Federal Trade Commission. (2011a). Cigarette report for 2007 and 2008.

Federal Trade Commission. (2011b). Smokeless tobacco report for 2007 and 2008. http://www.ftc.gov/os/2011/07/110729smokelesstobaccoreport.pdf. Accessed August 28, 2011.

Framework Convention Alliance. (2009). Tobacco industry targets social networking sites. http://www.fctc.org/index.php?option=com_content&view=article&id=316:tobacco-industry-targets-social-networking-websites&catid=235:advertising-promotion-and-sponsorship&Itemid=239. Accessed July 3, 2011.

Freeman B. (In press). New media and tobacco control. *Tobacco Control*.

Freeman B, Chapman S. (2010). British American Tobacco on Facebook: Undermining Article 13 of the Global World Health Organization Framework Convention on Tobacco Control. *Tobacco Control, 19*: e1–e9.

US Census. (2011). Population estimate: 2008. http://www.census.gov/popest/data/historical/2000s/vintage_2008/index.html. Accessed October 18, 2011.

US District Court for the District of Columbia. (2006). Final Opinion United States District Court for the District of Columbia – Civil Action No. 99-2496 (GK). http://www.tobaccofreekids.org/content/what_we_do/industry_watch/doj/FinalOpinion.pdf. Accessed July 28, 2010.

21 UNDUE INFLUENCE

Main Map

Action on Smoking and Health. (2010). The smoke-filled room: How big tobacco influences health policy in the UK. http://www.ash.org.uk/SmokeFilledRoom. Accessed August 12, 2011.

Argentina *Smoke-free Festivals*

Tobacco Free Kids. (2011). The Philippines: Advocates and government agencies work to combat industry interference. http://tobaccofreecenter.org/industry_watch/interference/legislation/philippines. Accessed October 20, 2011.

Australia *Plain Packaging and Quote*

Australian Government, Department of Health and Ageing, Your Health website. Plain packaging legislation receives the Royal Assent. Available at: http://www.yourhealth.gov.au/internet/yourhealth/publishing.nsf/Content/tobacco-label-passedleg. Accessed November 20, 2012.

World Trade Organization. (2011). News items: Concerns raised about tobacco and environmental measures. June 15 and 16. http://www.wto.org/english/news_e/news11_e/tbt_15jun11_e.htm. Accessed August 12, 2011.

News.com.au. (2011). Big tobacco buying influence: Roxon. May 26. http://www.news.com.au/breaking-news/big-tobacco-buying-influence-roxon/story-e6frfku0-1226063639476. Accessed August 12, 2011.

China *Elementary Schools*

NTD Television. (2010). Tobacco companies sponsor 69 elementary schools in China. January 26. http://english.ntdtv.com/ntdtv_en/ns_china/2010-01-26/907134456872.html. Accessed July 3, 2011.

Indonesia *Volcano*

Carless W. (2010). Indonesia: This volcano brought to you by Philip Morris. *Global Post*. November 4. http://www.globalpost.com/dispatch/indonesia/101104/indonesia-volcano-philip-morris. Accessed August 1, 2011.

Malawi *Chief of Health Services*

Report of the Committee of Experts on Tobacco Industry Documents. (2000). Tobacco company strategies to undermine tobacco control activities at the World Health Organization. July. http://www.who.int/tobacco/en/who_inquiry.pdf, p. 46. Accessed August 12, 2011.

Philippines *Ricafort Quote*

Group bears tobacco firms' efforts to stop anti-smoking policies. (2011). *Sun Star Manila*. July 17. http://209.59.190.9/manila/local-news/2011/07/17/group-bares-tobacco-firms-efforts-stop-anti-smoking-policies-167366. Accessed August 12, 2011.

UK *Tobacco Retailers Alliance*

Doward J. (2008). MPs fall foul of "dirty" tricks by tobacco giants. *The Observer*. December 14. http://www.guardian.co.uk/business/2008/dec/14/tobacco-industry-small-retailers. Accessed August 12, 2011.

US *Lorillard*

Solsman J. (2011). Lorillard hires ex-FDA analyst before possible menthol limits. *Fox Business*. June 7. http://www.foxbusiness.com/industries/2011/06/07/lorillard-hires-ex-fda-analyst-before-possible-menthol-limits/. Accessed August 12, 2011.

Federal Election Contributions

Center for Responsive Politics; OpenSecrets.org. (2011). Tobacco. http://www.opensecrets.org/industries/totals.php?cycle=2010&ind=A02. Accessed July 28, 2011.

Altria Group

Center for Responsive Politics; OpenSecrets.org. (2011). Tobacco.

Quote: Glantz

Parti T. (2011). Tobacco companies adjusting strategies to remain prominent political players. June 7. http://www.opensecrets.org/news/2011/06/tobacco-companies-adjusting-strategies.html. Accessed August 12, 2011.

Quote: Fooks et al.

Fooks G, Gilmore A, Smith K, Collin J, Holden C, Lee K. (2011). Corporate social responsibility and access to policy élites: An analysis of tobacco industry documents. *PloS Medicine, 8*(8): e1001076. http://www.plosmedicine.org/article/info%3Adoi%2F10.1371%2Fjournal.pmed.1001076. Accessed September 20, 2011.

Quote: Philip Morris

Morgan J. (1992). Legacy Tobacco Documents Library: Philip Morris. March 4. http://legacy.library.ucsf.edu/tid/qks81f00/pdf. Accessed August 12, 2011.

Text Panel

Center for Responsive Politics. OpenSecrets.org. (2011). Tobacco.

NTD Television. (2010). Tobacco companies sponsor 69 elementary schools in China.

Philip Morris International. (2010). Annual report 2010. http://media.corporate-ir.net/media_files/irol/14/146476/ar10.pdf. Accessed August 7, 2011.

Philip Morris International. (2011). Charitable contributions 2010. http://www.pmi.com/eng/about_us/corporate_contributions/documents/2010_charitable_contributions_total.pdf. Accessed July 3, 2011.

World Health Organization. (2003). WHO Framework Convention on Tobacco Control. Geneva: WHO Press. http://whqlibdoc.who.int/publications/2003/9241591013.pdf. Accessed August 5, 2011.

22 RIGHTS AND TREATIES

Main Map

World Health Organization. Full list of signatories and parties to the WHO Framework Convention on Tobacco Control. http://www.who.int/fctc/signatories_parties/en/index.html. Accessed November 30, 2011.

Symbol

World Health Organization. Sessions of the Conference of the Parties to the WHO FCTC. http://www.who.int/fctc/cop/sessions/en/. Accessed December 10, 2011.

Main Provisions of the WHO FCTC

World Health Organization. WHO Framework Convention on Tobacco Control. http://www.who.int/fctc/text_download/en/index.html. Accessed December 10, 2011.

WHO FCTC Parties

World Health Organization. Parties to the WHO Framework Convention on Tobacco Control.

International Treaties That Directly or Indirectly Address Tobacco Issues

United Nations Convention on the Elimination of All Forms of Discrimination Against Women. http://www.un.org/womenwatch/daw/cedaw/text/econvention.htm#article3. Accessed October 10, 2011.

United Nations International Covenant on Civil and Political Rights. http://www.hrweb.org/legal/cpr.html. Accessed May 1, 2011.

United Nations International Covenant on Economic, Social and Cultural Rights. Office of the UN High Commissioner for Human Rights. http://www2.ohchr.org/english/law/cescr.htm. Accessed May 1, 2011.

United Nations Universal Declaration on Human Rights. http://www.un.org/en/documents/udhr/index.shtml. Accessed May 1, 2011.

Minhas R. (2011). World Health Organization, Tobacco Free Initiative. Personal communication.

UN High-Level Meeting 2011

United Nations, (2011). UN High-Level Meeting on noncommunicable diseases. http://www.un.org/en/ga/president/65/issues/ncdiseases.shtml. Accessed December 1, 2011.

http://www.unhchr.ch/huridocda/huridoca.nsf/(Symbol)/E.CN.4.Sub.2.2003.12.Rev.2.En. Drafted in 2003. Accessed March 26, 2011.

The WHO FCTC Now Covers

Framework Convention Alliance. Updated status of the WHO FCTC ratification and accession by country. http://www.fctc.org/index.php?option=com_content&view=article&id=547:updated-status-of-the-who-fctc-ratification-and-accession-by-country&catid=173:general&Itemid=200.

Quote: Cicero

The quotations page. http://www.quotationspage.com/subjects/laws/11.html. Accessed November 1, 2011.

Text

Jha P, Chaloupka F. (1999). *Curbing the epidemic: Government and the economics of tobacco control*. Washington DC: World Bank.

Minhas R. (2011). World Health Organization, Tobacco Free Initiative. Personal communication.

23 PUBLIC HEALTH STRATEGIES

Main Map

World Health Organization. (2011). *WHO report on the global tobacco epidemic, 2011: Warning about the dangers of tobacco.* Geneva: World Health Organization.

For a complete explanation of the methods used to obtain the variables mapped here, please reference the technical notes and appendices for this report at http://www.who.int/tobacco/global_report/2011/en/.

Please note that the categories used on this map correspond with the following MPOWER *categories from the "Monitoring" data:*

"No Data" corresponds with the MPOWER *category, "No known data or no recent data or data that are not both recent and representative"*

"Minimal Monitoring" corresponds with the MPOWER *category, "Recent and representative data for either adults or youth"*

"Moderate Monitoring" corresponds with the MPOWER *category, "Recent and representative data for both adults and youth"*

"Complete Monitoring" corresponds with the MPOWER *category, "Recent, representative and periodic data for both adults and youth"*

Public Health Strategy

American Cancer Society, International Union Against Cancer. (2006). Strategy planning for tobacco control movement building: Tobacco control strategy planning guide #2.

Chapman S. (2004). Advocacy for public health: A primer. *Epidemiology and Community Health*, 58: 361–365. doi: 10.1136/jech.2003.018051.

Governments Collect Nearly $133 Billion

World Health Organization. (2011). *WHO report on the global tobacco epidemic, 2011: Warning about the dangers of tobacco.* Geneva: World Health Organization.

Insufficient Resources

World Health Organization. (2011). *WHO report on the global tobacco epidemic.*

Quote: Sun Tzu

Sun Tzu. (1982). *The art of war. A treatise on Chinese military science.* Singapore: Graham Brash (Pte) Ltd. (Compiled about 500 BCE.)

Text

Baris E, Brigden L, Prindiville J, da Costa e Silva V, Chitanondh H, Chandiwana S. (2000). Research priorities for tobacco control in developing countries: A regional approach to a global consultative process. *Tobacco Control, 9*(2): 217–223.

Gates and Bloomberg Unite in Global Fight Against Tobacco. (2008). *Medical News Today*. July 24. http://www.medicalnewstoday.com/articles/116039.php. Accessed September 2, 2008.

Bloomberg Initiative to Reduce Tobacco Use Grants Program. http://www.tobaccocontrolgrants.org/. Accessed November 30, 2011.

24 SMOKE-FREE AREAS

Main Map

SOURCES

World Health Organization. (2011). *WHO report on the global tobacco epidemic, 2011: Warning about the dangers of tobacco.* Geneva: World Health Organization.

METHODS

For a complete explanation of the methods used to obtain the variables mapped here, please reference the technical notes and appendices for this report at http://www.who.int/tobacco/global_report/2011/en/.

Smoking Bans in Restaurants

World Health Organization. (2011). *WHO report on the global tobacco epidemic, 2011: Warning about the dangers of tobacco.*

No Loss of Restaurant Sales

Distribution Services Statistics Section, Census and Statistics Department, Hong Kong. http://www.censtatd.gov.hk/hong_kong_statistics/statistical_tables/index.jsp?charsetID=1&tableID=088. Accessed November 15, 2011.

Effect of Smoke-Free Ban

Binkin N, Perra A, Aprile V, D'Argenzio A, Lopresti S, Mingozzi O, Scondotto S. (2007). Effects of a generalised ban on smoking in bars and restaurants, Italy. *International Journal of Tuberculosis and Lung Disease, 11*(5): 522–527.

Covered by Comprehensive Smoke-Free Laws

World Health Organization. (2011). WHO report on the global tobacco epidemic, 2011: Questions and answers. June 30. http://www.wpro.who.int/NR/rdonlyres/A78F9CF1-0DA8-4886-83AE-4823C063BCAE/0/QAs_GTCRIII_FINAL4July2011.pdf. Accessed October 1, 2011.

Quote: "Breathe," the Barman Replied

World Health Organization. (2006). Business as usual for smoke-free places. *Bulletin of the World Health Organization, 84*(6), 921–1000. http://www.who.int/bulletin/volumes/84/12/06-021206/en/index.html. Accessed April 15, 2011.

Brazil to Become World's Largest Smoke-Free Country

Campaign for Tobacco-Free Kids. (2011). Historic tobacco control law adds momentum to Latin America's progress in fighting tobacco use. Press Release, December.

Text

Americans for Nonsmokers' Rights. (2009). Patron surveys and consumer behavior. http://www.no-smoke.org/pdf/patronsurveys.pdf. Accessed July 1, 2011.

California Environmental Protection Agency. (2005). Proposed identification of environmental tobacco smoke as a toxic air contaminant, SRP approved version. Part B: Health effects. June 24. http://www.arb.ca.gov/toxics/ets/finalreport/finalreport.htm. Accessed November 30, 2011.

Callinan J, Clarke A, Doherty K, Kelleher C. (2010). Legislative smoking bans for reducing secondhand smoke exposure, smoking prevalence, and tobacco consumption. *Cochrane Database of Systematic Reviews, 14*(4): CD005992.

Hyland A, Higbee C, Borland R, Travers M, Hastings G, Fong G, Cummings K. (2009). Attitudes and beliefs about secondhand smoke and smoke-free policies in four countries: Findings from the International Tobacco Control Four-Country Survey. *Nicotine and Tobacco Research, 11*(6): 642–649.

Koong H, Khoo D, Higbee C, Travers M, Hyland A, Cummings K, Dresler C. (2009). Global air monitoring study: A multi-country comparison of levels of indoor air pollution in different workplaces. *Annals, Academy of Medicine, Singapore, 38*(3): 202–206.

Ludbrook A, Bird S, van Teijlingen E. (2005). *International review of the health and economic impact of the regulation of smoking in public places.* NHS Health Scotland.

Mage C, Goldstein A, Colgan S, Skinner B, Kramer K, Steiner J, Staples A. (2010). Secondhand smoke policies at state and county fairs. *North Carolina Medical Journal, 71*(5): 409–412.

New York City Department of Finance, New York City Department of Health & Mental Hygiene, New York City Department of Small Business Services, New York City Economic Development Corporation. (2004). The state of smoke-free New York City: A one-year review. http://www.nyc.gov/html/doh/downloads/pdf/smoke/sfaa-2004report.pdf. Accessed September 18, 2011.

Quinet M, Orban M, Philippet C, Riffon A, Andrien M. (2003). Non-smokers protection in restaurants and bars in Europe: A survey in five European countries, European Network for Smoking Prevention, Europe Against Cancer. http://www.fares.be/tabagisme/news/surveyHorecaFinalReport.pdf. Accessed June 20, 2005.

Raaijmakers T, van den Borne I. (2001). Cost-benefits of workplace smoking policies. In *Smoke-free workplaces: Improving the health and well-being of people at work, European Status Report, 2001.*

Fleitman S (ed), European Network for Smoking Prevention.

Repace J. (2003). A killer on the loose: An Action on Smoking and Health investigation into the threat of passive smoking to the UK workforce. Action on Smoking and Health. London. http://www.repace.com/pdf/killer1.pdf. Accessed September 9, 2011.

Vardavas C, Kondilis B, Travers M, Petsetaki E, Tountas Y, Kafatos A. (2007). Environmental tobacco smoke in hospitality venues in Greece. *BMC Public Health, 7*: 302.

Walsh R, Paul C, Tzelepis F, Stojanovski E, Tang A. (2008). Is government action out-of-step with public opinion on tobacco control? Results of a New South Wales population survey. *Australian and New Zealand Journal of Public Health, 32*(5): 482–488.

World Health Organization. (2007). Exposure to secondhand smoke: Policy recommendations. June 25. http://www.who.int/tobacco/resources/publications/wntd/2007/who_protection_exposure_final_25June2007.pdf. Accessed April 15, 2011.

25 QUITTING SMOKING

Main Map

World Health Organization. (2011). *WHO report on the global tobacco epidemic, 2011: Warning about the dangers of tobacco.* Geneva: World Health Organization.

For a complete explanation of the methods used to obtain the variables mapped here, please reference the technical notes and appendices for this report at http://www.who.int/tobacco/global_report/2011/en/.

Quitting Calendar

American Lung Association. (N.d.). The benefits of stopping smoking.

National Tobacco Dependence Treatment Services

Raw M, Regan S, Rigotti N, McNeill A. (2009). A survey of tobacco dependence treatment services in 36 countries. *Addiction, 104*(2): 279–287.

Quit Attempts

International Tobacco Control Policy and Evaluation Project. (2010). FCTC Article 14. Tobacco dependence and cessation. November. http://www.itcproject.org/keyfindi/itccessationreportpdf. Accessed December 1, 2011.

Kuwait

Memon A, Moody P, Sugathan T, el-Gerges N, al-Bustan M, al-Shatti A, al-Jazzaf H. (2000). Epidemiology of smoking among Kuwaiti adults: Prevalence, characteristics, and attitudes. *Bulletin of the World Health Organization, 78*(11): 1306–1315.

FCTC Article 14

World Health Organization. (2003). WHO Framework Convention on Tobacco Control. http://www.who.int/fctc/text_download/en/index.html. Accessed December 1, 2011.

Quote: Giovino

University of Buffalo. (2009). Major report on US tobacco-control policies and use finds stark contrasts in progress among states. June 10. http://www.buffalo.edu/news/10175. Accessed December 1, 2011.

Text

International Tobacco Control Policy and Evaluation Project. (2010). FCTC Article 14. Tobacco dependence and cessation. November. http://www.itcproject.org/keyfindi/itccessationreportpdf. Accessed December 1, 2011.

Peto R, Lopez A. (2001). The future worldwide health effects of current smoking patterns. In *Critical Issues in Global Health.* Eds. Koop E, Pearson C, Schwarz M. 154–161. New York: Jossey-Bass.

26 MASS MEDIA CAMPAIGNS

Main Map

World Health Organization. (2011). *WHO report on the global tobacco epidemic, 2011: Warning about the dangers of tobacco.* Geneva: World Health Organization.

For a complete explanation of the methods used to obtain the variables mapped here, please reference the technical notes and appendices for this report at: http://www.who.int/tobacco/global_report/2011/en/.

The Wheel of Mass Media Communications in Tobacco Control

World Lung Foundation. Mass media communications in tobacco control. http://www.worldlungfoundation.org/ht/a/GetImageAction/i/7828. Accessed May 31, 2011.

Adults Who Noticed Anti-Smoking Information on TV or Radio: 14 Countries

Global Adult Tobacco Survey. Multiple fact sheets and years. http://www.who.int/tobacco/surveillance/gats/en/index.html. Accessed September 11, 2011.

Radio vs. TV

Durkin S, Wakefield M. (2010). Comparative response to radio and television anti-smoking advertisements to encourage smoking cessation. *Health Promotion International, 25*: 5–13.

Quote: Mullin

Mullin S. (2011). Global anti-smoking campaigns urgently needed. *The Lancet, 378*: 970–971.

Text

Cotter T, Perez D, Dunlop S, et al. (2010). The case for recycling and adapting anti-tobacco mass media campaigns. *Tobacco Control, 19*: 514–517.

Durkin S, Biener L, Wakefield M. (2009). Effects of different types of antismoking ads on reducing disparities in smoking cessation among socioeconomic subgroups. *American Journal of Public Health, 99*(12): 2217–2223.

Durkin S, Brennan E, Wakefield M. (In press). Mass media campaigns to promote smoking cessation among adults: An integrative review. *Tobacco Control.*

Mullin S. (2011). Global anti-smoking campaigns urgently needed. *Lancet, 378*(9795): 970–971.

National Cancer Institute. (2008). The role of the media in promoting and reducing tobacco use.

Terry-McElrath Y, Emery S, Wakefield M, et al. (2011). Effects of tobacco-related media campaigns among 20- to 30-year-old adults: Longitudinal data from the USA. *Tobacco Control.* October 4. [Epub ahead of print]

Wakefield M, Bayly M, Durkin S, et al. (2011). Smokers' responses to television advertisements about the serious health harms of tobacco use: Pre-testing results from ten low- to middle-income countries. *Tobacco Control.* October 12 [Epub ahead of print]

Wakefield M, Spittal M, Yong H-H, et al. (2011). Effects of mass media campaign exposure intensity and durability on quit attempts in a population-based cohort study. *Health Education Research, 26*(6): 988–997.

World Health Organization. (2011). *WHO report on the global tobacco epidemic, 2011: Warning about the dangers of tobacco.*

27 PRODUCT LABELING

Main Map

World Health Organization. (2011). *WHO report on the global tobacco epidemic, 2011: Warning about the dangers of tobacco.* Geneva: World Health Organization.

For a complete explanation of the methods used to obtain the variables mapped here, please reference the technical notes and appendices for this report at: http://www.who.int/tobacco/global_report/2011/en/.

Symbol: First Ten Countries to Require Graphic Health Warnings

Canadian Cancer Society. (2010). Cigarette packet health warnings: International status report. October.

Percentage of Countries by Region With Product Labeling Laws That Prohibit the Use of "Light." "Mild," and Similar Misleading Descriptors

World Health Organization. (2011). *WHO report on the global tobacco epidemic, 2011: Warning about the dangers of tobacco.*

Centers for Disease Control and Prevention. (2011). Cigarette package health warnings and interest in quitting smoking: 14 countries, 2008–2010. *Morbidity and Mortality Weekly Report, 60*(20): 645–651.

Plain Packaging
Freeman B, Chapman S, Rimmer M. (2008). The case for the plain packaging of tobacco products. *Addiction, 103*(4): 580–590. doi:10.1111/j.1360-0443.2008.02145.x.

Health Warnings
World Health Organization. (2008). *WHO report on the global tobacco epidemic, 2008: The* MPOWER *package*. Geneva: World Health Organization.

China
Elton-Marshall T, Fong GT, Zanna MP, Jiang Y, Hammond D, O'Connor RJ, Yong HH, Li L, King B, Li Q, Borland R, Cummings KM, Driezen P. (2010). Beliefs about the relative harm of "light" and "low tar" cigarettes: findings from the International Tobacco Control (ITC) China Survey. *Tobacco Control, 19*(Suppl 2): i54–62.

Quote: Crow
House of Representatives Standing Committee on Health and Ageing. (2011). Tobacco Plain Packaging Bill 2011, Trade Marks Amendment. Canberra. August 4. http://www.aph.gov.au/hansard/reps/commttee/r197.pdf.

Quote: Roxon
Roxon N. (2011). Australia stubs out tobacco packaging. *Financial Times* (UK). November 21.

Text
ASH UK. (2010). The smoke-filled room: How Big Tobacco influences health policy in the UK. http://www.ash.org.uk/SmokeFilledRoom. Accessed November 15, 2011.

Physicians for a Smoke Free Canada. (N.d.). Picture-based cigarette warnings. http://www.smoke-free.ca/warnings/. Accessed October 13, 2011.

Roxon N. (2011). Address to the plenary session of the UN High-Level Meeting on noncommunicable diseases. September 19. http://www.health.gov.au/internet/ministers/publishing.nsf/Content/mr-yr11-nr-nr189.htm?OpenDocument&yr=2011&mth=09. Accessed December 1, 2011.

World Health Organization. (2005). Framework Convention on Tobacco Control. Geneva: WHO/TFI.

World Health Organization. (2008). *WHO report on the global tobacco epidemic, 2008: The* MPOWER *package*.

28 MARKETING BANS

Main Map
World Health Organization. (2011). *WHO report on the global tobacco epidemic, 2011: Warning about the dangers of tobacco*. Geneva: World Health Organization.

For a complete explanation of the methods used to obtain the variables mapped here, please reference the technical notes and appendices for this report at: http://www.who.int/tobacco/global_report/2011/en/.

Point-of-Sale Advertising Bans
World Health Organization. (2011). *WHO report on the global tobacco epidemic, 2011: Warning about the dangers of tobacco.*

Summary of Findings Against the Tobacco Industry
Tobacco-Free Kids. (2006). US District Judge Gladys Kessler's final opinion: Summary of findings against the tobacco industry, 2006. http://www.tobaccofreekids.org/content/what_we_do/industry_watch/doj/FinalOpinionSummary.pdf. Accessed April 10, 2011.

New Media
Elkin L, Thomson G, Wilson N. (2010). Connecting world youth with tobacco brands: YouTube and the Internet policy vacuum on Web 2.0. *Tobacco Control, 19*: 361–366.

A Comprehensive Ban on All Tobacco Advertising
World Health Organization. (2011). *WHO report on the global tobacco epidemic, 2011: Warning about the dangers of tobacco.*

Fifty-five Countries Have Banned Direct Advertising on the Internet
World Health Organization. (2011). *WHO report on the global tobacco epidemic, 2011: Warning about the dangers of tobacco.*

Quote: Phelps
DeParle J. (1989). Warning: Sports stars may be hazardous to your health. *Washington Monthly*. September.

Quote: Kessler
(2006). US District Judge Gladys Kessler's final opinion.

Text
Assunta M, Chapman S. (2004a). The tobacco industry's accounts of refining indirect tobacco advertising in Malaysia. *Tobacco Control, 13*(Suppl 2): ii63–70.

Assunta M, Chapman S. (2004b). "The world's most hostile environment": How the tobacco industry circumvented Singapore's advertising ban. *Tobacco Control, 13*(Suppl 2): ii51–57.

Campaign for Tobacco-Free Kids. (2008). Tobacco advertising, promotion and sponsorship. http://www.tobaccofreecenter.org/files/pdfs/en/APS_evidence_en.pdf. Accessed March 14, 2011.

Carter SM. (2003). New frontier, new power: The retail environment in Australia's dark market. *Tobacco Control, 12*(Suppl 3): iii95–101.

Chen Weihua. (2009). "I love China" ads are ridiculous. http://www.chinadaily.com.cn/opinion/2009-03/28/content_7626779.htm. Accessed August 27, 2011.

Freeman B, Chapman S. (2010). British American Tobacco on Facebook: undermining Article 13 of the Global World Health Organization Framework Convention on Tobacco Control. *Tobacco Control, 19*: e1–9.

Sargent JD, Beach ML, Dalton MA, et al. (2004). Effect of parental R-rated movie restriction on adolescent smoking initiation: A prospective study. *Pediatrics, 114*: 149–156.

Shanghai Daily. (2009). "Love China" campaign may be snuffed out. January 19. http://www.chinadaily.com.cn/china/2009-01/19/content_7408919.htm. Accessed August 27, 2011.

Wakefield M, Letcher T. (2002). My pack is cuter than your pack. *Tobacco Control, 11*: 154–156.

Wakefield M, Morley C, Horan JK, Cummings KM. (2002). The cigarette pack as image: New evidence from tobacco industry documents. *Tobacco Control, 11*(Suppl 1): i73–80.

World Bank. (1999). *Curbing the epidemic: Governments and the economics of tobacco control*. Washington, DC: World Bank.

29 TOBACCO TAXES

Main Map
Angola, Cuba, Equatorial Guinea, Fiji, Malawi, Morocco, Papua New Guinea
World Health Organization. (2009). *WHO report on the global tobacco epidemic, 2009: Implementing smoke-free environments.* http://www.who.int/tobacco/mpower/en/. Accessed May 23, 2011.

Austria, Belgium, Bulgaria, Cyprus, Czech Republic, Denmark, Estonia, Finland, France, Germany, Greece, Hungary, Ireland, Italy, Latvia, Lithuania, Luxembourg, Malta, Netherlands, Poland, Portugal, Romania, Slovakia, Slovenia, Spain, Sweden, UK
European Commission Directorate General Taxation and Customs Union. (2011). Excise duty tables: Part III: Manufactured tobacco. http://ec.europa.eu/taxation_customs/taxation/excise_duties/tobacco_products/index_en.htm. Accessed March 3, 2011.

All Other Countries World Health Organization. (2011). *WHO report on the global tobacco epidemic, 2011: Warning about the dangers of tobacco*. Geneva: World Health Organization.

WHO Member States Tax
World Health Organization. (2011). The Solidarity Tobacco Contribution, A new international health-financing concept prepared by the World Health Organization. http://www.who.int/nmh/events/un_ncd_summit2011/ncds_stc.pdf. Accessed January 3, 2012.

Cigarette Consumption Goes Down as Tobacco Taxes Go Up
NOMINAL CIGARETTE PRICES
Economist Intelligence Unit. (2011). World Cost of Living Survey, London.

CONSUMER PRICE INDEX
International Monetary Fund. (2011). World economic outlook database. April. http://www.imf.org/external/pubs/ft/weo/2011/02/weodata/index.aspx. Accessed May 4, 2011.

CIGARETTE CONSUMPTION PER CAPITA
ERC. (2010). World cigarette reports 2010. Suffolk, UK: ERC Group Ltd.

Tobacco Excise Tax Revenue as a Percentage of Total Tax Revenues
European Commission Directorate General Taxation and Customs Union. (2011). Excise duty tables: Part III: Manufactured tobacco.

Tax Revenue Goes Up as Tobacco Taxes Go Up
Cigarette Prices and Consumer Price Index
Central Statistical Office in Poland. (2011). Bank Danych Lokalnych. http://www.stat.gov.pl/bdl/app/strona.html?p_name=indeks. Accessed May 9, 2011.

Cigarette Tax Rates and Tobacco Tax Revenue
Ministry of Finances in Poland. (2011). Sprawozdania z Wykonania Budżetu Państwa. http://www.mf.gov.pl/index.php?const=5&dzial=36&wysw=2&sub=sub1. Accessed May 9, 2011.

Ministry of Finances in Poland. (2011). Ustawa o Podatku Akcyzowym. http://www.mf.gov.pl/dokument.php?const=3&dzial=333&id=164384. Accessed May 9, 2011.

Quote
Gates B. (2011). Innovation with impact: Financing 21st-century development. Report to G20 leaders. Cannes Summit, November. http://www.gatesfoundation.org/g20/Documents/g20-report-english.pdf. Accessed December 2, 2011.

Japan
Filipovic G. (2011). Japan Tobacco urges Serbia to align excise taxes with EU. June 17. http://www.bloomberg.com/news/2011-06-17/japan-tobacco-urges-serbia-to-align-excise-taxes-with-eu-1-.html. Accessed June 17, 2011.

New Hampshire
Sanborn A. (2011). Tobacco price increase offsets N.H. tax cut. July 24. http://www.seacoastonline.com/apps/pbcs.dll/article?AID=/20110724/NEWS/107240318/1/NEWSMAP. Accessed October 28, 2011.

Text Panel
Eberwine-Ullagran D. (2007). Best buys for public health: Good health need not be a luxury reserved for the world's rich. By investing in cost-effective interventions, developing countries can dramatically improve their populations' health. *Perspectives in Health, 11*(1): 2–9.

Franz GA. (2008). Price effects on the smoking behaviour of adult age groups. *Public Health, 122*(12): 1343–1348.

Gallus S, Schiaffino A, La Vecchia C, Townsend J, Fernandez E. (2006). Price and cigarette consumption in Europe. *Tobacco Control, 15*(2): 114–119.

International Agency for Research on Cancer. (2011). Effectiveness of price and tax policies for control of tobacco. In *IARC Handbooks of Cancer Prevention: Tobacco Control*. In press. Lyon, France: International Agency for Research on Cancer.

Jha P, Chaloupka FJ. (1999). *Curbing the epidemic: Governments and the economics of tobacco control*. World Bank Publications.

Jha P, Chaloupka FJ. (2000). *Tobacco control in developing countries*. Oxford: Oxford University Press.

Kostova D, Ross H, Blecher E, Markowitz S. (2010). Prices and cigarette demand: Evidence from youth tobacco use in developing countries. National Bureau of Economic Research Working Paper Series No. 15781. February. http://www.nber.org/papers/w15781. Accessed May 16, 2011.

Siahpush M, Wakefield M, Spittal M, Durkin S, Scollo M. (2009). Taxation reduces social disparities in adult smoking prevalence. *American Journal of Preventive Medicine, 36*(4): 285–291.

World Health Organization. (2010). WHO technical manual on tobacco tax administration.

30 LEGAL CHALLENGES AND LITIGATION

Main Map

Recently Decided or Pending Tobacco Industry Legal Challenges Against Governments' Tobacco Control Measures as of June 2011. List maintained by the International Legal Consortium at the Campaign for Tobacco-Free Kids.

File No. 0032-2010-PI/TC. http://www.law.georgetown.edu/oneillinstitute/publications/pdf/2011_PERU_TOBACCO_CONTROL_AMICUS.pdf. Accessed November 15, 2011.

History of Tobacco Tort Litigation Strategies in the US

Ontario Tobacco Research Unit. (2010). Litigation against the tobacco industry: Monitoring update. October 27. http://www.otru.org/pdf/16mr/16mr_litigation.pdf. Accessed November 30, 2011.

Sugarman SD. (2002). Mixed results from recent United States tobacco litigation. http://www.law.berkeley.edu/faculty/tobacco/mixed_results.pdf. Accessed December 13, 2011.

Cases Pending Against the Industry

British American Tobacco. (2010). Annual report 2010. http://www.bat.com/ar/2010/financial-statements/group-financial-statements/notes-on-the-accounts/note-30.html. Accessed June 28, 2011.

British American Tobacco. (2004). Directors' Report and Accounts 2004. http://www.bat.com/group/sites/uk__3mnfen.nsf/vwPagesWebLive/DO52AK34/$FILE/medMD6LRMA4.pdf?openelement. Accessed January 10, 2012.

Quote: Camilleri

Camilleri L. (2010). Presentation at Morgan Stanley Global Consumer and Retail Conference. New York. September 17.

Quote: Halton

Halton J. (2011). Tobacco battle lines form. *The* (Hong Kong) *Standard*. October 11. http://www.thestandard.com.hk/news_print.asp?art_id=115945&sid=. Accessed November 15, 2011.

Text

Ontario Tobacco Research Unit. (2010). Litigation against the tobacco industry.

World Health Organization. (2010). FCTC/COP4(5) Punta del Este Declaration on the implementation of the WHO Framework

Convention on Tobacco Control. http://apps.who.int/gb/fctc/PDF/cop4/FCTC_COP4_DIV6-en.pdf. Accessed November 15, 2011.

31 THE FUTURE

World Health Organization. (2011). Targets to monitor progress in reducing the burden of noncommunicable diseases. Recommendations from a WHO Technical Working Group on Noncommunicable Disease Targets. (Version dated July 15, 2011 for a web-based consultation with Member States.)

Beaglehole R, Bonita R, for *The Lancet* NCD Action Group and the NCD Alliance. Priority actions for the non-communicable disease crisis. *The Lancet*, Early Online Publication, April 6, 2011. doi:10.1016/S0140-6736(11)60393-0.

HISTORY

Centers for Disease Control and Prevention. (2010). Global Adult Tobacco Survey—Overview. http://apps.nccd.cdc.gov/gtssdata/Ancillary/Documentation.aspx?SUID=4&DOCT=1. Accessed December 1, 2011.

Lyons A, Petrucelli R. (1978). *Medicine: An illustrated history*. New York: Harry N. Abrams, p. 508.

Moyer D. (1998). The tobacco almanac: A reference book of fact, figures, quotations about tobacco. Self-published.

Routh H, Bhowmik K, Parish J, Parish L. (1998). Historical aspects of tobacco use and smoking. *Clinics in Dermatology, 16*(5): 539–544.

Tobacco Facts. (N.d.). Tobacco truth: From first drag to slavery—tobacco's beginnings.

Tobacco Milestones. (1996). *A brief history of tobacco*. Adapted from a chronology by the National Clearinghouse on Tobacco and Health. Ottawa.

Walton J, ed. (2000). *The Faber book of smoking*. London: Faber.

GLOSSARY

Centers for Disease Control and Prevention. (N.d.). Cancer fact sheet. Agency for Toxic Substances & Disease Registry. http://www.atsdr.cdc.gov/COM/cancer-fs.html. Accessed January 6, 2012.

Centers for Disease Control and Prevention. (2006). *The health consequences of involuntary exposure to tobacco smoke: A report of the Surgeon General*. Atlanta: US Department of Health and Human Services, Coordinating Center for Health Promotion, National Center for Chronic Disease Prevention and Health Promotion, Office on Smoking and Health.

SECTION DIVIDERS

Harm

Quote: King A. (2010). A statement by the Chief Medical Officer of Health—Towards a smoke-free Ontario. October 19. http://news.ontario.ca/mhp/en/2010/10/a-statement-by-the-chief-medical-officer-of-health---towards-a-smoke-free-ontario.html. Accessed November 22, 2011.

Statistic: Data derived from FCTC Death Clock. http://www.oxyromandie.ch/deathcalc.php. Accessed November 22, 2011.

Products and Their Use

Quote: Cauchon D. (2007). Smoking declines as taxes increase. *USA Today*. August 10. http://www.usatoday.com/news/health/2007-08-09-1Alede_N.htm. Accessed August 25, 2011.

Statistic: Data derived from ERC. (2010). *World cigarette reports 2010*. Suffolk, UK: ERC Group Ltd.

Costs

Quote: Yurekli AA. (2001). A public health priority: Curbing the epidemic. World Bank. http://www.bruneiresources.com/pdf/istob_ayda_curbingacademic.pdf. Accessed December 2, 2011.

Statistic: Yang L. et al. (2011). Economic costs attributable to smoking in China: Update and an 8-year comparison, 2000–2008. *Tobacco Control, 20*, no. 4 (July 1): 266–272.

Tobacco Industry

Quote: Report of the Committee of Experts on Tobacco Industry Documents. (2000). Tobacco company strategies to undermine tobacco control activities at the World Health Organization. http://www.who.int/tobacco/en/who_inquiry.pdf. Accessed August 12, 2011.

Statistic: Data derived from ERC. (2010). *World cigarette reports 2010*.

Solutions

Quote: World Health Organization. (2008). *WHO report on the global tobacco epidemic, 2008: The* MPOWER *package*. Geneva: WHO.

Statistic: World Health Organization. (2011). *WHO report on the global tobacco epidemic, 2011: Questions and answers*. June 30.

WORLD TABLE SOURCES AND METHODS

SOURCES FOR DATA NOT PRESENTED IN MAIN MAPS AND METHODS

World Bank Income Groups: The World Bank. (2011). Countries and economies. http://data.worldbank.org/country. Accessed July 28, 2011.

World Bank classifies countries as low-income economies, lower-middle-income economies, upper-middle-income economies, high-income economies. For the purpose of the *Atlas*, "lower-middle" and "upper-middle" economies have been classified as middle-income countries.

Male and Female Currently Smoking ANY Tobacco Product: World Health Organization (2011). WHO report on the global tobacco epidemic, 2011. Australia: Australian Institute of Health and Welfare. (2011). 2010 National Drug Strategy Household Survey Report. http://www.aihw.gov.au/publication-detail/?id=32212254712. Accessed November 20, 2012.

Male and Female Crude Tobacco Use Prevalence: World Health Organization (2011). WHO report on the global tobacco epidemic, 2011: Warning about the dangers of tobacco. Geneva: World Health Organization. Australia: Australian Institute of Health and Welfare. (2011). 2010 National Drug Strategy Household Survey Report. http://www.aihw.gov.au/publication-detail/?id=32212254712. Accessed November 20, 2012.

Total of Boys' and Girls' Tobacco Use Prevalence: Sources match those listed in the Sources section of the Main Map of the Boys and Girls chapters. A simple average was calculated for the following countries: **Côte d'Ivoire, Denmark, France, Germany, Guatemala, Honduras, Japan, Kiribati, Marshall Islands, Netherlands, San Marino, Sweden, Switzerland, UK**.

The values for **West Bank and Gaza Strip** were provided separately and averaged together.

Tobacco Production (tonnes): Food and Agricultural Organization. (2011). FAOSTAT Data, Tobacco unmanufactured: Production Quantity, 2000, 2009. http://faostat.fao.org/site/567/DesktopDefault.aspx?PageID=567#ancor. Accessed October 10, 2011.

PHOTO CREDITS

02 Harm from Smoking

CT scan: McMullan, DM, and Cohem, GA. (2006). Radiographic evidence linking tobacco use and lung cancer. *New England Journal of Medicine 354*: 397.

04 Types of Tobacco

Kreteks: Tony de Feria

Dissolvable smokeless tobacco products: Associated Press

05 Nicotine Delivery Systems

Nico Water: Associated Press

Sticks, Strips, Orbs, and Snus: Roswell Park Cancer Institute, Buffalo, NY

Snus ad: http://www.snuscentral.org/latest-snus-news/camel-snus-quit-cigarettes-stop-smoking-2011.html. Accessed August 2, 2011.

08 Female Tobacco Use

Suffragette: Museum of Public Relations

10 Girls' Tobacco Use and 20 Tobacco Marketing

Kiss: Katarina Radovic, Branding Magazine, February 2012.

21 Undue Influence

China: Tsinghua University International Center for Communication

Indonesia: Fauzan Ijazah © 2010 GlobalPost

23 Public Health Strategies

Field worker: Centers for Disease Control and Prevention

26 Mass Media Campaigns

"Sponge": Cancer Institute NSW, Australia

27 Product Labeling

Smoking Harms Unborn Babies: © Commonwealth of Australia.

28 Marketing Bans

Shanghai Tobacco Company: Michael Eriksen, April 2011

History

Baroness de Dudevant (aka George Sand): Print collection, Miriam and Ida D. Wallach Division of Art, Prints and Photographs, The New york Public Library, Astor, Lennox and Tilden Foundations.

Lucky Strike building: Manuscripts and Archives Division, The New York Public Library, Astor, Lennox and Tilden Foundations.

Marlboro cowboy: Illustration by Kakha Begiashvili

Cigarette executives: Associated Press

WHO FCTC poster: World Health Organization, WHO Make every day World No Tobacco Day

MPOWER logo: World Health Organization

INDEX

h 4/2014 P